Mesoamerican Healers

Mesoamerican
Healers

edited by Brad R. Huber
and Alan R. Sandstrom

UNIVERSITY OF TEXAS PRESS, AUSTIN

Copyright © 2001 by the University of Texas Press
All rights reserved
Printed in the United States of America
First edition, 2001

Requests for permission to reproduce material from this work
should be sent to Permissions, University of Texas Press,
P.O. Box 7819, Austin, TX 78713-7819.

ⓧ The paper used in this book meets the minimum requirements
of ANSI/NISO Z39.48-1992 (R1997) (Permanence of Paper).

Library of Congress Cataloging-in-Publication Data

Mesoamerican Healers / edited by Brad R. Huber and Alan R.
Sandstrom.—1st ed.
    p.   cm.
Includes bibliographical references and index.
ISBN 978-0-292-73456-2

    1. Indians of Mexico—Rites and ceremonies.   2. Indians of
Mexico—Medicine.   3. Indians of Central America—
Guatemala—Rites and ceremonies.   4. Indians of Central
America—Guatemala—Medicine.   5. Shamans—Latin
America.   6. Healers—Latin America.   7. Midwives—Latin
America.   I. Huber, Brad R. (Brad Richard), 1954–
II. Sandstrom, Alan R.
F1219.3.R38 M47   2001
306.4'61—dc21   2001033103

Note: No part of this manuscript may be quoted or referenced
without the express permission of the editors.

It is with great pleasure and respect that we dedicate this book to George Foster, Mary Foster, Claudia Madsen, William Madsen, Benjamin Paul, and Lois Paul. Their many important contributions to anthropology are an inspiration to us all.

Contents

List of Tables

List of Figures

Foreword

by Bernard Ortiz de Montellano

As a nation, we spend billions of dollars on unproven nostrums, nonexistent "energies," and various therapeutic touches and massages. The Federal Drug Administration has been rendered impotent by the thinly disguised subterfuge of labeling these substances as "food supplements." These remedies are legitimized by pseudoscientific claims for "quantum healing" or "hydrinos," or by ultra-relativistic postmodernist claims that "all theories are equally valid" or that scientific evidence is not relevant because "there are different ways of knowing." The result is that "natural" or "alternative" methods and remedies are held to be superior to those of Western biomedicine, which is accused of being impersonal and reductionist. This has led to wasting billions of dollars on ineffective remedies, severe diseases not being treated until it is too late, and unforeseen adverse drug interactions. On the other hand, the attitude of most biomedically trained health personnel—who consider traditional healers quacks or superstitious charlatans —is just as unfortunate. In developing countries this attitude means that millions of people do not get either effective biomedicine or the possible benefits of an effective cooperation between traditional and biomedical healers. There is much that traditional healers can offer medicine, not only in physiologically active compounds derived from herbal medicine, but also in treating illness as a holistic entity with interacting cultural, psychological, and physiological components.

This volume represents medical anthropology at its best. It strikes a balance between the hubris of biomedicine and an uncritical postmodernism. It is a state-of-the-art survey of healers, and will be a mandatory reference because of its breadth of coverage, the authoritativeness of its authors, and the excellence of its bibliography. The chapters on midwives, as well as Paul and McMahon's treatment of bonesetters, are particularly good. The inclusion of physicians, nurses, and social workers among healers studied is a novel and welcome feature.

Much has been written on medicine in Mesoamerica, but it is widely dispersed and in need of updating. The range and timeliness of this volume fills this need and makes it a welcome and indispensable addition to the literature.

Acknowledgments

Putting together this volume was a very enjoyable and rewarding experience. We would like to take the time to thank all of the authors for their outstanding contributions. In addition, thanks go to Dr. James Dow for creating Figures 1.1 and 1.2, to Professor David Oberstar (Modern Foreign Languages, Indiana University-Purdue University Fort Wayne) for his work in helping translate Carlos Viesca's chapter, to Dee Dee Luff and Alonia White (College of Charleston) for their many acts of kindness and their help with the bibliography, and to Mendi Benigni and Jannette Finch (Academic Computing, College of Charleston) for sharing their knowledge of computers. Special thanks go to Theresa J. May, Leslie Doyle Tingle, and Sue Carter at the University of Texas Press, to the two scholars who carefully reviewed and commented on this manuscript, to Pamela Effrein Sandstrom for her work on the index, and to Eliza Glaze, Shirley Jeffries, Vickey Nelson, and Michael Phillips of the College of Charleston's Robert Scott Small Library for their assistance with interlibrary loan requests.

Mesoamerican Healers

CHAPTER 1

Introduction

Brad R. Huber

Overview of the Study of Mesoamerican Healers

Mesoamerican healers are captivating people to watch at work, assist, listen to, read about, and study. Anthropologists have been fascinated with them for well over fifty years. Many outstanding ethnographers (e.g., Bennett and Zingg 1986; Bunzel 1952; La Farge and Byers 1931; Nutini 1968; Oakes 1969; Redfield and Villa Rojas 1934; Vogt 1969b; Wagley 1949; Wisdom 1940) have provided important information about Mesoamerican healers as part of a more general discussion of the life cycle, occupational specialization, religion, or culture change. And a fairly large number of scholars have published books and articles that have as their main focus one or more kinds of Mesoamerican healers, for example, bonesetters, curers, midwives, nurses, pharmacists, phlebotomists, physicians, spiritualists, social workers, or surgeons.

Fortunately, several excellent bibliographies can be used to locate these works as well as others that discuss topics related to Mesoamerican healing and medicine, for example, Argueta and Zolla (1994), Cosminsky and Harrison (1984), Ramírez (1978), and Vargas Melgarejo (1994). There is also an outstanding two-volume encyclopedic dictionary of traditional Mexican medicine by Soledad Mata Pinzón et al. (1994) as well as the single best source for descriptive data on traditional Mexican healing, the three-volume, 977-page book by Virginia Mellado Campos et al. (1994). Other useful sources of general information are Adams and Rubel (1967); Freyer-muth Enciso (1993); Lozoya Legorreta, Velázquez Díaz, and Flores Alva-rado (1988); Mendelson (1965); Méndez Domínguez (1983); Vargas and Casillas (1989); and Wisdom (1952).

Some of the earliest publications that focused on Mesoamerican sha-mans were produced by Parsons (1931), Bower (1946), Gillin (1956), and Madsen (1955). William Madsen's comparative piece was very influential because it showed that shamanism was widespread in Mesoamerica and that the divine call of Mexican shamans was similar to that of shamans in other parts of the world. His work was followed by more detailed or problem-oriented investigations. Scholars working with Guatemala shamans have produced exceptionally rich accounts. They include Campos (1983) and Carlsen and Prechtel (1994), and especially Colby and Colby (1981), Doug-las (1969), Metzger and Williams (1972), and Tedlock (1992a). Barbara Tedlock's work is remarkable for a number of reasons, including her atten-tion to detail, use of cross-cultural comparisons, and innovative research methods.

In Mexico, there is a large body of work on shamans, including Alvarado (1991), Álvarez Heydenreich (1992), Bonfil Batalla (1968), Dow (1986a), Fabrega and Silver (1970, 1973), Farfán Morales (1988), Gallegos Deveze (1996), Hamburger (1963), Huber (1990a, 1990b), Huber and Anderson (1996), Incháustegui (1994), Kunow (1996), Larme (1985), Lipp (1991), Claudia Madsen (1968), William Madsen (1983), Myerhoff (1974), Nutini and Forbes de Nutini (1987), Ruz (1983, 1992), Sandstrom (1975, 1978, 1991), Sandstrom and Sandstrom (1986), Vogt (1966), and Zayas (1992).

Evon Vogt does a superb job of describing the organization of shaman-ism and the wide variety of rituals shamans perform in the Maya village of Zinacantan (Chiapas). Dow's work is noteworthy for its intimate, firsthand account of a respected Ñähñu (Otomí) shaman's power, practices, and code of ethics, and for his theory of symbolic healing. This theory is insightful and widely applicable (see also Dow 1986b). Lipp's (1991) work is a com-prehensive and detailed ethnographic account of Mixe cosmology, ethno-medicine, and shamans. When Dow's and Lipp's work is compared to that of scholars who have worked in the Yucatan, Chiapas, and Guatemala, it is clear that there are similarities between Mixe, Ñähñu, and Maya shamans in terms of their recruitment, training, and initiation, but marked dissimilari-ties in terms of the use of cut paper figures, plant hallucinogens, divining bundles, and social organization, with Mayan shamans entering the religious hierarchy to a greater degree.[1]

Mesoamerican midwives have received almost as much anthropological attention as shamans. León (1910), McKay (1933), and Kelly (1956) published pieces on Mesoamerican midwifery during the first half of the twentieth century. Their work was followed by a flurry of publications in the 1970s, when women entered anthropology in larger numbers. Some of the more notable publications during this decade are those by Harrison (1977) and McClain (1975), and especially those by Sheila Cosminsky (1976a, 1976c, 1977a, 1977b), Lois Paul (1975), Lois and Benjamin Paul (1975), and Brigitte Jordan (1993). In a series of articles that span twenty-five years, Cosminsky has detailed the various roles midwives undertake as well as how their roles, beliefs, and practices have changed over time. Lois and Benjamin Paul do an outstanding job of describing the recruitment of Maya midwives and of explaining their relatively high but ambiguous status. One of Brigitte Jordan's most important contributions is her development and application of the concept of "authoritative knowledge." The study of Mesoamerican midwives gained additional momentum in the 1980s and 1990s with the work of Bortin (1993); Day (1996); Faust (1988); Greene (1988); Güémez Pineda (1989, 1997); Hurtado (1984, 1997a, 1997b); Maust (1995, 1997); Mellado Campos, Zolla, and Castañeda (1989); O'Rourke (1995b); Parra (1989, 1991, 1993); and Sesia (1992).

Until recently, interest in Mesoamerican bonesetters has been minimal. This is unfortunate because bonesetters are widespread (Mellado Campos et al. 1994) and effective. Benjamin Paul (1976) wrote the first article dedicated entirely to the study of the Maya bonesetter. It remains the best and most interesting discussion of the bonesetter's recruitment and the empirical and spiritual aspects of bonesetting. Paul's article was followed by Robert Anderson's (1987) analysis of a Mexican bonesetter's treatments and their safety. Nearly twenty years after the appearance of Paul's article, Clancy McMahon completed a 260-page master's thesis on bonesetters from the same community that Paul has worked in since the early 1940s. McMahon's (1994) thesis is notable for his detailed firsthand account of a bonesetter reducing a fracture. McMahon's work was followed by an article on bonesetting in a Nahua community by Huber and Anderson (1996). Another work that contains substantial information on bonesetters, as well as curers, midwives, and spiritualists, is Perez's (1978) dissertation.

Very little is known about spiritualists in Guatemala. In Mexico, a number of scholars, such as Sylvia Ortiz Echániz (1977), Soledad Mata Pinzón et al. (1994), and Kaja Finkler (1994b), provide detailed discussions of Spiritualism as a religion. Isabel Lagarriga Attias (1975, 1978b) was among the first to have written extensively about the healing role of Spiritualists. Her work was followed by that of Kaja Finkler (1984, 1994b, 1994c), whose *Spiritualist Healers in Mexico* was first published in 1985. It is a remarkable book for many reasons, not the least of which is Finkler's assessment of the therapeutic effectiveness of Spiritualist healing. The works by Baytelman (1986), Kearney (1977), and Reyes Gómez (1992) also contain valuable information on Mexican Spiritualists.

Physicians have not been extensively studied in Guatemala. However, Eduardo Guerrero Espinel et al. (1992) provide a nice overview of Guatemala's health sector and include some basic data on various kinds of biomedical "human resources," including the spatial and organizational distribution of doctors in Guatemala. Wellington Amaya Abad (1994, 1995) provides succinct biographical accounts of Guatemalan doctors, past and present, including those who specialize in ophthalmology (see also Granados Ortiz 1983). Enge and Harrison (1988) discuss Guatemalan doctors as maternal health care providers and Dolores Acevedo and Elena Hurtado (1997) evaluate in detail the relationship among doctors, nurses, and midwives. The latter article is noteworthy in that it shows the importance of class and ethnicity among healers in Guatemala's health care system.

Quite a bit more has been published about physicians in Mexico than in Guatemala. Collado Ardón and García Torres published a ground-breaking article on Mexican doctors in 1975. This was followed by the interesting work of Finkler (1991), Frenk and his colleagues (1985, 1990, 1991, 1995), Garduño-Espinosa (1995), Nigenda (1995), and Nigenda and Solorzano (1997). Margaret Harrison's work (1995, 1998) focuses on the personal and family circumstances of female physicians, their identification with place, the development of their careers, and migration and mobility through the life-course. In addition to this work, there is information on a successful group of elite healers from Tijuana who mix scientific knowledge with ancient curing-techniques (Schroeder 1990), physicians working in rural Mexico (Módena 1992), Mexican epidemiologists (Ruiz-Matus et al. 1990) and psychologists (Durán-González et al. 1995), and the contributions of Spanish doctors who immigrated to Mexico in the late 1930s (Guarner Dalias 1993).

Compared to doctors, nurses and social workers working in Mexico and Guatemala have received less scholarly attention. Eduardo Guerrero Espinel et al. (1992) provide good basic data on Guatemalan nurses and Eva García Pastor de Domínguez et al. (1988) describe a self-tutorial system that has been used to train auxiliary nurses in Guatemala since 1978. María Matilde Martínez Benítez et al. (1993) analyze nursing in Mexico from a sociological perspective; Marilyn Douglas et al. (1996) examine auxiliary nurse stressors, satisfiers, and coping strategies. Margaret Harrison (1994) used questionnaires and interviews to understand how nurses (and female doctors and social workers) view their job and how their status is shaped by the structure of Mexico's public health care system, family and personal needs, and *machismo*. Her approach as a medical geographer is worthy of emulation by other social scientists.

Harrison (1994) and Schmid-Dolan (1995) provide some basic data on social workers and their training in Mexico. We are not aware of any books or articles that discuss social workers in Guatemala in any detail. However, there are a number of publications that describe other kinds of health workers (e.g., health promoters, rural health technicians, volunteer collaborators) who have been recruited from indigenous Guatemala communities (Cabrera 1995; Colburn 1981; Heggenhougen 1976; Long and Viau 1974; Ruebush and Godoy 1992) and from Tarahumara communities in Mexico (Hubbard 1990). There is also some information on pharmacists in Guatemala (De Valverde 1989) and in Mexico (Logan 1983).

Sandra L. Orellana's book, *Indian Medicine in Highland Guatemala* (1987), is the single best modern, secondary source of information on different kinds of indigenous Guatemalan healers during the pre-Hispanic and colonial periods. This book and those mentioned below have excellent bibliographies that readers can use to discover primary and secondary sources of information on Mesoamerican healers prior to the twentieth century. For pre-Hispanic and colonial Mexican healers, consult León (1910), Hobgood (1959), and Rodriguez Baciero et al. (1987), and especially the groundbreaking work of Aguirre Beltrán (1963), Anzures y Bolaños (1989), Hernández Sáenz (1997), López Austin (1967), Quezada (1989, 1991), Sepúlveda (1988), and Viesca Treviño (1984, 1990). Carlos Viesca Treviño's work is remarkable for its detailed treatment of Mexica medical specialties and their transformation during the colonial period. Luz María Hernández Sáenz's (1997) book is the most comprehensive publication on all major types of colonial

Mexican healers at the time of independence. Both Hernández Sáenz and Viesca Treviño note the importance of race, class, and gender, and make meticulous use of primary archival documents.

George Foster's contributions to medical anthropology (e.g., 1953, 1987, 1994) are diverse and quite extensive. Like Benjamin Paul, he is the author of several very influential publications and has worked in the same community for more than fifty years. Foster's work helps us to better understand Mesoamerican healers because he clearly recognizes the important influence Spanish healers and their theory of humors had on Mesoamerican folk medicine. The well-documented example of the diffusion of humoral medicine to the New World is all the more remarkable because it was preceded by the centuries-long spread of Greco-Persian-Arab humoral medicine to Spain.

Scope of the Book

Throughout this book, comparisons are made regarding the socioeconomic status of Mesoamerican healers (e.g., gender, age, family of origin), their recruitment and training, compensation and workload, diagnosis of illness, conceptual models, and their relationship to other types of medical practitioners and religious and political leaders. My use of the term "Mesoamerican" (literally, Middle American) needs to be clarified because it means different things to different people (see Carmack, Gasco, and Gossen 1996:5–6). Those who think of Mesoamerica primarily in geographic terms may find the scope of this book more limited than the title suggests. As Table 1.1 and Figures 1.1 and 1.2 indicate, comparisons are made of healers from a relatively large number of indigenous groups, but only those from Mexico and Guatemala. Practical considerations preclude discussion of healers from Belize, El Salvador, Honduras, Nicaragua, Costa Rica, and Panama.[2] Considerations of length also meant some kinds of healers working in Mexico and Guatemala could not be examined (e.g., dermatologists, ophthalmologists, dentists, psychologists, radio doctors, epidemiologists, volunteer health promoters, acupuncturists, homeopaths, fortune tellers). In any case, there is relatively little written about these kinds of healers.

"Mesoamerican" is often used to refer to a particular historical tradition of aboriginal cultures. For readers who generally think of Mesoamerica

TABLE I.I: LIST OF NAMES OF INDIGENOUS MESOAMERICAN GROUPS

Major Maya Groups in Mexico and Guatemala

ALMG Name[1]	Other Commonly Used Names
Achi	Achí
Akateko	Acateco
Awakateko	Aguacateco, Aguacatec
Chikomuselteko	Chicomucelteco
Chontal	
Chuj	Chuh
Ch'ol	Chol
Ch'orti'	Chortí
Itza'	Itzá
Ixil	Ixil
Jakalteko	Jacalteco, Jacaltec
K'aqchikel	Cakchiquel, Cakchikel
K'iche'	Quiché, Kiché
Lakandon	Lacandón, Lacandon
Mam	Mame
Mocho'	Mochó, Motozintleco, Motozintlec
Mopan	Mopán
Poqomam	Pokomam, Pocomam
Poqomchi'	Pokomchí, Pocomchí, Pokonchi
Q'anjob'al	Kanjobal, Kanhobal
Q'eqchi'	Kekchí, Kekchi
Sakapulteküo	Sacapulteco
Sipakapense	Sipacapeño
Tektiteko	Teco, Tectiteco
Tojolab'al	Tojolabal, Toholabal
Tzeltal	
Tzotzil	
Tz'utujil	Tzutujil, Tzutuhil
Uspanteko	Uspanteco, Uspantec
Yukateko	Yucateco, Yucatec
Wasteko	Huasteco, Huastec, Teenek

TABLE I.I (cont.)

Major Non-Mayan Groups in Mexico

HMAI Name[2]	Other Commonly Used Names
Amuzgo	
Chatino	
Chichimec	Chichimeca, Chichimeca-Jonaz, Ézar
Chinantec	Chinanteco
Chocho	
Cora	Nayeri
Cuicatec	
Guarijío	
Huave	Huazanteco, Juave, Mareño
Huichol	
Ixcatec	Ixcateco, Ichcatec
Kickapoo	Kikapu, Kikapoo
Kiliwa	Ko'kew
Mazahua	
Mazatec	Mazateco
Mixe	
Mixtec	Mixteco
Nahua	Nahuatl
Ñähñu	Otomí
Opata	
Pame	
Pápago	
Pima	
Popoloca	
Popoluca	
Purépecha	Tarascan
Rarámuri	Tarahumara, Tarahumar
Seri	
Tepehua	
Tepehuani	Tepehuanes del Sur, Tepehuan, O'dam

TABLE 1.1 (cont.)

HMAI Name[2]	Other Commonly Used Names
Tlahuica	
Tlapanec	
Totonac	Totonaca
Trique	Triqui
Yaqui	
Zapotec	Zapateco

[1] Orthographic conventions used for names of Maya groups in the left-hand column are based upon those recommended by the Academia de Lenguas Mayas de Guatemala (ALMG). They emerged out of the work of Adrian Inez Chavez (see Lewis 1993).

[2] For the most part, names for non-Maya groups in the left-hand column are those used in Volumes 7 and 8 of the *Handbook of Middle American Indians* (HMAI) (Vogt 1969a).

in these terms, the scope of the book may be more inclusive than they anticipated. Healers who are mestizos or who view themselves as descendants of Spaniards are discussed in detail. Contributors look at healers from Native American groups in north Mexico as well. Many scholars would group them with the North American Southwest (e.g., Ortiz 1983). These groups and types of healers were included because the authors of the chapters wanted to highlight the historical and contemporary interrelationships among them.

In addition to the above limitations in scope, this book does not treat in great detail the use of medicinal plants by Mesoamerican healers. Interest in Mesoamerican medicinal plants has a long history and the literature on this topic is voluminous. A minimum of several hundred pages would be necessary to treat this topic in an appropriate manner. Some of the more important resources on medicinal plants and their use by healers in Mexico and Guatemala are mentioned below.

One of the best places to learn about medicinal plant use in Guatemala is Orellana's 1987 book. It also has a nice nineteen-page overview of historical and current botanical, ethnobotanical, and ethnographic sources on medicinal plant use in this country as well as in Mexico. Another source to consult to learn about medicinal plant use in Guatemala is Armando Cáceres's (1996) *Plantas de uso medicinal en Guatemala*. Julia Frances Morton's *Atlas of Medicinal Plants of Middle America: Bahamas to Yucatan* (1981) is one of the best single sources about medicinal plants in Mexico. Espe-

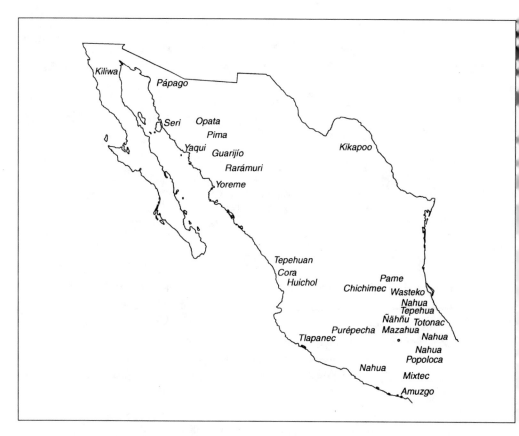

FIGURE 1.1: Western Mesoamerica.

cially worthy of mention are two 1994 books whose six volumes collectively contain nearly 3,400 pages of information on medicinal plants in Mexico: (1) Emes Boronda, Ochurte Espinoza, Castañeda Silva, and Peralta González' *Flora medicinal indígena de México: Treinta y cinco monografías del Atlas de las plantas de la medicina tradicional mexicana*; and (2) Argueta Villamar, Cano Asseleih, and Rodarte's *Atlas de las plantas de la medicina tradicional mexicana*. The latter has an extensive bibliography of sources that deal with anthropological, botanical, chemical, ecological, ethnobotanical, geographical, historical, pharmacological, and toxicological aspects of medicinal plants. Also worthy of special mention are Alcorn (1984); Berlin and Berlin (1996); Bye (1986); Bye and Linares Mazari (1987); Frei, Baltisberger,

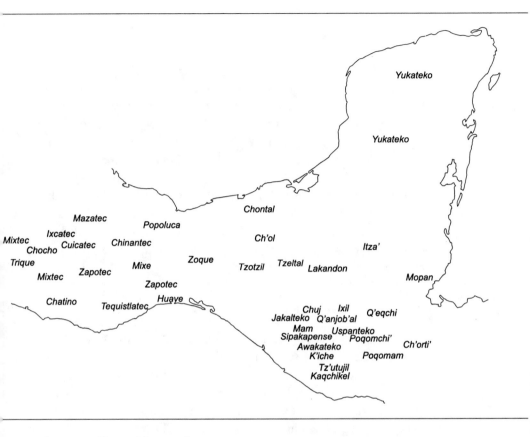

FIGURE 1.2: Eastern Mesoamerica.

Sticher, and Heinrich (1998); Frei, Sticher, Viesca Treviño, and Heinrich (1998); Ortiz de Montellano (1975); and Weimann and Heinrich (1998).

Methodological Approaches

The approach taken in Chapters 2 and 3 is ethnohistorical. The authors make extensive use of archival materials and supplement them with published, secondary sources. Physicians, surgeons, pharmacists, phlebotomists, nurses, midwives, and *curanderos* are compared to each other. The authors also make regional comparisons and show how a healer's role has changed over time.

The next eight chapters concern themselves with contemporary practitioners. They are examples of regional controlled comparisons of healers from neighboring, culturally similar groups. All of the authors have first-hand experience working with healers in one or more Mesoamerican communities and have conducted an extensive review of the literature. Several have worked with two or more kinds of healers. As Dow and Lipp note, comparisons present a number of problems, for example, lack of information and imprecise definitions of some healers. Nevertheless, they are worthwhile because they lead to an appreciation of the amount and kinds of variation that exist among different types of healers. Equally important, regional controlled comparisons stimulate the development of midlevel theories. Since healers come from groups that are similar in many respects, differences in a small number of variables often "form integrated clusters, or systemic variations, whose functional or causal interdependence [holds] explanatory power" (Johnson 1991:4).

Theoretical Perspectives

Although there is more cross-fertilization and overlap now than in the past, economists, historians, political scientists, medical anthropologists, geographers, psychologists, and sociologists traditionally focused on different kinds and aspects of medical practitioners. For example, medical anthropologists have looked extensively at midwives and magico-religious healers such as shamans, often in relatively small non-Western societies. Medical sociologists frequently studied doctor–patient interactions and the organization, educational experience, and socioeconomic status of doctors and nurses in Europe and North America. Medical geographers have often focused on the accessibility, utilization, and spatial distribution of medical personnel and facilities in nations throughout the world. Scholars from these disciplines also tended to employ different theories. Four theoretical perspectives and how they can be applied to Mesoamerican healers are discussed below.

Interpretive theories explore the meaning and "metaphors of health and illness and the symbolic uses of the human body in various cultures" (McElroy and Townsend 1996:64). Finkler uses an interpretive approach at times in her chapter on Spiritualist healers. For example, she discusses a patient with heart palpitations to illustrate the way Spiritualist symbols are transmitted from healers to patients. The patient's Spiritualist healer suggested her heart palpitations were like crystalline drops falling into an empty glass. The drops symbolized God's words and the empty glass represented the patient. After the patient recovered, she became a Spiritualist healer herself and often referred to this metaphor when she talked to other patients about illness. Finkler also suggests spirit possession trance allows Spiritualist healers to experience their bodies in a new and sacred way, and that this may be health promoting.

There are different and competing theories of feminism. Following Sherwin (1996: 188–189), feminist theory is understood here as the recognition that women are oppressed by sexism, and that this oppression may involve one or more of the following conditions: exploitation, marginalization, powerlessness, cultural imperialism, and violence. Harrison's chapter is in part an application of this theory. She discusses the increasing number of women entering the medical profession in Mexico, an increase that took place when a shift occurred from physician scarcity to excess. In turn, there was a corresponding decrease in job security, pay, and status. Women physicians were affected more negatively by these changes than were male ones. They are more likely than male physicians to work part time in the public sector. In addition, the percentage of women physicians working in less desirable sectors of Mexico's health system is greater than the percentage of women working in more desirable sectors. Harrison also discusses the fact that women physicians are expected to fulfill the same family obligations they have in the past, and how this makes it difficult for female doctors to take annual renewal courses, especially when travel is necessary.

The authors of several other chapters note that gender and type of healing role are correlated in Mesoamerica. During the colonial period, physicians, surgeons, pharmacists, and phlebotomists were generally men, while midwives and nurses were overwhelmingly female (Hernández Sáenz and Foster). The contemporary period is similar in the sense that higher status, better remunerated medical occupations are undertaken by men while lower status, lower paid ones are filled by women (Harrison, and Hurtado and Sáenz de Tejada). Dow and Lipp note that both men and women can become shamans. However, only male shamans tend to combine healing with the higher status role of priest. Female shamans have relatively little to do with the public aspects of religion and politics in Mesoamerican communities.

The political economy perspective is often used to critically look at how the world economic system and broad social and political forces shape illness and healing (McElroy and Townsend 1996:65–69). This theory helps scholars to appreciate the important role funding from foreign countries and nongovernmental organizations (NGOS) plays in Guatemala's health system, including the type and distribution of healers (see Hurtado and Sáenz de Tejada's chapter as well as Bossert 1987, Cardona and Campos 1995, Guerrero Espinel et al. 1992, and La Forgia and Couttolenc 1993). The institutional violence directed toward some of Guatemala's medical practitioners during the late 1970s and 1980s can also be understood within a political economy perspective. The American Association for the Advancement of Science (1992), Cabrera Perez-Arminan (1995), and Liebman (1994) document cases in which rural and urban health promoters, nurses, doctors, and medical students had to drastically curtail their activities because of widespread violence and their presumed antigovernment sympathies. Some were imprisoned, disappeared, and killed.

Political economy is especially useful in understanding how power, social class, and ethnicity are determinants of medical practice, and of the social relations among healers. One of the main contributions of Hernández Sáenz and Foster is to show how the organization and characteristics of colonial healers reflected the social, economic, and ethnic stratification of the society in which they practiced. At the top of the medical hierarchy were wealthy, university-trained "pure blooded" Spaniards and Creoles. At the bottom were poor, uneducated, "racially mixed" practitioners: phlebotomists, midwives, nurses, and *curanderos*. Numerous mechanisms of social control, secular and religious, formal and informal, regulated Mesoamerican healers and medical practices during the colonial period. The Royal Protomedicato was charged with licensing medical personnel and enforcing legislation. Medical faculty within a university were ranked below the faculty of canons, theology, and law. Rural missions had hospital annexes.

Medical ecological theory views the health of a group as a reflection of the quality and kind of relationships within the group, with neighboring groups, and with plants, animals, and nonbiotic features of the environment (McElroy and Townsend 1996:2, 12, 67). Paleopathologists, social epidemiologists, and medical anthropologists have successfully used this theory to understand links among birth, fertility, nutrition, stress, death, and illness on the one hand, and the environment, subsistence patterns, and population size on the other. Although healers have not been extensively examined from a medical ecological perspective, the authors of two chapters suggest how this approach can be applied to them. Huber and Sandstrom found a moderately strong positive correlation between population size and the likelihood that midwives will be found in an indigenous group, degree of medical specialization, and presence of a traditional medical organization. Dow found that shamans from sparsely populated north Mexican groups use fewer ritual objects than those from the east, west, and central regions. Medical ecological theory continues to shows promise. We suspect it can be used to account for other aspects of Mesoamerican healers, such as the number and types of medicinal plants healers use, the kinds of conceptual models employed, and the degree of competition among healers.

The above four theories shed light on different aspects of Mesoamerican healers, and for that reason they will continue to be useful. Nevertheless, these theories have limitations and problems with which scholars are still struggling. For example, some ecological explanations in medical anthropology are justifiably viewed as reductionist, "leaving out too many cultural variables, and not giving adequate emphasis to the forces of politics, economics, and history" (McElroy and Townsend 1996:67). However, scholars are developing an approach—political ecology—that merges ecological theory and political economy (Baer, Singer, and Susser 1997; Brown 1988). We are encouraged by this synthesis. The medical ecological perspective can accommodate political ecological theory as well as feminist and interpretive analyses. Accommodation is more productive than the wholesale rejection of this theory. It is consistent with anthropology's holistic and multidisciplinary approach (see also Anderson 1996; Biersack 1999; Kottak 1999).

Organization of This Volume

This volume contains ten topical chapters. The first two offer ethnohistorical perspectives on Mesoamerican healers, emphasizing their indigenous, Hispanic, and African origins and influences. The next eight focus on contemporary healers: shamans, Spiritualists, midwives, bonesetters, physicians, nurses, and social workers. Many of the authors of these chapters are well known to Mesoamericanists. I am pleased that they contributed to this volume. Their chapters represent the state of the art in the study of Guatemalan and Mexican healers.

Hernández Sáenz and Foster's chapter provides the best documentary support yet for the theory that the humoral component of Spanish American folk medicine came from elite colonial healers—physicians, surgeons, pharmacists, phlebotomist-barbers, and missionary friars. Viesca shows how indigenous, mestizo, African, and "mixed-race" healers at the lowest levels of the medical hierarchy were increasingly denigrated and persecuted as the number of physicians and missionaries increased. For example, Maya curers during the early colonial period grew reluctant to practice for fear of being accused of witchcraft. The Inquisition condemned the use of peyote, which was much more widespread in the past than it is at the present time among indigenous healers. When hearing Indians confess, friars regularly included questions to determine if they had been going to indigenous healers or believed in predictions based on dreams or omens.

Opposition to indigenous healers continued in Mexico and Guatemala well into the nineteenth century, and, as Dow, Lipp, Cosminsky, and Hurtado and Sáenz de Tejada show, it continues in various forms up to the present time. Dow notes that some Mesoamerican groups have shamans who participate in public religious ceremonies while other groups have shamans who limit their work to healing illness. The latter are found among groups where Roman Catholic and evangelical Protestant influence has been comparatively long and sustained.

Lipp examines the various ways shamans organize themselves and how their organization is related to other aspects of a community's social organization, finding that shamans from many Maya groups are formally and publically recognized, ranked in a hierarchy, and come from societies with lineage-based social organizations. In contrast, Oaxacan shamans generally lack an ancestor-based vertical arrangement and come from groups with a bilateral and generational kinship pattern. Finkler explains why the majority of Spiritualist temple leaders, healers, and patients are women, taking into account the exclusion of most women from full participation in social and political affairs, the subjugation of women to men, and their husbands' acts of violence during drinking binges.

Huber and Sandstrom, Cosminsky, and Hurtado and Sáenz de Tejada look at different aspects of Mesoamerican midwives. Huber and Sandstrom found that midwifery is more varied in northern and central Mexico than in southern Mexico and Guatemala. In addition to finding that ecological and demographic factors are systematically related to midwifery organizations, training, and gender, these authors discovered that the way midwives are recruited (sacred or secular) predicts the likelihood that they will cooperate with doctors and nurses. This is a finding with potential practical significance.

Cosminsky leaves no doubt that Maya midwives are still one of the most important types of healers working in Mexico and Guatemala today, delivering most births in most rural communities. They have also been the type of healer most subjected to medicalization. As a by-product of this process, their authoritative knowledge has been contested and their role has been increasingly secularized. In addition, they have been placed in a hierarchy in which they are subordinate to doctors and nurses, and in a dominant position with respect to their clients.

Hurtado and Sáenz de Tejada compare Guatemalan physicians and nurses to midwives working with Guatemala's Ministry of Health Services. This brings into sharp focus the importance of class, educational level, gender, and ethnicity. Physicians and nurses are mostly *ladino*, speak Spanish, and have a university or high school degree. Midwives are generally illiterate Mayan woman who live and work in impoverished rural communities. These authors find that control is exercised in a variety of ways such as requiring a license to practice, training at monthly health services meetings, scoldings and reprimands, denigration of their supposed abuse of liquor, and criticism of their alleged misuse of massages and sweat baths. As a result, midwives may resist licensing, practice in secret, and avoid referring pregnant women to health centers. Ethnic discrimination is deeply rooted in Guatemalan society, and discrimination against traditional healers is common. Nevertheless, Hurtado and Sáenz de Tejada provide considerable evidence that the situation is beginning to improve as doctors, nurses, and midwives learn more about each other, become more tolerant, and begin to work together to produce positive health outcomes.

Paul and McMahon undertake the considerable task of comparing various subgroups of bonesetters in Mexico and Guatemala. One of their most interesting findings is that supernaturally called bonesetters are found primarily in the Yucatan, Chiapas, and Guatemala. Their status in the community is higher than that of secular bonesetters even though they use fewer medicinal products and do not charge a fee for their services.

In the last topical chapter, Harrison compares contemporary, formally educated healers—physicians, nurses, and social workers—to each other and examines their distribution throughout Mexico. As in several other chapters in this volume, gender and class stand out as two very important variables. However, Harrison also analyzes the importance of *place* in understanding some of the problems Mexico is experiencing with respect to access to biomedical health care.

Notes

1. I thank Frank Lipp for this insight.
2. The inclusion of healers from these six countries would have more clearly revealed the contemporary and historical significance of African and Caribbean medicine.

CHAPTER 2

Curers and Their Cures in Colonial New Spain and Guatemala

The Spanish Component

Luz María Hernández Sáenz and George M. Foster

Introduction

At the time of the discovery and conquest of the New World, European medicine was basically classical Greek humoral pathology, as set forth in the *Hippocratic corpus* (fifth century B.C.), systematized by Galen (second century A.D.), and augmented and codified in Persia (sixth and seventh centuries) and in Baghdad (ninth to eleventh centuries) by Moslem scholars such as Rhazes, Haly Abbas, and Avicenna (980–1037), whose *Canon of Medicine* is considered to be the definitive statement of Greco-Persian-Arab medicine.

The Greeks believed the four humors were fluids that freely circulated through the body's more solid tissues. Each of the humors was assigned a pair of qualities that characterized the four primary elements of which the earth was thought to be composed: *fire* (Hot), *air* (Cold), *water* (Moist), and *earth* (Dry). Thus, the humor *blood* was Hot and Moist, *phlegm* Cold and Moist, *yellow bile* (or *choler*) Hot and Dry, and *black bile* (or *melancholy*) Cold and Dry. By the time of Christ the concept of the humoral qualities had been extended to include foods and herbal and other remedies as well. To illustrate, garlic was classified as Hot and Dry, chickpeas Hot and Moist, barley Cold and Dry, and mallow Cold and Moist. It must be emphasized that these characteristics—or *calidades* (qualities), in Spanish—are metaphoric and not thermal. Thus, in contemporary Mexico a cup of coffee may be thermally hot, cold, or lukewarm, but metaphorically it is always Hot. (We indicate metaphoric temperature by capitalizing the first letter of the word; lowercase first letters indicate thermal values.)

An equilibrium model explained health: with the four humors in relative balance, an individual enjoyed good health; illness occurred when humors were diminished or increased beyond their optimum points. Thus the physician's task was to determine which were the offending humors, and take steps to restore the lost equilibrium. This was accomplished through diet, herbal and other internal medications, and therapies such as bleeding, purging, administering enemas, and applying plasters. Since hot and cold environmental insults were the principal causes of loss of humoral equilibrium, herbs and foods of opposite quality to the insult were prescribed according to the formula "a Cold remedy for a hot illness, and a Hot remedy for a cold illness." This "principle of opposites" has prevailed as the basic humoral therapeutic strategy through more than two millennia.

Carried by the Moslems through north Africa into Spain and Italy, the ancient Greek writings, first translated into Syriac and then Arabic, as well as the Arabic medical legacy itself, gradually became known to medieval Christian scholars through Latin translations—often badly done—made in such places as Salerno (Sicily), Monte Casino (Italy), and Toledo (Spain). By the mid-fifteenth century, copies of original Greek texts also began to appear in western Europe. Latin translations of these copies, while more accurate than those of Arabic manuscripts, arrived on the scene too late to replace the latter as the most important influence on European medicine (Sarton 1954:89).

Thus the ancient doctrine of humors became the basis of medieval Christian medicine, remaining dominant until near the end of the seventeenth century, when the discoveries of such men as Vesalius (1514–1564), Harvey (1578–1637), and Sydenham (1624–1689) forced a reexamination of the prevailing assumptions about health and illness, which ultimately led to the rejection of humoral theory and its replacement by the biomedical paradigm that has guided the development of medicine ever since. Yet from the writings of Vesalius, Harvey, Sydenham, and their contemporaries, and from the content of medical training in universities, we see that the humoral doctrines of Hippocrates, Aristotle, Galen, and Avicenna continued to be the major source of medical theory and practice until well into the eighteenth century.

This was the elite medical system brought to the New World by Spanish physicians, pharmacists, botanists, and members of the religious sodalities. In the ethnographic literature it usually is called the "hot–cold syndrome," or the "hot–cold dichotomy." Even longer than in Europe it remained the dominant formal medical paradigm, although, as will soon be noted, it maintained an increasingly uneasy alliance with contemporary biomedicine.

The Diffusion of Spanish Medicine to the New World

When the Spaniards arrived in America they found indigenous curers skilled in a variety of therapeutic treatments including herbal remedies, the setting of broken bones, administering of enemas, and the like. Hernán Cortés was so impressed by Aztec medicine that he is said to have urged the Emperor Charles V not to send Spanish doctors because indigenous curers were so competent. Although this story may well be apocryphal,[1] it serves as a metaphor for the astonishment of the conquistadores at the skill of Aztec curers. Among the medical wonders of Mexico noted by the Spaniards were the botanical gardens of the Emperor Moctezuma in Oaxtepec (in the modern state of Morelos) and near Tenochtitlán (Mexico City). In these repositories of medicinal herbs from all parts of the empire, Spanish botanists and doctors familiarized themselves with the New World pharmacopeia.

The Spaniards were anxious to learn the medical practices of doctors, priests, and sorcerers in New Spain for at least two reasons. First, insofar as magic and witchcraft were a part of curing rituals, members of the missionary orders recognized that to extirpate the (to them) idolatrous beliefs and practices, they must first know them. And second, there was a genuine intellectual curiosity about the medicinal herbs and other substances previously unknown to Europeans, that were assumed to have medicinal virtues. It was hoped, and widely believed that, hidden in New World pharmacopeias were remedies to treat new plagues (such as syphilis) that were appearing during this age of discovery.

By far the most important study of Aztec medicine was undertaken by the Franciscan friar Bernardino de Sahagún at the Colegio de Santa Cruz, founded by members of this order in 1536 in the town of Tlaltelolco, at that time a suburb of the City of Mexico, and today a part of the city proper. Here, over a period of more than forty years, Sahagún, who had arrived in New Spain in 1529, worked with a variety of Aztec informants, including elders of the society, merchants, priests, and *curanderas* knowledgeable about herbs and other therapies. Aided by a group of Aztec scribes trained to write their language in Latin letters, he systematically recorded the data brought together in his *General History of the Things of New Spain.*[2] This monumental work, of course, deals with many aspects of Aztec culture in addition to medicine.

For seventeenth-century Spaniards the theoretical basis for prescribing herbs was their humoral value—the Hot/Cold qualities in relationship to the perceived cause of the illness. Thus, Spanish doctors, pharmacists, and the clergy, who began incorporating New World herbal remedies into their medical practice, were concerned to know the humoral qualities of these heretofore unknown herbs. Their classificatory efforts were well under way by the time the Emperor Philip II sent his personal physician, the naturalist Francisco Hernández, to New Spain in 1570 to make a complete inventory of the natural history of the country. Before he returned home in 1577, Hernández had described more than three thousand plants, to almost all of which he had assigned humoral values (Del Pozo 1965:66).

"Of this work," writes López Austin (1975:107), "one immediately sees that it is the intention of the European scientist to classify the American natural world within his framework, deducing from the *calidades* he assigns to these plants the effects he believes they have on the human body." The "principle of opposites," a cold remedy for a Hot illness and a hot remedy for a Cold one, is clearly spelled out. Thus, of the herb *Acxoyatic*, Hernández writes that it is cold and humid; the root, drunk cold, cures fever (Hernández 1942:34). And of squash, all varieties are cold and humid, "good for those suffering from fever or heat in the kidneys" (Hernández 1959, 1:51).

The transmission of Spanish medicine to the New World conformed to the same dynamic that characterized the diffusion of other elements of Iberian culture to the New World: an *elite*, or *formal*, level, and a *popular*, or *informal* level. The formal medical establishment was headed by the Royal Tribunal of the Protomedicato, or medical board. Of medieval origin, the Protomedicato was established in New Spain in the sixteenth century ("about 1527," according to González-Ulloa 1959:38) to license doctors and pharmacists, to inspect pharmacies, and to prevent "medical crimes" such as the practice of medicine by unlicensed personnel and the sale of nonauthorized or unfairly priced drugs. A 1646 royal decree sanctioned the local custom of appointing two senior faculty members as first and second *protomédicos* and left the appointment of the third board member to the viceroy. Despite legislation, the limited number of licensed practitioners, the ineffectiveness of colonial medicine, the cultural heterogeneity of the population, and the inability of most people to afford the services of licensed practitioners made the task of the Mexican Protomedicato unrealistic and impossible to carry out according to its charter. The situation of the medical practitioner in Guatemala was even more chaotic as this captaincy lacked a formal Protomedicato until 1793 (Asturias 1958:167–169).

The informal level of transmission of Spanish healing practices to the New World was that of *medicina casera*, the domestic medicine of the conquistadores and those who followed them. As Aguirre Beltrán (1963:261) reminds us, "The conquistadores and settlers, with few exceptions of low social status in origin, were the carriers of ideas and practices of popular Spanish medicine." Fear of the evil eye, and the strategies used to treat illness thought to be caused by *el mal de ojo*, as well as the belief that medicinal herbs were most effective if gathered during Lent or on the Eve of St. John (June 24) are illustrative of this level. Still other Spanish curing practices doubtless represent diffusion at both elite and popular levels: hagiolatry— the invocation of saints to help the sick person, and the associated use of votive offerings—comes to mind.

Unlike in Spain, however, where humoral medicine appears never to have been an important part of folk medicine, in the New World it filtered down to the popular level to provide the rationale not only for mestizo folk medical beliefs and practices but also, through the acculturative process, for many indigenous peoples as well. Until the recent past, a great deal of Spanish American folk medicine has been based on the classical Greek concept of the four humors, and the "principle of opposites" model for treatment of illness. About the elite level of transmission the historical record is very good indeed, although much remains to be done in archival research. About the transmission to Mexico of Spanish folk medicine, the record is much less complete, leading to considerable disagreement among scholars as to the point of origin of many practices, especially the modern occurrence of the hot/cold dichotomy as a part of popular medicine (for a comprehensive discussion of the diffusion of humoral medicine to the New World, see Foster 1994:147–188).

Elite Medicine in New Spain

By the end of the seventeenth century in New Spain,[3] four categories of elite curers were recognized by, and—theoretically at least, and to varying degrees—were under the jurisdiction of the Protomedicato (Quezada 1989: 15–27). In order of their rank and prestige they were as follows:

1. Physicians. *Médicos* were university graduates, formally examined and licensed to practice internal medicine.
2. Surgeons. *Cirujanos latinos* were university graduates, examined and licensed to practice external medicine. *Cirujanos romancistas* studied at least four years under an "approved professor." They were licensed not only to operate but also to bleed patients, remove cataracts, treat hernias, set broken bones, and attend difficult parturitions.
3. Pharmacists. *Boticarios* acquired their skills as "on-the-job" apprentices. Although not university-trained, they were educated men who could read Latin and were licensed following successful passing of the Protomedicato examination.
4. Phlebotomists-barbers. *Sangradores-barberos* were examined by the Protomedicato and were licensed to extract teeth, to bleed patients and to "cup" patients (i.e., apply *ventosas*). Many of them were also barbers in the usual sense of the word, shaving and cutting the hair of customers.

In addition to these four groups, there were the missionary friars—Franciscans, Dominicans, Augustinians, Jesuits, and others—who, although not recognized as part of the formal medical system, played a very important role in the care of the sick and poor by establishing hospitals. In cities, patients in their hospitals were attended not only by them, but also by physicians and surgeons, and pharmacists as well, who supplied prescribed medications. In rural hospitals they themselves supplied most of the care for indigenous and mestizo patients.

Two other categories of caregivers—in colonial times the most numerous of all—must be noted:

Midwives. Most *parteras* were, like their patients, Indian or mestiza in race. Lacking formal training, they delivered babies and provided pre- and postnatal care according to the customs of the ethnic or tribal group to which they belonged.

Curanderos, who were illegal practitioners, constituted the largest and most varied of all categories of curers. They were (and are) the specialists to whom most urban poor and rural Mexicans first turn for medical help. Some were *hueseros*, skilled in setting dislocations and broken bones; others were *masajistas* skilled in massage techniques used to relieve the pain of sprains and strains, as well as restoring a "fallen fontanel" (*caída de la mollera*); still others treated *bilis*, a hot illness calling for Cold remedies, and children afflicted with the evil eye (*mal de ojo*).

Physicians and Their Training

The first New World medical education that was largely Spanish in content was begun in 1536 at the Franciscan Colegio de Santa Cruz in Tlaltelolco. Here, in the same institution where Fray Bernardino de Sahagún gathered the data for his *General History of the Things of New Spain*, Indian students were, in addition to medicine, taught reading and writing in Spanish and Latin, as well as the fundamentals of Christianity, rhetoric, philosophy, and music.

The formal medical training of Spanish and Creole students as physicians in New Spain did not begin until after the founding of the Real y Pontificia Universidad de México in 1553. Although formal *cátedras* (professorships) were not established for another twenty-five years, the teaching of medicine began almost immediately, and by 1775 had become "a very important part of the university curriculum" (González-Ulloa 1959:42). The first "chair," the Prima de Medicina (First of Medicine), was established in 1578, followed in 1598 by that of Vísperas (Vespers—so-called because the professor met the students in the early evening). The addition of a chair of Methodo Medendi, and a *cátedra* of anatomy and surgery in 1621, completed the medical offerings of the university until the eighteenth century.

From 1621 onward the curriculum of the Mexican university was based on these four courses. All lectures were conducted in Latin, except when the difficult nature of the topic required Spanish. Students attended classes five days a week, two hours in the morning and two in the afternoon, and met every other Saturday to discuss the material covered in the lectures. In 1643 Virrey Palafox ordered that both teachers and students should attend the three dissections that were to be performed each year (González-Ulloa 1959:43). University records reveal, however, that for a variety of reasons, such as lack of cadavers and salary disputes, this requirement was often ignored.

In Guatemala, the Universidad de San Carlos was established in 1681 and, because of a lack of local candidates, held its first *oposiciones* for the chair of medicine in Mexico. The only Mexican applicant, José Salmerón y Castro, was offered the professorship, but failed to appear in Guatemala to take up the appointment. Consequently the post was filled provisionally by a local physician until 1688 when Miguel Fernández, recently arrived from Spain, was appointed the first tenured professor of medicine at San Carlos. More than a century later, in 1796, "a supernumerary chair" in surgery (without salary) was added (Lanning 1956: 210–211, 291–292).

A great concern with health problems is evidenced by numerous medical works published in Mexico City from 1570 on. The earliest was *Opera medicinalia*, by Francisco Bravo, a physician born in Spain and a migrant to Mexico City prior to 1570, when his work appeared. Jarcho describes the *Opera* as "the work of an experienced and widely read physician in whom learning preponderates heavily over observation" (1957:429). This characterization of Mexican medicine appears to hold true until the late eighteenth century. "The Greek and Arab writers were studied in great detail. . . . Modern authors were not excluded but were usually refuted in favor of the Greeks" (Jarcho 1957:431).

Other important colonial publications include Juan de Cárdenas' *Primera parte de los problemas y secretos maravillosos de las Indias* (1591), Gregorio López' *Tesoro de medicinas* (Guerra 1982; written and edited from 1580–1588 but not published until 1672), Agustín de Vetancurt's *Teatro mexicano* (1698), and, most important of all, at least in transmitting Spanish humoral beliefs and practices to the popular level, Juan de Esteyneffer's *Florilegio medicinal* (Anzures y Bolaños 1978; originally published in 1712).

In New Spain the monopoly of the Real y Pontificia Universidad on medical education remained unbroken until 1787 when the Audiencia approved the Medical Academy of Puebla. Five years later, the University of Guadalajara opened a third program. Nonetheless, Mexico City continued to attract the majority of medical students and through the university maintained control over examinations and licensing.

It is important to emphasize that in stratified societies such as those of colonial New Spain and Guatemala, to attend a university conferred upon the student a high status that separated him from other practitioners of medicine, as well as most of the other members of society.[4] In Mexico, as in the rest of the Spanish empire, this special status was safeguarded by academic and racial exclusivity. To be accepted into the medical program, the applicant had to present proof not only of his academic qualifications (a bachelor of arts degree or equivalent), but also of his *limpieza de sangre* (blood line untainted by Jewish, Moslem, or black ancestry), as well as the financial ability to maintain a standard of living (including attire, lodging, and textbooks) commensurate with his university status.

Students could aspire to three degrees: bachelor's, *licenciado*, and doctoral. After attending the required courses (which after 1788 also included botany) and performing in a satisfactory manner, the student applied for his final examination for his *bachillerato*. This oral examination took place before a board of eight examiners of the faculties of medicine and either philosophy or arts. If approved, the student received the degree of bachelor of medicine. Two further years of internship in a hospital under the supervision of a licensed physician completed his training. The new physician was then examined by the Protomedicato and licensed as a practitioner.

The next academic step for a physician was the degree of *licenciado*, equivalent to a present-day master's degree. This implied further years of study, an *acto de repetición*, or exposition and debate on the works of a classical authority, and an examination on a theme from the works of Hippocrates or Avicenna, chosen by the examiners. During the eighteenth century the examination cost 600 pesos, a hefty sum that made it impossible for many students to aspire to the *licenciado* degree.

The doctoral degree required yet another examination, with attendant expense for the graduation ceremony, but no further formal studies. According to surviving university records, from 1734 to 1826 at least seventy-three graduates received the degree of bachelor of medicine in Mexico. Of these five went on to become *licenciados* and fifty-five obtained a doctoral degree. In Guatemala, from 1704 to 1821, the Universidad de San Carlos granted thirty baccalaureates, twelve *licenciaturas*, and twelve doctoral degrees (Lanning 1956:210).

By the eighteenth century, the official curriculum of the Real y Pontificia Universidad de México (and therefore that of the Universidad de San Carlos), issued in 1645, lagged years behind the curricula of Spanish, French, and Scottish medical faculties. However, recent studies indicate that by the second half of the eighteenth century, large numbers of contemporary European medical books legally entered New Spain, and this new knowledge was reflected in medical education (Hernández Sáenz 1997:28–30). "The availability of and demand for modern medical texts and the public debates taking place at the university indicate that a large number of Mexican physicians were up to date with modern developments" (Hernández Sáenz 1997:40). To illustrate, in 1774, a year before he received his bachelor's degree, Joaquín Pío Antonio de Eguía y Muro Morales took part in a debate on Albrecht Von Haller's work *De Sensibilite* (1759) and Santorio Santorio's *Medicina Statica* (1614). Eleven years later in a similar debate, Eguía y Muro Morales, by then a doctor of medicine, discussed Friedrich Hoffman's *Pathology* (1740), Boerhaave's *De lue venerea* (1727), and Johannes de Gorter's *De medico dogmático*. On both occasions, the lectures included the views of contemporary European authors, indicating the speaker's knowledge of their medical theories.

Eguía y Muro Morales was by no means the only authority on contemporary medicine. In *Mercurio Volante*, a journal he edited, Dr. José Ignacio Bartolache displayed impressive knowledge of contemporary European medical developments by listing the publications of European medical authors such as the anatomist Jacob Winslow (1669–1760) and the physicians Gerhard Freyherr Van Swieten (1700–1772) and Johannes Gorter (1689–1762). Both Eguía y Muro Morales and Bartolache were graduates of the University of Mexico, and neither had traveled abroad. Hernández Sáenz concludes, "The treatment a patient could receive in Mexico City was not much different from that of Edinburgh, one of the most renowned centers of medical education at the time" (1997:43–44). But, despite their familiarity with modern authors, their *actos de repetición* and examinations were all on traditional topics, and their university records reflect only their knowledge of Hippocrates, Avicenna, and Galen. Similarly, the University of San Carlos graduates were well acquainted with authorities such as Benjamin Bell (1749–1806) and his work on tumors and ulcers, the Italian physiologist Felice Fontana (1730–1805) and his work on wounds and poison complications, and Pierre Lassus (1741–1807), an authority on typhoid (Lanning 1956:286).

Such evidence suggests that new medical knowledge added to rather than displaced old assumptions and practices. Thus, while the theories of the most knowledgeable physicians were based on clinical observation and contemporary European medical principles, in practice most therapies continued to involve traditional practices such as bloodletting and purging, which produced tangible physical responses. Age-old assumptions such as the Hippocratic doctrine of "critical days" (that is, the belief that a disease ran its course within a particular time frame, ending in a crisis that occurred on a specific day after onset), and the belief that the digestive system must be cleansed of residual food or fecal matter that might result in fermentation or petrification or otherwise obstruct the natural processes of the organism, were also important factors in determining therapies.

Thus, prescribed treatments sought "to conduct the patient through disease," and not to oppose nature. In his *Mercurio Volante*, Bartolache warned readers not to try to "shorten nature's work by adding and varying medicines." The characteristic symptoms of fevers and other illnesses (lack of appetite, nausea, vomiting, and diarrhea) were believed to be caused by the weakening of the muscular fibers of the stomach. The removal of its contents was thought to prevent the spread of such weakness to the rest of the body. When illness caused vomiting, practitioners used emetics such as *ipecacuanha*, white vitriol (zinc sulphate), mineral turpeth (sulphate of mercury), and tartar emetic (antimonial potassium tartrate) "to unload the breast" and "to imitate nature." Emetics were often complemented by a cathartic mixture of tobacco, water, and honey. By not regarding medicine as an applied science, the establishment emphasized the distance between theory and practice, thus limiting the role of medical theory to etiologies and justification of treatment (Risse 1986:179, 284).

Yet the intellectual ferment of the late eighteenth century could not be denied. It was a time of renewed interest in botany, zoology, and mineralogy, studied in a more methodical and scientific fashion than previously. Formal botanical training began in 1787 with the establishment of the *cátedra de botánica*; this was made a prerequisite for licensing physicians, surgeons, and pharmacists (Lanning 1985:230–231; Tanck de Estrada 1982: 45–48). The same year, the crown approved the important Royal Scientific Expedition of New Spain and Guatemala, headed by the Spanish physician Martín Sessé. Its members reached Upper California in the north, and Central America in the south and provided a detailed description of the customs of the people encountered and classified the flora and fauna of the area according to the Linnean system (Engstrand 1981:7–17). The increasingly analytical mentality of the times promoted a more scientific study of the properties of various medicinal substances. The Mexican botanist José Mariano Moziño complemented his research on the *planta escobosa*,[5] a supposed cure for rabies, with the observation of actual hospital cases (Moziño 1795). Similarly, Sessé obtained permission from the government to conduct drug experiments at the Royal Indian Hospital. A ward was set aside with specialized personnel (a nurse and a head intern) who carefully monitored and recorded the effects of the various medicinal preparations on the patients (Howard 1980:70). As bizarre and useless remedies began to be discarded by the medical establishment, the gap between scientific and folk medicine widened.

The Training of Surgeons

If the late colonial physician was struggling to shake off the shackles of tradition and overcome its shortcomings, the surgeon was seeking recognition as a professional. Spain distinguished between the *cirujano latino*, who, like the *médico*, was university-trained and had studied Latin, and the *cirujano romancista*, who did not speak Latin and whose training was acquired through apprenticeship. Although both were certified to treat the same cases, better job opportunities and more privileges were available to the few *cirujanos latinos*. However, the realities of life in New Spain and the scarcity of qualified surgeons made this distinction academic; in case of emergency anyone present with the slightest knowledge of surgery operated.

Due to the low status of the early colonial surgeons, there were few works printed on surgery. Probably the first medical work with special references to Mexico was *Secretos de Chirugía*. Published in 1567 in Valladolid, Spain, by Arias de Benavides, it contains a discussion on medieval authors such as Guy de Chauliac and a long section on syphilis based on the author's experiences in a Mexico City hospital (Somolinos d'Ardois 1978, 4:21–25). Alonso López de Hinojosos's *Summa y recopilación de chirugía*, the first medical text to be published in New Spain, appeared in 1578. A second edition (1595) includes the first gynecologic-obstetric treatise to appear as well as a "book" on children's illnesses (Somolinos d'Ardois 1978, 4:59–67; 103–111). Another notable work was Agustín Farfán's *Tractado breve de anathomía y chirugía*, published in 1579. A second edition (1592) offers practical information for *romancista* surgeons and barbers. Its pragmatism—a contrast to López de Hinojoso's academic approach—makes it the best surgical work of the time (Somolinos d'Ardois 1978, 4:69–75; 85–101). The second edition is also interesting for what it tells us about the Americanization of the humoral pharmacopoeia: in contrast to the first edition, "there is a notable increase in the mention of Mexican products such as matlaliztic uli, and istafulatl" (*istafiate* [*Artemisia filifolia*]; Jarcho 1957:437).

Also worthy of mention is Juan de Barrios' 1607 *Verdadera medicina, cirugía, y astrología,* a book that covered all medical knowledge of the time, with sections on pediatric medicine and anatomy, and a chapter on gynecology-obstetrics much superior to that of López de Hinojoso. Later in the century, the need for a surgical text for university-trained surgeons prompted Diego de Osorio y Peralta to write *Principia Medicinae Epitome, et Totius Humani Corporis Fábrica* (1685), the first anatomy text to be published in New Spain. It summarized Galen's work on fevers, Hippocrates' *Aphorisms,* and an "anatomy" written in Spanish and based "on the experiences" of its author (Fernández del Castillo 1982, 1:183–187).

The development of surgical skills in Mexico was abetted by dissections performed in the hope of learning more about the recurrent and devastating epidemics of the sixteenth century. The first mention of a dissection dates back to 1576, when Dr. Juan de la Fuente, professor of medicine and anatomy at the university, dissected the corpse of an Indian, hoping to determine the causes of a serious epidemic of *cocoliztle* (probably smallpox) raging in the colony (Fernández del Castillo 1982, 1:321–327). The first *protomédico,* Francisco Hernández, along with López Hinojoso, also promoted dissections for the same purpose (Somolinos d'Ardois 1978, 3:230). The most notable of all dissections during the colonial period was that of the scientist Don Carlos de Siguenza y Góngora, who donated his body for research. According to the wishes of the donor, the results were made public to other practitioners for the welfare of the community (Fernández del Castillo 1982, 1:321–327).

Despite the valuable contributions of various surgeons and the formal division between *latinos* and *romancistas,* in the early nineteenth century surgery continued to be considered inferior to medicine. This is hardly surprising. With his liberal education, rhetorical abilities, and his privileged university status, the physician was trained to cater to the needs of the elite. In contrast, most surgeons were poorly educated craftsmen whose bloody work, coupled with the filthy conditions prevailing in hospitals of the time, hardly lent itself to occupational prestige. Furthermore, until the mid-eighteenth century the division between surgeons, bleeders, and, even worse, barbers, was far from clear-cut, and contemporaries often used the terms incorrectly or interchangeably. For example, in 1779 Nicolás de Navas was appointed "ministro sangrador y chirugico" (bleeder and surgical *minister*) of the Inquisition, while his successor was described merely as "barbero de presos" (prisoners' barber), although the position appears to have included providing medical attention as well as barber services.

In Mexico, as in Europe, it would take crown intervention to professionalize surgery. The reform of surgical education in the Spanish Empire started in the early eighteenth century with the establishment of surgical colleges and a curriculum that combined medical theory and practice. Despite their success, the new institutions were unable to satisfy the urgent demand for naval and military surgeons, and the authorities had to search for a solution overseas.

In 1763, Antonio Arroyo, administrator of the Royal Indian Hospital in Mexico, petitioned the crown for the right to establish an anatomical amphitheater where dissections comparable to those performed at the Royal Hospital of Madrid could be carried out. Arroyo believed that such an amphitheater, in addition to the training of medical and surgical students, would promote medicine by helping them to understand "the epidemics that originate among the Indians." After some hesitation, Madrid endorsed Arroyo's ideas, but with important modifications. Instead of the proposed amphitheater, the crown ordered the establishment of a Real Escuela de Cirugía patterned after the Spanish surgical colleges, to create a pool of surgeons to cater to the needs of the colony's army and navy personnel (Howard 1980:4–6). The school's program included courses of anatomy (illustrated with wooden or wax anatomical figures and complemented with dissections), experimental physics and general pathology, hygiene (similar to preventive medicine), surgical pathology, physiology (a combination of anatomy, chemistry, and physics), chemistry, botany, "the art of bandages," and a course on surgical procedures. The textbooks employed, such as John Gorter's *Quirurgia repurgata* and Diego Velasco y Villaverde's *Curso teórico de práctica de operaciones*, attest to the school's innovative curriculum, which would ultimately legitimize this branch of medicine. After completing the four-year course, aspiring surgeons served a second four-year internship in a hospital, where they acquired firsthand experience (Burke 1977:100; Serrano 1946b:369–375).

Surviving documents indicate that, although an average of only ten to twelve surgeons graduated yearly, more than one hundred students of different levels attended each year. The Escuela de Cirugía was responsible for the total or partial training of hundreds of surgeons, many of whom immediately joined the army. The urgent demand for qualified surgeons resulted in the admittance of candidates of mixed ancestry. Judging by its director's statement that the school was "the refuge of many young men of modest means," surgery became the avenue by which those unable to fulfill university racial or socioeconomic requirements could legally join the profession (Hernández Sáenz 1997:85–92; Reales Ordenanzas 1804). Formal education led to legitimization and marked the beginning of surgical professionalization in Mexico, offering its practitioners the chance of professional and socioeconomic advancement.

The opportunities opened to Mexican surgeons did not extend to their Guatemalan colleagues. As the Captaincy General of Guatemala did not attract the attention of military authorities, the establishment of the Real Colegio de Cirugía in the General Hospital of Guatemala City (1804) was a local effort that received little encouragement from Madrid. The new institution, modeled after the Royal Surgical College of San Carlos in Madrid, boasted three professorships and, the first year, six students. Unfortunately, the institution was never properly funded. In 1811, it was still "provisional," its faculty and personnel had not been paid, and its financial future was uncertain. The Royal Surgical College continued its hand-to-mouth existence, but by 1819, only one professor remained (Lanning 1985:296–303).

Pharmacists and Pharmacies

Like physicians and surgeons, pharmacists fell under the jurisdiction of the Protomedicato. To obtain a license, the future pharmacist served four years as apprentice under a licensed master, from whom he learned to recognize, weigh, measure, store, and prepare simple and compound substances as prescribed by the *Pharmacopea Matritense*, a manual published in 1739 to standardize the prescriptions sold in all pharmacies of the Spanish Empire. The apprentice also learned to read Latin (essential because physicians' prescriptions were written in this language) and to familiarize himself with the different preparation methods, such as infusions, sublimation, and distillation, and was taught to prepare lozenges (Pérez y López 1791–98:247–248). The license was granted following a successful theoretical and practical examination and, after 1787, completion of a course in botany. Once licensed, a pharmacist could legally own his place of business.

The colonial drugstore, or *botica*, had at least three rooms. The front area, usually in better condition than the rest, was used to dispense prescriptions to the public; sometimes it was provided with a bench, and also served as a meeting place where patients, clients, and neighbors socialized, and where *curanderos* sometimes offered their services. The second room was fitted with small stoves for preparing multi-ingredient *compuestos* and other remedies, while the back room, used for storage, might be fitted with the necessary shelving (Antonio Garfías 1801). The nature of contemporary remedies was such that they were easily available. Ingredients such as sarsaparilla, tobacco, or *epazote* could hardly be controlled through a monopoly.

In New Spain a great variety of remedies were available to physicians, their patients, *curanderos*, and to the public in general. In addition to the offerings of well-stocked pharmacies, herbal and other remedies could be obtained from vendors in public markets, and from itinerant *yerberos*, who sold their *remedios* in streets or town squares. Two basic categories of remedies, known as *simples* and *compuestos*, were offered for sale. *Simples* included any single organic or inorganic substance used as medicine, while *compuestos* were drugs compounded of simples or, as contemporary documents describe them, "compounded by art."

Contemporary pharmacy inventories were organized in different categories. The Royal Indian Hospital, for example, lists a total of 711 items divided into thirty-six main classes, subdivided according to mode of preparation. Chamomile or *manzanilla* (*Artemisia capillaris*), used as a stomachic, antispasmodic, and febrifuge, appears as a simple stored under the category "flowers," but was also kept as a powder and prepared as both simple and compound water, while, according to Gregorio López' *Tesoro de Medicinas*, rose flowers and their seeds (used to cure headaches, earaches, and diarrhea) were prepared either as water or pulp (Guerra 1982:54, 67; Zedillo Castillo 1984:272–284).

In addition to *simples* and *compuestos*, drugstores sold prepared medicines such as the "new and improved" *pastillas marciales* (iron pills) developed by Dr. Bartolache from a European formula. Bartolache advertised the pills in his *Mercurio Volante*, recommending them for intermittent fevers, gout and rheumatic pains, lack of appetite, and dropsy, as well as for preserving health and retarding aging. Despite these remarkable qualities, this preparation was not for everybody. The advertisements cautioned pregnant women and those suffering from smallpox, pneumonia, epilepsy, or dysentery against taking it, and advised readers to first seek their physician's advice. The fact that instructions for their use were printed in both Spanish and Náhuatl clearly indicates that medical preparations were routinely purchased by Mexico City's Indian as well as Creole and mestizo populations (Bartolache 1979:177–179; 183–189).

Pharmacists obtained their supplies from many sources: wholesale merchants known as *especieros*, who did not fall under the jurisdiction of the Protomedicato and who dealt in spices and aromatic drugs (Lanning 1985: 233), as well as from other *boticas*. The intricate worldwide network that joined producers and middlemen with consumers is illustrated by the 1808 supply proposal of the Hospital Real de San Carlos of Veracruz. Commercial agents in key ports such as Barcelona and Cádiz or Manila served as brokers for the surrounding areas. Drugs from the Levant were obtained either through Spain or from a French port such as Bayonne; Oriental substances such as Chinese rhubarb, camphor, and cinnamon were imported from Manila via Acapulco and the annual Manila galleon, while Peruvian bark (quinine), cocoa butter, and other South and Central American products were shipped from Guayaquil, Havana, Guatemala, Cartagena, and Campeche. Transportation costs, taxes, and the markup of middlemen dramatically increased the prices paid by local consumers. A *libra* (345 grams) of the emetic *ipecacuanha* selling in Havana for 2 to 3 pesos cost as much as 22 pesos in Mexico City. The cost of *compuestos* varied according to that of their components. A *libra* of seeds, an ingredient in a tonic known as *bálsamo del obispo*, available in Guatemala at 2 reales, sold in Mexico City for 8 reales an ounce (Cervantes 1808:68–72).

Phlebotomists

Surgeons were continually aware of the need to differentiate themselves from other practitioners of lower status. Among the latter were the phlebotomists, or bleeders. Belonging to the same socioeconomic class as most of the local population and characterized by the same mixed racial ancestry and cultural background, they were in much closer contact with the general public than their higher ranking colleagues. Phlebotomy formed an integral part of Greek humoral theory. Its purpose was not only to cure illness by

ridding the patient of excessive or unhealthy humors, but also to maintain
health by insuring their proper balance. Type of ailment and the affected
area determined the patient's preparation for the procedure, including time
and point of the incision (Voigts and McVaugh 1984:1–6).

Although by the late eighteenth century bleeding was becoming increasingly controversial, it continued to be used by recognized medical authorities.[6] Following eighteenth-century mechanistic and neuropathologi-
cal theories, practitioners resorted to bleeding as an antiphlogistic method
that also reduced tension and spasms. Its popularity as the best treatment
for inflammatory ailments can easily be explained by its immediate and visible effects on the symptoms that characterized fevers (thought to be due
to an excess of blood, a Hot and Moist humor): it lowered pulse rate and
temperature and dispelled congestion (Risse 1986:203–207). Blood was extracted by surgically opening a vein, by the application of leeches, and by
cupping.

Phlebotomists were trained at a master's shop or *tienda*, marked outside
by an official sign indicating that the establishment operated in compliance
with the law. The size and interior arrangement of shops varied; at a minimum they included the practitioner's professional certificate displayed on
the wall, his *herramientas*, or "tools," and probably a chair. A lattice separated the shop proper from the living quarters of the phlebotomist and his
apprentices (Hernández Sáenz 1997:192, 197). It was here that the young
aspirants learned the veins and arteries, how to bleed, and how to apply
leeches and cupping glasses, as well as the "art" of extracting teeth. They
were also instructed on how to avoid causing any harm to the patient and to
correct any "mistakes" made during the procedure. To obtain a license a
phlebotomist had to prove his theoretical knowledge to the *protomédicos*,
naming specific veins and arteries, explaining how to bleed, and indicating the type of lancet required and the reasons to refuse bleeding even if
prescribed by a physician. He also had to prove his practical ability by demonstrating a procedure on a hospital patient (Fernández del Castillo 1982:
277–279).

Legislation clearly delineated the requirements for licensing and the limits of the phlebotomist's practice, but reality dictated a different course. Surviving documents indicate that the enforcement of regulations was usually
loose in the case of "lower" practitioners. Licensing files reveal incomplete
applications, inability to fulfill training requirements, and mixed racial an-

cestry. As to practice, phlebotomists often enjoyed considerable freedom of action. Remote areas usually lacked medical practitioners and, even when physicians and surgeons were available, most patients could not afford their services. Aware of these problems, the Spanish authorities allowed two exceptions to the regulations. First, if no other practitioner was available, a phlebotomist was allowed to perform any medical or surgical treatment necessary, or to act as a forensic expert. Second, legislation exempted Indian pueblos from the regulations when the lack of physicians and surgeons made the bleeder the only one with any surgical expertise, and when the Spanish authorities lacked the necessary jurisdiction to enforce the rules (Consulta 1798). The case of a Juan Timoteo Cárdenas Espinosa, an unlicensed bleeder in the town of Otumba, well illustrates this situation. His practice included sewing up deep wounds as well as treating other serious injuries. Although some of his diagnoses were incorrect, his services were greatly appreciated by the community, and he was praised both by his patients and the local authority (Cárdenas Espinosa 1805).

Although in theory part of the formal medical system of the colony and subject to the Protomedicato, most bleeders operated illegally and, as in the case of Cárdenas Espinosa, often practiced surgery.

Hospitals and the Missionary Orders

From the earliest years of New Spain the average patient, whether Indian, mestizo, or Creole, was most likely to receive care based on Spanish medical practices in a hospital. The first, the Hospital de Jesús, was founded by Cortés himself in 1522 (Guerra 1969: 184). The Hospital Real de Indios, for the care of indigenous inhabitants of Mexico, and the Hospital Real de Españoles opened their doors in 1534 (González-Ulloa 1959:41). By the end of the seventeenth century, Mexico had over 150 hospitals, a number that had risen to more than two hundred by the eighteenth century (Guerra 1969: 184).

The founding of hospitals was of equal importance in Guatemala. A decree issued in November 1527 ordered that a site be selected for a hospital "where the poor, and *peregrinos* [pilgrims, wanderers] could be succored and cured," and that it be named El Espital de la Misericordia (Asturias 1958: 65). Bartolomé de las Casas recalled in 1534 that when the hospital opened, it accepted not only sick patients but also "old men no longer able to work," as well as orphaned children. One finds in this practice the first idea of an asylum for the aged and of a hospice (Asturias 1958).

Shortly thereafter the Dominicans founded the Hospital de San Alexo, "destined solely and exclusively for treating and succoring Indians" (Guerra 1969:66). Following this lead, in 1553 Don Francisco Marroquín, the first bishop of Guatemala, using personal resources, built the Hospital de Santiago for Spaniards, "since the Indians [already] have that of San Alexo" (Asturias 1958). The Hospital de la Misericordia was in use until it was destroyed by an earthquake in 1717. The hospitals of San Alexo and Santiago, and others built in subsequent years, were all—save one—destroyed by the devastating earthquake of 1773. Antigua Guatemala was all but abandoned, and hospitals were gradually rebuilt in the present city of Guatemala (Asturias 1958:69).

Although in both countries some hospitals were civil, the vast majority owed their existence to the missionary orders, especially the Franciscans, Dominicans, Augustinians, Jesuits, and Carmelites. Patients in urban hospitals were attended not only by religious personnel but also by "licensed practitioners" who, during the colonial period, "divided their activities between private practice among the high class of Spaniards and Creoles and the hospital wards for the sick and poor and the Indians, who were regularly provided with pharmacies and European drugs" (Guerra 1969:185).

In contrast, in small towns and rural areas almost all care was by the friars of the missionary orders. Thus, in Mexico, "Spanish missionaries fanned out across the provinces and far into the sparsely inhabited north, bringing both a new religion and a new medical care to remote and primitive tribes at the padres' isolated adobe missions. The priests, friars and missionaries also operated the many hospitals the Spaniards constructed. So it was the clergy who were chiefly responsible for introducing and promulgating Spanish concepts of medicine among the natives and persuading them to accept alien standards" (Schendel 1968:86).

Midwives

Almost all *parteras* were formally untrained women, racially Indian or mestizo, who practiced according to the traditional ways of their local cultures. Not until the late eighteenth century, when licensing became (at least in theory) a requirement to practice, were they officially incorporated into the medical establishment. Despite the new regulations, the large majority of midwives continued to practice without a license, to the dismay of the Protomedicato. Nonetheless, contrary to traditional belief, police records indicate that the *parteras'* professional opinions were highly regarded by the authorities and proved vital in court trials (Hernández Sáenz 1997: 204–212). The attitude of the judicial authorities contrasts and contradicts the disdainful and condescending attitude of the medical elite, who criticized the women's lack of formal training and accused them of practicing "to the detriment of humanity" (Serrano 1946a: 310). Unfortunately, modern authors have taken such criticisms at face value.[7] The "sudden" concerns (absent before the eighteenth century) and hostile attitude of the medical practitioners stemmed from their own interest in obstetrics. By formally accepting obstetrics as part of medicine, the establishment appropriated its practice, reducing licensed midwives to a secondary role and marginalizing *parteras* without credentials. Nonetheless, tradition persisted and many midwives continued various pre-Conquest practices, such as giving opossum-tail broth to a parturient to hasten labor and saving the newborn's umbilical stump for medicinal purposes. Practices such as these have survived in both Indian and mestizo communities, although with decreasing vigor, to the present.

Nurses

In colonial times, nurses were not recognized as part of the medical profession and therefore were not subject to uniform legislation; they were ruled only by the regulations of the hospital where they worked. Their exclusion from the jurisdiction of the Protomedicato meant that *limpieza de sangre* and gender requirements did not apply. Furthermore, with the exception of the Royal Indian Hospital, nurses did not require any previous training to work in a hospital but learned their trade through experience. Their duties included "external medical applications" such as ointments and enemas ordered by the physician, and the purification of the wards by burning of aromatic herbs in order to rid the air of miasmas. They were also present during the physician's or surgeon's daily rounds, probably playing an active role, and served as aides to the interns (Constituciones 1778). Thus, nursing was the only area that not only accepted but also trained mixed-blood personnel of both genders who were not able to enter other branches of the medical profession.

Despite the opportunities that hospital work and training offered, nursing occupied a wide, undefined area between the lower echelons of the medical profession and the common hospital servant. Regulations describing nurses as "servants" as well as "nurses" reflect their ambiguous position. Their humble position is corroborated by their poor wages, which were among the lowest of the hospitals' pay scale. The female nurses of the Royal Indian Hospital earned 3 pesos a month (1 peso less than the kitchen aid), while the head nurse, also a female, received 6 pesos a month. The amount received by the male head nurse, 12 pesos a month, indicates that females, at least in this institution, suffered discrimination. Other hospitals, such as San Pedro in Puebla, paid slightly better and more equitable wages. In 1811, San Pedro paid its female nurse 13 pesos a month, the same amount it paid to an intern who had, at least in theory, some formal training. As a point of comparison, the salaries of the Hospital de San Pedro surgeons ranged between 25 and 41 pesos a month (Gastos del Hospital de San Pedro 1811; Lista de Sueldos 1800).

The nurses' racial heterogeneity, the nature of their duties, and their marginalization from the medical profession reinforced their inferior social status in the eyes of their contemporaries and prevented nursing from being recognized as a branch of medicine. However, despite its stigma, nursing was the only occupation open to those who, because of race, gender, or lack of training, were otherwise excluded from the health care field.

Curanderos

In spite of—or perhaps more accurately because of—the legal requirements characterizing formal medicine in New Spain until independence in the early nineteenth century, most people were forced by economic necessity to resort to popular, technically illegal, curers: the *curandero* (male) or *curandera* (female). As Quezada makes clear, "Spanish, Indian, Negro, Mestizo and Mulato patients turned to the *curandero*" for medical needs (1989: 122). Initially there were at least two (and perhaps three) distinct popular medical traditions: the Native American, the Spanish, and the African. The

Native American and Spanish systems are well documented, while the African is largely surmised.

Native American medicine explained serious illness in supernatural or magical terms, as punishment by angry deities for violations of religious taboos, as spirits entering (or "possessing") the bodies of victims, as loss of the *sombra* or *tonalli* (soul) caused by *susto* (a fright) or stolen by a witch, and the like. Other perceived causes of illness included accidents (broken bones, lacerations, burns from cooking fires), as well as emotional insults from experiences such as anger, shame, disillusion, and jealousy.

As in all complex medical systems, various kinds of curers were known in pre-Conquest Mexico. Priests and shamans endowed with supernatural powers were turned to when a patient was suspected of having violated a taboo or of having angered a neighbor who then resorted to witchcraft to avenge the perceived trespass. There were curers who divined by throwing grains of maize into water, or by feeling the pulse (*pulsadores*). Other curers knew how to capture a wandering or stolen *sombra*. *Chupadores* sucked out intruded disease objects or poison, and *sobadores* massaged. Still others treated illness by *limpiando* (cleansing) a patient by lightly rubbing her or his body with such things as the herb *istafiate*. Obviously these are classificatory categories, and in practice there was much overlap: a shaman might also be a skilled herbalist, and a bonesetter might have shamanistic talents. Moreover, it is important to note that, given the absence of government regulations and of licensing in the New World, no sharp line can be drawn between elite and popular medicine in pre-Spanish Mesoamerica.

In Spain the folk medical curer usually was (and is) called a *saludador*, while the curer with clairvoyant power—the diviner—is referred as a *zahorí*. Their power often is the consequence of circumstances surrounding their birth: those who "cry in the womb" of their mother or who have *una cruz en el paladar* (a cross on the hard palate), or who are the seventh consecutive son are thought to have *un don* (a gift [from God]) or *gracia para curar* (grace [from God] to cure). Some divined by scrying (looking for reflections in a pan of water) or by breaking eggs in water. Many considered Tuesdays and Fridays to be especially efficacious days for treatments. Herbal and other internal treatments were often prescribed *en ayunas*, that is, while fasting, on an empty stomach.

With the passage of time Spanish and American traditions syncretized to form a remarkably homogeneous folk medicine common both to Indian and mestizo populations. It is significant that the humoral component in this new hybrid medicine came from the elite, and not the popular, Spanish context. At first thought it seems surprising that the "Hot–Cold syndrome" played a very limited role in Spanish popular medicine, since in all Spanish America it became a dominant element in the *curandero*'s diagnosis and treatment of illness. We believe the following hypothesis accounts for this apparent enigma.

The devastating effects on population occasioned by smallpox, tuberculosis, malaria, yellow fever, and measles, against which the indigenous peoples had no natural immunity and against which their medications had little if any effect, created a fertile ground in which Spanish humoral explanations and practices speedily took root. In contrast, Spanish popular medicine was already vigorous and well entrenched at the time humoral theory became known from Latin translations of Arabic manuscripts. Since popular medicine was meeting the expectations of its adherents (which is not to say that in a clinical sense it really cured), there was little incentive to adopt new medical explanations and treatments, increasingly available from trained physicians.

There were many places, such as pharmacies, urban hospitals, and the *conventos* of the religious orders, where the indigenous and mestizo populations of New Spain were exposed to the therapies of practitioners of Spanish elite medicine and their underlying rationale. With respect to the role of pharmacies, Quezada (1989:21) puts it thus: "As is done in our days, pharmacists prescribed medications according to the patient's symptoms and freely sold everything prohibited." Again, patients in hospitals were in direct contact not only with the friars (whose medical knowledge was basically humoral) but also, at least in urban centers, with medical doctors whose training had been based on Hippocrates, Galen, and Avicenna. Through such contacts, as well as other exposures to European medicine, Indians and mestizos alike absorbed humoral concepts.[8]

Conclusions

Colonial curers reflected the hierarchical and miscegenous society in which they practiced. Physicians and "Latin" surgeons were university trained, while *romancista* surgeons, pharmacists, and phlebotomists learned their trade as apprentices. The theoretical basis for the training of both groups was Greco-Persian-Arabic humoral medicine from the works of Hippocrates, Galen, and Avicenna. The organization of these several branches of medicine followed the Spanish pattern, with a government supervisory board, the Protomedicato, in charge of licensing medical personnel, of enforcing legislation, and of safeguarding professional rights and privileges. These elite practitioners served the select few who were able to afford their services, largely Spaniards and Creoles, and, in urban hospitals, Indian and lower class mestizos. In rural hospitals patients under the care of members of the religious orders were treated according to the same humoral principles.

Alfred Crosby has coined the term "Columbian Exchange," to describe the biological and cultural consequences of the meeting of the Old and New Worlds (Crosby 1972). The concept of the "Columbian Exchange" can also serve as a model for the fusion of Spanish and American medicine. In broad outline, the New World contributed a rich store of herbal and other remedies, while Spain contributed the basic explanatory theory to which the specific therapies of the two systems increasingly conformed. Thus, colonial Mexican medicine may be described not only as a synthesis but also as an exchange between two different worlds.

In this exchange the Europeans were the clear winners. Not only did they obtain knowledge of and access to a great many herbal and other remedies previously unknown to them, but even more important, the new sources of food, such as maize, potatoes, beans, squash, tomatoes, manioc, chocolate, and peanuts—to mention only the most important—by improving European diets, did far more to improve the health of people than all of the therapeutic practices of the two worlds combined. Even if syphilis was brought back by Columbus from the New World—and the jury is still out—on balance the health of Europeans benefited enormously from the discovery of America.

The picture is just the opposite for the indigenous peoples of the New World. Lacking natural immunity to the diseases brought from the Old World, entire populations were decimated on a scale unparalleled elsewhere in human history. The most sophisticated medicine of both Europe and America was powerless to combat the epidemics of the colonial period. Old World cultigens, and especially domestic animals, undeniably improved New World diets, but their benefits hardly became apparent before the late nineteenth century, and certainly humoral medicine can claim none of the credit for the gradual growth of population beginning a century before.

With most people too far removed from direct contact with elite medical practice to adopt it in its clinical forms, they selectively adapted Hippocratic and subsequent humoral teachings to their own cultural context. Traditional New World *remedios* and treatments were reclassified according to Spanish Hot-Cold beliefs, thus producing a unique popular system, carried both by *curanderos* and the population at large.

This syncretic process can be illustrated by many examples, of which only two are given here.

First, in Spanish America it is widely believed that *frialdad en la matriz* (cold in the womb) is the cause of sterility. As late as the second decade of the nineteenth century, regulations of the Real y Pontificia Universidad de México specified that the lectures of the incumbent in the chair of Vísperas should be based on the Hippocratic Aphorisms. Aphorism LXII, Section 5 states, "Those [women] whose uterus is cold and dense do not conceive . . ." (Izquierdo 1955:98), while Aphorism CXXIII states that " . . . cold produces sterility . . ." (1955:208). This classic explanation of why some women have difficulty in conceiving, or remain barren all of their lives, has been accepted by Spanish Americans of all social classes. Common treatments are consistent with this humoral etiology: for example, poultices of tobacco leaves (a New World plant, humorally classified as Very Hot) are applied to a woman's abdomen, or she drinks teas of Hot herbs both native American and Old World in origin, such as tenurite, *amargosos*, and *garañona* (a mint).

Second, the synthesis of indigenous pre-Conquest medicine with Spanish elite and popular medical therapies is illustrated by Fray Juan de Esteyneffer's smallpox treatment. He first reminds his readers that San Marcial, San Francisco Xavier, and Santa Rosalía are spiritual intercessors for smallpox sufferers. He next advises keeping a sheep in the same room as the patient "inasmuch as this animal easily draws unto itself the evil of the illness." He then recommends specific remedies such as "lentil water" to which is added bezoar stones, coral, or pearls, well pulverized, or scrapings of deer antlers, or powder of the root of the Mexican herb *coanenepilli* (*Passiflora jorullensis*). To protect her or his throat, the patient is advised to gargle a decoction of barley water to which is added *llantén*, oak leaves, dried roses, or pomegranate blossoms. Bleeding and purging, he suggested, should be used sparingly (Anzures y Bolaños 1978, 1:503–508).

This treatment is consistent with humoral theory: smallpox, obviously a fever, is treated with both New and Old World herbs and other medications, a majority of which are metaphorically cold. Popular hagiolatry is recognized by the saints who are advocates for smallpox sufferers. A sheep in the sick room represents the "principle of opposites": mutton usually was classified as Cold. Finally, barley water is the Cold drink par excellence in humoral medicine, in this case made even more effective by the addition of the metaphorically cold native Mexican *llantén* (*Plantago major*), used to the present day according to the Mexican botanist Maximino Martínez, for mouth ulcers (1944:163).

Esteyneffer's medical ideas reflect the degree of synthesis achieved in less than two centuries. Thus it can be said with assurance that by the time of independence, humoral beliefs had become a dominant theme in not only the *curandero*'s armamentarium but also in much of the *medicina casera*, the home remedies used by mestizo housewives and other lay persons. Humoral beliefs and practices have continued to play a major role in folk medicine almost to the present. Only now—at the beginning of the twenty-first century—is this syncretic medicine really being challenged by a mixture of other systems, including not only biomedicine but also homeopathy, Spiritualism, *medicina naturista* ("naturalist" medicine), and other alternative forms.

Notes

1. As Kay (1996:22) points out, no one seems to know a specific citation for this statement.
2. Aztec medical beliefs and practices as described by Sahagún are found in the *Florentine Codex*, the *General History of the Things of New Spain*, translated into English by Arthur J. O. Anderson and Charles E. Dibble and published in fourteen volumes as monographs of the School of American Research, Santa Fe, New Mexico, 1950–1970. Particularly relevant to medicine are Anderson and Dibble 1954, Book 8; Dibble and Anderson 1957, Books 4 and 5; 1961, Book 10; and 1963, Book 11. See also Edmonson 1974.
3. In Guatemala the almost total lack of licensed practitioners and the absence of a formal Protomedicato prevented the same categorization and the development of a formal medical establishment until the nineteenth century.
4. "Within the university, the Medical Faculty had a lower rank than those of Canons, Theology and Law, . . . Only the Faculty of Arts, in which there were no doctoral degrees, was considered below that of medicine" (Hernández Sáenz 1997:46).
5. Probably the *Centaura* or *Millettia reticulata*.
6. It may be remembered that European and American medicine of this period was by

no means free of humoral shackles: Benjamin Rush, a signer of the Declaration of Independence and one of the country's most distinguished medical doctors, through heroic bleeding hastened the death of countless patients during the Philadelphia yellow fever epidemic of 1793 (Powell 1949).

7. See, for example, Serrano (1946a) and Noemí Quezada (1989).

8. Foster (1994: 147–164) devotes an entire chapter to the many avenues of access open to humoral theory to filter down to the *curandero*'s level.

CHAPTER 3

Curanderismo in Mexico and Guatemala

Its Historical Evolution from the Sixteenth to the Nineteenth Century

Carlos Viesca Treviño

Introduction

Traditional medicine in Mesoamerica is based upon knowledge and practices that originate from systems of thought and worldviews that are different from those of the West. This knowledge and these practices both derive from and provide the rationale for the daily activities of professional healers. These professionals vary in their characteristics from culture to culture, but throughout the ancient lands of Mesoamerica they are known as *curanderos*. The word *"curandero"* does not have a precise meaning. It refers to an individual's role as a healer while at the same time implying that this individual is not a medical doctor in the Western sense. A *curandero* is a person who cures, or who tries to cure, in accord with the ancient pre-Hispanic indigenous pattern, adding knowledge that has accrued for nearly five centuries since the Spanish Conquest.

The Birth of the Curandero

The Mesoamerican *curandero* first appears in the sixteenth century, although the precise time cannot be determined because the specific role was not created by a decree or a commemorative act. Rather, the *curandero* is the product of the Conquest; indigenous medical specialists such as the Nahua *tícitl*, the Huastec *ilalix*, the Tzeltal *h'ilojel* and Tzotil *h'ilol*, the Mayan *h-men*, the *ah cut* of the Pokoman, and its Quiché equivalent, the *ah cun*, became diluted and homogenized. All of these pre-Hispanic healers gradually became *curanderos*, with the single Spanish term serving to overshadow cultural differences among them. Previous to the Conquest, all of these healers had been doctors in the complete sense of the term: specialists who solved the health problems of their own people through activities ranging from attending to relations with the sacred to the preparation of medicines.

These pre-Hispanic doctors prepared themselves diligently from childhood for their future roles. In large cities such as Mexico-Tenochtitlán, both males and females were tutored at the sides of their fathers or mothers (Ocaranza 1934a:25). To this instruction was added a systematic apprenticeship in the *calmécac*, where the student acquired knowledge of the *tonalpohualli*, the divinatory calendar in which the destiny of persons was read. Students also received knowledge of religious ceremonies related to health and of the preparation of some medicines (Viesca Treviño 1984:218). The *calmécac* was the institution of higher learning for Mexica (Aztec) nobles, although it has been pointed out that there may have been schools with the same name located in the artisan neighborhoods where various trades, including medicine, were taught (López Austin 1973:72). In Mexico-Tenochtitlán the doctors lived in the districts of Atempan and Tzapotlaltenan, the latter named for the goddess of medicine. It is a logical assumption that medicine would be taught in the school connected to the temple dedicated to this goddess.

It is interesting that an Indian doctor like Martín de la Cruz, to be discussed later, was known to be a noble and *principal*, statuses not consistent with the craft of medicine. However, it is known that among the Mayas of the Verapaz region of Guatemala there were noble doctors called *ah cut* who attended fellow members of the nobility. These doctors learned their trade from their parents, as well as how to read and write, which helped them considerably in the acquisition of knowledge. At the same time, among the Maya, there existed other doctors for the common people, called *ahicom*, opening the possibility that a similar distinction existed among the Nahuas (Miles 1957:768; Orellana 1987:60–61).

Documents from a few years after the Conquest speak of Indian doctors. The conquistadores, who were not well educated, saw how effective indigenous professionals were in the healing arts. They called them doctors in their writings, and were themselves treated by them. This was certainly the case for Hernán Cortés and his soldiers. Wounded after the battle of Otumba in 1520, he and his men were treated by indigenous doctors after they took refuge in the city of Tlaxcala (Cortés 1991:128; Díaz del Castillo 1955 1:404; López de Gómara 1552, fol. 65).

Because of the scarcity of European doctors and surgeons, the Spaniards, many of whom were victims of diseases about which they knew little or which took new and aggressive forms in subtropical Mexico, resorted to Indian healers, whom they still classed as doctors. The example of Viceroy Antonio de Mendoza is well known. Suffering from a serious infirmity, called apoplexy in some sources (a cerebral vascular problem), and in others *mirarchia*, a meningeal condition, he turned to an Indian from Cuernavaca who finally cured him (Benavides 1992, fol. 61r). The viceroy had been near death, and before he was cured by the Indian doctor, he had consulted all of the Spanish doctors then living in Mexico.

Another Indian doctor in Mexico City during the colonial period, Martín de la Cruz, is the well-known author of *Libellus de Medicinalibus indorum herbis*, a book of prescriptions written in 1552 and popularized under the name *Cruz-Badiano Codex*. The excellent documentation available on de la Cruz permits us to infer the activities of other indigenous doctors who were active in the viceregal capital. De la Cruz was the doctor for the indigenous children who studied and lived at the Colegio de Santa Cruz in Tlaltelolco (Gómez Canedo 1982:134–215; Ocaranza 1934b). It is thought that he taught indigenous medicine there, although documentation is lacking. He obtained a position at the Colegio with the help of Viceroy Mendoza, worked closely with him, and possibly participated in the treatment of his serious illness of 1550.

It is important to note that because of the high levels of mortality among Indians caused by epidemics of smallpox, measles, whooping cough, and particularly the *huey cocolitzli*, or great disease of 1545 (probably a virulent form of typhus), the Spaniards thought that the basic physiological nature of Indians was different from that of Europeans. Just as Indians were accustomed to and required particular forms of government, just as they dressed differently from the Europeans and ate distinct types of food, so they were thought to require medical treatment designed specifically for them. Indian doctors were in the perfect position to provide that special care. When the "Indian Republic" was established in Tlaltelolco, Spanish officials thought an Indian school and Indian doctors were a necessity.

Nevertheless, by about 1550, the idea of developing a "university" for Indians in the Colegio de Santa Cruz de Tlaltelolco was abandoned. With Spanish dominance well established, an effort was made to found a university along European lines. Thus, in 1553, the Royal and Pontifical University was established, and although at the beginning professorial chairs in medicine were not created, ranks of doctors and surgeons, trained in various universities in Spain, were incorporated into the university at this time. The diverse backgrounds of the medical personnel caused the *protomédicos* to develop the policy of checking documents and examining men who wanted to practice medicine or to become surgeons or pharmacists.

The belief that Indian doctors should care for Indians, coupled with the system that regulated the medical profession, led to the requirement that Indian doctors must seek authorization to promote medicine. I have limited myself to studying documentation coming from Mexico City and its neighboring areas, so I do not know if authorization was required for indigenous doctors to practice in other parts of New Spain or Guatemala. For the present, authorizations have been found that were signed by the viceroy. Once their requests had been analyzed and their status and curing methods had been investigated, native doctors like Martín de la Cruz and Antón Hernández were free to practice *their* kind of medicine (Velasco 1551, fols. 148v and 149r). This license was valid for Mexico City, Tlaltelolco, "and any other place," but was limited in the sense that it expressly said "they can cure Indians" only. The distinction was clearly and explicitly drawn between Indians and Spaniards, and between the doctors appropriate for each type of person (Viesca Treviño 1995:489–490). Two-and-a-half years later, Martín de la Cruz is mentioned as the examiner of Indian doctors. Antón Martín and Graviel Santiago were appointed to join him in that duty in October of 1553 (Luis de Velasco 1553, fol. 332v). The latter two indigenous doctors are classified as *amantecas*, or artisans—practitioners of a manual art. This puts them closer, if a parallel can be drawn, to the status of a practical surgeon than to that of a doctor.

The presence of indigenous doctors can be documented in various other regions. A doctor of the Tarascan chief Calzontzin saved the guardian of the convent of San Francisco from death, purging him with a Michoacán root and introducing to New Spain's pharmacopoeia one of the popular medicines whose renown spread to Europe (López Piñero 1990:28–30; Monardes 1988:29).

The bishopric of Michoacán was unusual in that Franciscan convents that would take in the sick were scattered throughout the region, and hospitals were built alongside chapels in all the towns organized by Vasco de Quiroga. There were always portals for the sick and in many cases more formal infirmaries, and it is possible that local indigenous doctors took care of patients in these places of healing (Venegas 1973:74, 107). The *Relaciones geográficas*, mandated by Philip II in the 1570s, reveals that in Tancítaro the natives had a hospital where all of the poor of the town were treated (*Relación de Tancítaro* 1987:290). Similar hospitals were found in Pinzandaro Arimao, Tlapalcatepeque (*Relación de Tancítaro* 1987:302), Tingüindín (*Relación de Tingüindín* 1987:327), and Tuchpan (*Relación de Tuchpan* 1987:389). In addition, there was a very humble hospital in Zapotlán, and likewise in Tamazula (*Relación de Tingüindín* 1987:395, 401), these last two founded by Franciscan friars. In Xiquilpan there was a hospital also founded by a Franciscan about which it was stated explicitly that natives "were treated with herbs they know" (*Relación de Xiquilpan* 1987:417). On the other hand, in Tiripitío several old women served as doctors.

By 1579, which is when the *Relación de Tiripitío* was written, it is affirmed that most patients in the hospital founded by the encomendero Juan de Alvarado were treated using Spanish practices, including bleeding and purging with Michoacán root. This hospital was run by Augustinian friars (*Relación de Tiripitío* 1987:351). These Indian doctors displayed their knowledge publicly regarding the diagnosis of illnesses. They spoke of changes in warmth and coldness, a method of understanding illness that was compatible with the Galeno-Hippocratic humoral medicine that Spanish doctors practiced. They also used medicinal plants, products or parts of animals, and minerals in their cures that could be tested objectively. What they hid with great care were ritual practices that recalled the close relationship of their medicine with the religion of their ancestors. In the *Relación de Chilchotla*, concerning a Tarascan settlement, it is pointed out that the people had confidence in their doctors. This confidence is noted even though indigenous curers are labeled in the document as "impostors who pass themselves off as doctors." They are called imposters because of their practice of blowing into a jug full of water, looking toward the sky for a diagnosis, and saying "some words that cannot be understood," surely prayers and magic incantations (*Relación de Chilchotla* 1987:109).

It is interesting to note that in Chilchotla as well as in the great majority of small settlements within its jurisdiction there existed hospitals connected to churches, all founded by Don Vasco. Many are described as being very good. A question arises: What was the relationship between the Tarascan "doctors" who served in these hospitals and the "impostors" criticized as superstitious? Were some of the doctors and impostors the same people? It is important not to lose sight of the fact that Michoacán was a region of great cultural development in pre-Hispanic times. There were doctors of great renown in the region and doctors of the *cazonci*, the Tarascan leader, who had their own responsibilities and leadership, like other groups of artisans. It was not unusual for them to convene meetings of the *xurimecha* when a sick person was of high social rank and the illness was dangerous (*Relación de las ceremonias y ritos y población y gobierno de los indios de la Provincia de Michoacán* 1977:178; Sepúlveda 1988:101). It is thus not surprising that a medical organization sui generis in the Tarascan region and distinct from other medical organizations of the viceroyalty persisted for many years within the colonial structure.

The presence of Indians familiar with illnesses and medicinal herbs in Guatemala is recorded from the sixteenth century. In the texts of the *Relaciones geográficas* commissioned by Philip II in the 1570s, healers are mentioned in various contexts. In the *Relación de Zapotitlán*, a lack of doctors is noted except in the large cities. But the author affirms that there existed "learned Indians who know remedies and use them and know many medicinal herbs" (*Relación de Zapotitlán* 1982:143). This is irrefutable proof of the presence of indigenous "doctors," even though the author of the *Relación* denied them that title. In the accounts of Santiago Atitlán and surrounding settlements, the author mentions only that the natives made use of medicinal plants, without distinguishing between popular knowledge and specialized knowledge of the *curanderos* (*Relación de Santiago Atitlán* 1982:90, 108, 130, 143).

Further south, in the region known then as Verapaz, divided from Guatemala by the Sacapula River, indigenous medicine as well as the entire population and culture faced a serious crisis. The region suffered from a high mortality rate due to misfortunes and epidemics triggered by radical changes in people's lives, especially the concentration of Indians in settlements. In the face of this disaster, older people no longer wanted to cure for fear of being accused of sorcery. While in fact there is practically no record of people actually being accused of sorcery, magic, or witchcraft, the ancestral knowledge of prayers, herbs, and other remedies was slowly being lost (Francisco Montero 1575?:243). However, in a letter to the king, a judge (*oidor*) of the Audiencia, García de Palacio, does mention superstitious activities of various types and the activity of the indigenous midwives (García de Palacio 1576:281). In the case of populations that maintained their ancient dispersed settlement patterns and that were far removed from Spanish authorities, it is reasonable to believe that the indigenous peoples maintained their doctor-priests. It is also clear why they did not reveal them to outsiders since they would face the threats of the tribunals of the Holy Office of the Indies and the Royal Protomedicato.

In general terms, one can imagine that in the mountainous and forested regions of southeast Mexico, in Guatemala, and Verapaz, *curanderos* working in secret among the local people established themselves very early on. The statement of Fray Bartolomé de las Casas in this regard is unequivocal: "they had doctors, great herbalists, and perhaps [even] better sorcerers" (De las Casas 1967, 2:514). It is very probable that the *curandero* acted as diviner and vehicle of the gods similar to the roles played by doctors before the Conquest. To these roles were also added some priestly functions such as commending the sick person to the lords of the hills, or taking confessions, a practice that continued to be reported during the eighteenth century (Orellana 1987:61–62). Doctors combining prayer, divination, and medical treatment based on herbs soon became widespread throughout Mexico.

However, there were a few notable exceptions. For example, in Santiago Atitlán, Guatemala, two types of doctors, those who divine and those who treat illness, continue to practice up to the present time (Douglas 1969:147; Orellana 1987:62). The near total annihilation and subsequent concealment of surviving priests and upper class doctors led to the appearance in rural areas of *curanderos*, whose numbers remained unknown. Midwives were much more apparent, as were the herbalists (*yerbateros*), whose presence, especially in Yucatan, has continued up to the present.

It is likewise logical that in the new cities founded by the Spaniards after the Conquest, indigenous doctors were limited in number because they would have had few patients, whether Indian or European. For example, we know that in the 1570s the city of Guatemala had only five hundred inhabitants composed of Creoles and Spaniards. Oaxaca, founded with eighty inhabitants in 1529, had only slightly more than five hundred inhabitants during the same period, in addition to approximately three hundred Indian

service people (*Relación de Antequera* 1984:33). The absence of data on the
use of indigenous herbs and medicines, and even on the *curanderos* themselves, in this size of a town is thus not surprising. However, we do know
that in nearby Mitla, an important pre-Hispanic site, indigenous doctors
and their professional activities persisted and that they cured "fevers and
smallpox" with "herbs from the wild" that they had collected (*Relación de
Tlacolula y Miquitla* 1984:261). The situation would not have been much
different in Guatemala, even though we lack information about *curanderos*.
We do have information available about a doctor who is not named in the
document. We know he was authorized in 1542 to cure sick people who
consulted him, in spite of being forbidden to do so the previous year because
his patients were dying at such a high rate. The lack of doctors, especially in
Guatemala, forced extreme measures (Remesal 1966:274).

This leads us to another problem: the ambiguous, paradoxical attitude
of the colonial authorities toward indigenous doctors who were being
transformed into *curanderos* and losing their professional legitimacy in the
new social context. While some of them were officially recognized and
consulted, others, perhaps the majority, were banished, and some were
persecuted.

Discrediting indigenous doctors began with the ever-increasing number
of Spanish doctors arriving in New Spain, and above all, as a result of the
founding of the Royal and Pontifical University in 1553 and the establishment of professorships of medicine in 1578. Discrediting *curanderos*, along
with denials of the efficacy of indigenous medicine, was a way to eliminate
the competition of indigenous medicine that had been so successful up to
that time.

The fierce diatribe that Francisco Hernández, chamber doctor of
Philip II and *protomédico* of the Indies, directed against indigenous medicine
is found in his *Antigüedades de Nueva España*. This work, finished in 1574,
sets down the principal reasons from the perspective of a Renaissance Spanish doctor for rejecting indigenous doctors. Hernández spoke of their lack
of specialization, of finding neither pharmacists nor surgeons among them,
"but rather only doctors who practiced all of medicine." He also accused
them of mere empiricism; "they neither study the nature of the illnesses and
their differences," nor prescribe medicines in accordance with the cause of
the illness, or accident. They do not bleed nor adapt treatments "to the

various humors that have to be expelled," nor do they know the crises or judicious days (Hernández 1984:100–101). Hernández' criticism was that the medicine practiced by the indigenous doctors was not the same as that taught by European faculties of medicine. In short, it did not follow the doctrines of Hippocrates and Galen. As a result, indigenous doctors officially became *curanderos*, even though their numbers and the number of their patients were large, and they were often effective (Ortiz de Montellano 1975). Hernández later reconsidered his opinion in light of the practical knowledge of some indigenous doctors.

In spite of Hernández' criticisms, we continue to find evidence of indigenous doctors officially practicing in Tlaltelolco. Tlaltelolco was an Indian neighborhood where Fray Bernardino de Sahagún, during these same years, gathered his data about indigenous doctors, whom he cites by name: Gaspar Matías, Pedro de Santiago, Francisco Simón, Miguel Damián, Felipe Hernández, Pedro de Requena, Miguel García, and Miguel Motolinia (Sahagún 1969 3:326). Indigenous doctors were present some fifty years later, as is evident in the 1618 complaint of Diego Cisneros, doctor of the viceroy marquis of Guadalcazar. He reported that Indian doctors who prescribed hot maize drinks (*atoles*) broke all dietary rules, and that herbalists, who were quite numerous in Mexico City, had far more clients, both Indian and Spanish, than any accredited doctor (Cisneros 1618, fol. 138; Viesca Treviño 1996:199). Indigenous doctors are mentioned time and again in later years. Fray Agustín de Vetancurt speaks in 1689 of "herbalists and native doctors" who practiced publicly, that is, with some type of official recognition. In Tlaltelolco, he consulted twenty of them about the properties of plants, which he cites in his *Teatro mexicano* (De Vetancurt 1982, pt. 1, fol. 64). This situation extends to the end of the colonial period. There is no lack of documents referring to the existence of *curanderos* practicing their trade with the knowledge and recognition of the local authorities. The latter recognized that the *curanderos* were less ignorant of medicine than people who knew nothing about such matters, and that in the absence of Spanish doctors, the authorities preferred that people go to them. The same conclusion is drawn by the mayors of Querétaro and Guanajuato in the last years of the eighteenth century (AGN, Protomedicato, vol. 2, exp. 8, fol. 272; vol. 3, fol. 65).

It is clear that the first regulations of the Spanish government retaining indigenous doctors in office to treat indigenous patients (and later blacks, mestizos, and other "races") remained in force due to the lack of doctors who had graduated from universities or who had been educated in the medical system of the conquerors. It is also clear that this circumstance constituted—and still constitutes—a tacit recognition of the failure of government health policies and programs to eradicate indigenous medical culture. The prevailing tolerance was definitely undesirable from the Spanish viewpoint. It was compelled by health needs, deferring the legal elimination of *curanderos* to a future that has never arrived (Quezada 1989:28).

Tolerance of *curanderos* occurred in Spanish cities like Querétaro, which had fifty thousand inhabitants in 1791 and only two doctors, and in Puebla, which was even larger, and which found itself in desperate straits in 1798 because a smallpox epidemic made the paucity of doctors evident. This tolerance is indicative of the situation that prevailed in New Spain at the very height of the development of colonial institutions. The edict promulgated by Viceroy Branciforte in 1799, declaring that "there is no prohibition against *curanderos* helping the sick in Indian areas," recognized the work of indigenous doctors treating the non-Spanish population of New Spain (AGN, Protomedicato, vol. 3, exp. 8 fol. 159). Therefore, the Spaniards tolerated the existence of "superstitious" practitioners, who were suspected of hiding their faith in the ancient gods and cults and of manipulating that reality as an important and secret aspect of their cures. The Spaniards needed their knowledge and understanding of medicines as well as the means to administer them (Anzures y Bolaños 1989; Quezada 1989:29; Viesca Treviño 1991:135). These practitioners pursued a particular method of treatment which is well illustrated in one of the first prosecutions of *curanderismo* that has come down to us, that of Ana, a *curandera* of Xochimilco, who was accused and sentenced to receive one hundred lashes in April of 1538. She was accused not because she treated patients, but because of *how* she treated them. The report indicates that she had come to treat an Indian woman who was ill in the house of the person filing the report. After incensing and sprinkling the sick woman with water, she pinched her body and "with each pinch she pulled out a wad of paper the size of her thumb," which she later confessed she had in her fist. She also said that "the devil Tezcatlipoca" was the cause of the evil from which the patient suffered. The part of the *curandera*'s treatment relating to the pre-Hispanic cult is what was officially prohibited by colonial authorities. More precisely, the dominant groups forbade what the subjugated groups favored. The latter group had a hybrid culture, incorporating elements of the most diverse kind, from the scientific language of the conqueror to the popular vulgar language of bile, envy (*muina*), and the shadow, a concept brought by African slaves that was combined with the pre-Hispanic *tonalli*. To this mix was added European magic, with all its paraphernalia.

Forty years ago, Aguirre Beltrán recognized the importance of a process he called acculturation, by which he meant the interchange of concepts, practices, and beliefs in a bilateral fashion moving from the dominant culture to the dominated and from the indigenous to the European (Aguirre Beltrán 1963). The large proportion of blacks, mulattos, and mestizos who took part in the proceedings of the Inquisition that dealt with *curanderismo* is historically important for two reasons. First, Aguirre Beltrán notes that only a small number of Indians were accused by the Inquisition because they were the object of special treatment and could be judged only by the Tribunal for Indians. Second, it was well known that blacks, mestizos, and Spaniards had access to *curanderismo* both because of the existence of *curanderos* and because of the extensive use of *curandero* practices by these groups. Members of these groups shared a wide range of beliefs, from the use of herbal treatments to sorcery (Aguirre Beltrán 1963:362–416; Quezada 1989:123–131). The presence of *curanderos* of Spanish, black, and mestizo origin led to the creation of a new medical system whose indigenous elements varied with the number of natives living in a particular region of New Spain as well as with the growth of other ethnic groups. A small minority of the people distanced themselves from all types of "superstitious" beliefs. However, the long list of Spaniards and Creoles accused in Querétaro in 1614 of using the powder of turkey buzzard heads, mule brains, turtledove heads, lice, and worms to win the love of another person shows how many people were involved in magical "superstitions" (AGN, Ramo Inquisición, vol. 278, exp. 20).

It should be pointed out as well that the existence of documents accusing people of superstitious practices and sorcery, and the lack of documents that give information about procedures for administering medicines or for surgical procedures, skew our vision of *curanderismo* in New Spain. *Curanderismo* appears to be based more on elements of magical belief than it really was. As Quezada points out (1988:29, 108), the written emphasis on magical procedures should not prevent us from seeing that there was more to *curanderismo*.

The Preparation of Curanderos

Although the indigenous doctor received a solid tutorial preparation within his own family and from the group of *titici* who lived in established neighborhoods, the breakup of traditions after the Conquest marked the appearance of significant differences in training techniques, some of which signal a return to earlier practices. Despite the efforts of Spanish authorities to maintain control of natives dedicated to healing, for example, the requirement that candidates be examined by established indigenous doctors with some standing, these efforts were limited to the large cities, and especially those in which an indigenous system of government was maintained parallel to that of the conquerors. The most frequent method of transmitting rational medical knowledge of illness and therapeutic resources was from fathers and mothers to children. However, the decline in the number of *curanderos* with a clear family lineage led to new forms of initiation and access to knowledge. It was common for acolytes to present themselves to an Indian *curandero* to learn the healing arts, and this influenced the kinds of knowledge acquired. The example of Roque de los Santos, who practiced in Zacatecas and was accused of being a "superstitious *curandero*" before the Holy Office, is illustrative. Roque came from a family of *curanderos*, where he learned to heal, but in order to legitimize his initiation, he presented himself to Francisco López, an established Indian *curandero* (Quezada 1988: 39; AGN, Ramo Inquisición, vol. 848, fols. 1–63).

The call by supernatural powers to become a *curandero* was expressed in different ways. First, some people simply declared that they had the power to heal. This situation was not unusual in the context of Spanish culture of the sixteenth century and was not necessarily seen as aberrant. For example, Fray Lucas de Almodóvar had this gift (Mendieta 1971:626, 588). In the inquisitorial proceedings, numerous people declare the same thing, that is, that God made them *curanderos*, and even sorcerers, before they were born. Examples of this are the testimonies of the anonymous Indian of Opaxnalá in 1626 (AGN, Ramo Inquisición, vol. 354, fol. 506), of Petra de Torres, a Spaniard living in Tlanepantla who said flatly in 1766 that she healed by the grace of God and had not learned from anybody (AGN, Ramo Inquisición, vol. 1028, fol. 265), and of Cristóbal de Ontiveros, who in Taxco, in 1626, proclaimed that he had been born a diviner (AGN, Ramo Inquisición, vol. 362, fol. 87). Other records include that of García, a black man who told of having cried from within his mother's womb, thus announcing his gift (AGN, Ramo Inquisición vol. 333, fol. 50). We also find this sign in contemporary *curanderos* like Ciro Cabañas from the area of Matías Romero, Veracruz (Lagarriga and Viesca Treviño 1981). Finally, we have the account of Pedro Joseph, who said that he knew what he knew because his heart beat rapidly from joy, an experience that caused him to be accused of being a fortune teller (AGN, Ramo Inquisición, vol. 849, fol. 312).

More obvious still was the appearance of a cross and wound on the left ankle of Pedro Astasio, a black doctor from the house of the Duke of Linares. These signs intensified every Friday, according to charges filed against him as recorded in Zitácuaro in 1717 (AGN, Ramo Inquisición, vol. 800, fol. 15). José Antonio Hernández had a cross visible on his palate. A Galician, he was said to have cried in his mother's womb, and was born on Good Friday at three in the afternoon. He could heal on Friday only and treat only twelve patients per week, a number symbolic of the twelve apostles (AGN, Ramo Inquisición, vol. 1235, fol. 1; Quezada 1988:36). The list could be expanded, but the examples given cover very different parts of the territory of New Spain and date from the beginning of the seventeenth century to the end of the eighteenth, demonstrating the temporal and spatial extent of a similar mode of recruitment. The mode of recruitment varied depending upon the cultural and ethnic origin of the *curanderos*, ranging from the Spaniard Petra Torres, who spoke of the grace of God, to the presence of diviners with an African background, to the call of the indigenous *nahual*, a Mesoamerican tradition dating back millennia.

One important mode of recruitment is the call to become a *granicero*. These possessors of the power to control rain and hail and to destroy or insure a good crop trace back to the ancient priests of Tláloc. Their presence is documented from the time of the old priest of the Sacred Mountain, today called the Sacromonte de Amecameca, to the present time (Chimalpahin Cuauhtlehuanitzin 1965). The defining experience of these specialists is being struck by lightning. After surviving this trauma, they receive a call in a dream, and once the call is accepted, they undergo an apprenticeship through visions in which the future *granicero* comes to know the spirits who make lightning, the house of the gods of rain, and the way to control the elements of nature. Healing practices are an important addition to this complex. Even to the present day, these practices are often oriented to the control of sorcery or offenses by invisible beings sent through shamanic activities. They also may include the use of medicinal plants.

Like the lesions due to contact with lightning, being cured of illness or being saved from dying heralds access to the capacity to heal. These are shamanic signs present in a large number of cultures, including those of pre-Hispanic Mexico. There are many examples documented throughout the whole colonial period. Circumstances of each case are usually modified, however, such that the ancient gods are identified with the devil, or the curer enters into various kinds of pacts with the devil. In short, elements of European sorcery are incorporated into the accounts.

Another kind of initiation is the call from some deity or spiritual power in the form of convulsions. This pattern is of African origin and recalls the presence of *orishas* possessing the chosen person in order to act through him or her. For example, Lucas Ololá, a black slave who came from Portuguese Guinea and lived in the Huasteca, became the spokesman of the indigenous god Paya and transmitted his messages while in a trance state. This is a magnificent example of the process of syncretism that fuses an African substratum with traditions from the indigenous population that becomes his clientele (Aguirre Beltrán 1963:65). The example and the region from which it comes shows an uninterrupted tradition leading to the *santería* religion that exists there today. *Santería* is widely diffused along the coasts of the Gulf of Mexico and is centered in Tamaulipas and Veracruz.

An important characteristic of the *curandero* is his or her capacity to cause harm. This power creates an ambiguous feeling of dependence and distrust on the part of the users of his services. Distrust and fear arise from two circumstances. First, the *curandero* possesses knowledge of drugs. Drugs in the sense used by ancient Greeks include both medicines and poisons. Thus, they can be used to heal as well as to cause illness or even death. Distrust is also created in many cases by the belief that the curer has entered into a pact with the devil and with the ancient gods. In accusations and other documents from the Inquisition, even though these usually downplay the presence of indigenous *curanderos* in New Spain, "superstitions" and the use of sorcery are consistently mentioned (Aguirre Beltrán 1963:362–416). The territory corresponding to these reports is likewise extensive, stretching from the mining regions of the north to Guatemala. In 1620 Durango, for example, the use of the classic text of European magic, *Las clavículas de Salomón,* is documented (AGN, Ramo Inquisición, vol. 328, fol. 129), and in Guatemala, at the beginning of the seventeenth century, accusations of sorcery are widespread (AGN, Ramo Inquisición, vol. 285, fols. 29 and 36). In Honduras, the dean and bishop wrote letters in 1614 about sorcery used by black and Indian women (AGN, Ramo Inquisición, vol. 301, fol. 12). In Atlixco, Puebla, the mulatta Catalina de la Llosa experienced hardships and illnesses as the result of her refusal to maintain relations with a black *curandero,* an in-law of hers. Having returned to his side, she spewed from her vulva "thorns and small worms" (AGN, Ramo Inquisición, vol. 751, fol. 24; Aguirre Beltrán 1953:94). This case demonstrates that *curanderos* were thought to have the capacity to harm people through spells.

Of particular interest is the conservation and diffusion of a wide range of divinatory practices whose purpose is to find out the cause or outcome of illnesses as well as to learn the future and to discover the cause of misfortune. All types of divination were viewed with suspicion by the orthodox Spaniards because they incorporated elements connected with the pre-Hispanic religion. It is not by accident that in the confessional tracts written for use by friar catechists, there was always a question about whether the Indian who was making his confession had resorted to sorcerers or believed in predictions based on dreams and omens of various kinds (Molina 1975, fol. 20).

The belief that gods and supernatural beings are present inside of plants and animals was widespread, supporting the identification of the divine entity with its multiple disguises. In that way, sacred plants like *peyotl* or *ololiuhqui* were seen as gods and venerated as such, and that is how they were understood by those persecuting idolatries. The use of hallucinogenic substances by *curanderos* was as common as it was secretive, given the risk that was run if the authorities discovered a *curandero* using them. In 1620 the Inquisition issued an edict condemning the use of peyote (AGN, Ramo Inquisición vol. 333, fol. 35), which was used not only by the Chichimec people but also daily by people in more centrally located areas. The authorities had to renew the condemnation in 1684 (AGN, Ramo Inquisición vol. 758, fol. 105). In 1622 accusations of its use appear in Mexico City (AGN, Ramo Inquisición vol. 335, fol. 96 and vol. 341, fol. 4), Texcoco (AGN, Ramo Inquisición vol. 335, fol. 6), and Atlixco, where the indigenous mayor was accused of using hallucinogenic plants (AGN, Ramo Inquisición vol. 342, fol. 3). The peyote complex in the northern and northwestern territories, where it has been most studied today, was in place by the seventeenth century. Documents dated 1632 also confirm its presence in Santa Fe, New Mexico (AGN, Ramo Inquisición vol. 304, fol. 26). In Chihuahua, in 1726, a mulatto *curandero* named Juan Calderón, besides drinking peyote, had *al demonio* (to the devil) painted on his back (AGN, Ramo Inquisición vol. 1116, exp. 5, fols. 243–246). In Real de Suaqui, Sonora, an Indian was prosecuted in 1776 for performing the peyote song and dance (AGN, Ramo Inquisición vol. 1104, fol. 24). All of these cases demonstrate clearly the continuity of the rituals "discovered" by Lumholtz (1904) at the beginning of the twentieth century, which are still the focus of research on Indian culture by anthropologists and other researchers.

Ololiuhqui and *pipitzintli* are two other plants with psychedelic effects that are mentioned throughout the colonial period. The latter plant was studied in 1772 by Antonio Alzate, who showed that its effects were due to natural causes and not to the work of the devil (Alzate 1985: 53–62).

Specializations of Curanderos

The various Spanish documents refer to *curanderos* generically, using that term or a similar one from an indigenous language or dialect. However, it should not be overlooked that specialized knowledge and skill in certain kinds of treatments were kept in closed groups or within families that then transmitted them from generation to generation. These modes of transmission led indigenous healers toward increased specialization. Similarly, the Europeans, who sharply divided medicine from surgery, and surgeons from bloodletters, barbers, and bonesetters, imposed their own model on new Spain. *Curanderos* took pride in showing that they had adapted, at least superficially, to the new pattern. However, it should not be forgotten that in pre-Hispanic times medical and surgical activities were not contrasted in principle. Rather, the exercise of one or the other or both depended more on personal abilities or the healer's particular training in accordance with specific family traditions (Viesca Treviño 1984: 220–222).

In a document dated 1629, Hernando Ruíz de Alarcón speaks generically of the Nahuatl *tícitl* and refers to midwives as female doctors. Ordinarily, says the author, *tícitl* is understood to mean "what in Spanish is implied by the term doctor." But in reality, it connotes doctor, wise man, fortune teller, and sorcerer—and even having a pact with the devil. It was believed that the *tícitl* can have remedies against any illness, since he knows medicines, knows how to placate "our Lord God or the Blessed Virgin," and likewise handles *ololiuhqui*, peyote, or gods of nature (Ruíz de Alarcón 1987:195). In accordance with the type of activities carried out by a *tícitl*, he or she might well take on the appearance of a specialist, perhaps in the same manner that individual ability was recognized in the pre-Hispanic period (Viesca Treviño 1984:222). Sometimes the specialist was referred to by a name that reflected the divinatory techniques he used. For example, the *atlantlachixque* looked at the reflection of a sick child's face in water to determine if his *tonalli* was present (Ruíz de Alarcón 1987:197; Ponce de León 1987:10). There was also the *tetonalmacani*, skilled at returning the *tonalli* to those who had lost it due to fright or a serious illness (Ponce de León 1987:10).

In contrast, bonesetters are not differentiated specifically by Ruíz de Alarcón (1987:212), nor by other early authors. However, this specialist, called *tepoztecpahtiani*, was recognized from ancestral times. And Ruíz de Alarcón does record the spells uttered to help manipulations aimed at setting fractures or treating dislocated bones. He also mentions the potions with needles used to heal the pain of "bones of the back" (Ruíz de Alarcón 1987:214). Reference is also made to the existence of *curanderos* who "sucked" areas near dislocated or fractured bones and who magically removed the evil. This was the case of José Luis, a famous black bonesetter who treated people by combining sucking with a physical procedure to remove spells (Quezada 1988:97). In addition, references in the *Popol Vuh* to the original ancestors, Grandfather and Grandmother, have them setting bones as one of their tasks. In the Maya area of the highlands of Guatemala and Chiapas, veiled references to bonesetting are found throughout the colonial period and this specialty is well documented in contemporary ethnographic studies (e.g., Orellana 1987:65–66).

Similar to the bonesetters are the massagers, or *sobadores*. There is also mention of *zurujanos* (surgeons), including those who treat hernias, based on a model that is essentially Spanish (Ponce de León 1987:7). Quezada, in a study of colonial *curanderismo*, recognizes the existence of the ancient technique of the *teiczalizatli*, a specialist who treads on the back of the ill person with his heated callused feet (Quezada 1988:97; De la Serna 1902: 418). There are also descriptions of *curanderos* who used suction, those who let blood similar to the European pattern, and still others who sucked on the belly or head of the patient and extracted bizarre objects that they identified with evil. The latter technique can be identified as much with the indigenous *techichinami* as with the European sorcerer (Quezada 1988:90). Cleansings, breathing on the ill person, including the variation of spraying some liquid from the mouth of the healer, and censing are all used by most *curanderos*.

It is also important to note that causing someone to become ill or suffer misfortune appeared to be the work of a specialist. Making pacts with evil powers and having the capacity to do harm can be linked to characteristics of the majority of indigenous deities and of gods of African origin. I believe that the use of dolls or images that represent the person one wishes to make ill is an element of African origin. The practice appears with relative frequency in the documents of the colonial period and is still used in Mexican *curanderismo* (Quezada 1988:65).

The Nineteenth Century

The independence of New Spain and the Captaincy General of Guatemala did not provide advantage to people who practiced *curanderismo*. Even though social conditions did not change much, medical practice did. Due to discoveries and the development of a new human biology, medicine strove to make itself more scientific in the early-nineteenth-century sense of the term. It became the object of regulations that became more rigorous as each day passed. If the Protomedicato had turned a blind eye to *curanderos* of all types and ignored their activities covering many areas of health care, the Medical School of the Federal District and later the Consejo Superior de Salubridad (Higher Council of Health) prohibited the practice of medicine by anyone who did not have a professional degree issued by an institution of higher learning recognized by the corresponding public authorities. In 1841, the Consejo requested that those who practiced medicine present a diploma and certification issued by mayors and magistrates verifying they were indeed recognized doctors. However, this attempt at regulation failed since these authorities confused "legally authorized professors with the charlatans and *curanderos*" who abounded in the national territory (Martínez Cortés 1993:42).

The laws promulgated by the authorities of the Second Empire sought the same thing in 1865. They prohibited the practice of medicine by those who were not approved in accordance with the existing laws (Martínez Cortés 1993:144). The obligatory registration of professionals before the Council was aimed at greater control and the gradual elimination of those who practiced without having had the corresponding education, among them all the *curanderos* of indigenous and popular tradition. Article 220 of Mexico's first public health code in 1891 advocated the same policy.

Nevertheless, *curanderos* of all types continued working and solving many health problems, even when the advances of medicine made obvious the errors in some aspects of their work. Just as the Visitador de la Serna was unsuccessful in the middle of the seventeenth century when he requested that indigenous doctors and *curanderos* be identified and forbidden from practicing (De la Serna 1902:464), so too was the Ministry of Justice when it stipulated in 1842 that *curanderos* who practiced without a degree were to be pressed to serve in the military (Álvarez Amézquita et al. 1960, 1:252). In 1875, the National Academy of Medicine published in its journal a note which pointed out the risks of the *curanderos'* unscientific or marginally scientific practices and the abundance of charlatans of all kinds.

Curanderismo was shaped by an ethos that joins *curanderos* closely to their patients. This is especially true within indigenous groups that live in relative isolation, and among those people such as mestizos, who continue to defend their ancient culture. *Curanderismo* was also conditioned by a scarcity of doctors who had graduated from schools, as well as the concentration of these doctors in larger cities. Ever present, *curanderos* and all their social functions began by the early twentieth century to be the object of interest of anthropologists, and eventually the idealized image of the indigenous doctor, the *tícitl*, came to form an idealized part of national identity.

CHAPTER 4

Central and North Mexican Shamans

James W. Dow

Shamanism

The definition of "shaman" is far from precise. Some people argue that there are many types of shamans. Lipp (see Chapter 5) examines some of these arguments. It is a vast subject, but, in order to identify the people that it examines, this chapter needs only to define shamans in the context of Mexican cultures. One simple way of defining shamans is by what they do. In general, shamans are healers who specialize in symbolic healing, effects of the mind on the body. The primary tool of Mexican shamans is magical ritual. However, every magical healer in Mexico is not a shaman. There are magical healers, such as Spiritualists or psychic surgeons, whose work is not part of a native tradition and, hence, they are not called shamans. In Mexico, "shaman" designates a magical healer who works within a modern Native American cultural tradition.

Yet, not all healers in the native communities are shamans. There are other, nonmagical, healers. For example, the Cora have herbalists, bonesetters, midwives, and prayer makers (Mellado Campos et al. 1994:69). Curers in Pichátaro, a Purépechan community, are primarily herbalists whose main function is to restore a bodily equilibrium that has been upset by diet, external factors such as weather, or emotional disturbances (Garro 1986:352). The Chichimec-Jonaz have midwives, herbalists, and bonesetters. The primary difference between these healers and the shamans is that they do not make use of magical ritual, although they work within a modern Native American cultural tradition.

Another common means of defining shamans in Mexico is by the way in which they receive their power to cure. Madsen (1955:48) defines a shaman as an individual who has received the power to cure directly from supernatural beings through dreams, visions, or spirit possession. This opposes them to the bonesetters, herbalists, and so on, who derive their power to cure from a naturalistic knowledge of curative substances and techniques. The existence of these other types of curers in the native tradition shows that naturalistic philosophies are part of native Mesoamerican thought (Cosminsky 1976b; Ortiz de Montellano 1975) and that shamans are just one type of healer. Yet, because they deal with an emotionally charged world beyond ordinary perception, they are often regarded as the most powerful healing specialists.

Shamans may also use nonmagical treatments such as herbal medicines, but these are used within the context of an overall magical treatment. Although the patient may benefit from the biomedical effects of the herbs, he or she is led to see them as part of an overall magical solution to the problem. Shamans may be midwives, too, such as among the Tepehua. Both Tepehua shamans and Tepehua midwives are called *hat'aku·nu'*. When they are semidivine and highly revered, they are called *lak'ainananín* (Williams García 1963:141). If a Tepehua woman who is a midwife is married to a shaman, she is called a shaman too.

Variations in the Descriptions of Shamanism

Variations in the literature on shamanic belief and practice in central and north Mexico are due either to (1) real subcultural differences or (2) different ways that anthropologists have of interpreting and describing the same thing. Typically, a cultural anthropologist concentrates on faithfully describing a culture and does not worry about the comparability of his or her description with the description of other cultures made by other anthropologists. Unfortunately, there are many ways of describing similar beliefs and rituals; thus anyone trying to compare patterns of magic and religion must work hard to separate what is truly different in each culture from what is simply an artifact of ethnographic style. Take for example the following two descriptions of the "cleaning" in a Purépecha culture first and then in a Totonac culture.

> Purépecha: The "cleaning" is a common ritual in the Purépechan region. In these zones, it refers to a magico-religious practice aimed not only at preventing, curing, and diagnosing an illness in a manner similar to other traditional medical practices in Mexico, but also at "curing the house," where the procedure has the purpose of taking out of the house the elements that have contaminated it or "bewitched" it. In other words, the concept that underlies this ritual has not been changed since in both cases the end of the cleaning is the same, whether or not the entities treated are animate or inanimate such as houses, *milpas*, etc. (Mellado Campos et al. 1994:684, my translation)

> Totonac: The sweeping, or cleaning properly called, consists of passing around the body of the individual, especially around the head, face, and then the back, very rapidly an animal (chicken or pullet), a plant (branches of certain ritual plants) or an object (candle), that will pick up the air.—If it exists, the cleaning could be preventive—The objects employed in the cleaning will be thrown in a remote place, far from the house. (Ichon 1973:251, my translation)

Comparing such ethnographies is a difficult task for which there is no easy method. One must estimate what is common and what is different from a thorough reading of the material. In making comparisons between villages and peoples one must take into account the focus of the ethnographer, who seldom uses standardized forms for observation and measurement. One ethnographer may overlook something that another is fixated on, and vice versa. One cannot make fine comparisons, because the lack of a feature in a report does not mean that it does not exist.

The Extent of Shamanism in Central and North Mexico

Influenced by the writings of the late Carlos Castañeda, the popular image of the Mexican shaman in the United States has been of a lonely, socially marginal person who believes he can transform himself into an animal and who is little concerned for the people of his or her community. The reality is quite different. Mexican shamans are respected people in their communities. Their dedication and spirituality are admired. They can fail to cure, they can disappoint some people, but, by and large, they are respected like medical doctors in Western culture.

Not all the native cultures of central and north Mexico support the same type of shaman. A cursory analysis has led me to propose two types: a *traditional* type and a *curandero* type.

Traditional Shamans base their work on a coherent non-Christian religious belief system. They work with traditional myths that have pre-Columbian connections. The traditional shaman is a religious leader and may be graded with others in a hierarchy of spiritual attainment. The traditional shaman is also a pastor who leads a flock of devoted followers and may also be called on by the community to officiate at religious gatherings or to perform other public services. The mark of the traditional shaman is that he or she is regarded as an authority of an unseen spirit world known to almost everybody through myth.

Curandero Shamans practice magical healing without the authority and prestige of being religious leaders in their communities. They draw on a wide range of folk belief including colonial Spanish and modern rural beliefs. The mythical basis of their rituals is more diffuse. *Curandero* shamans are often subdivided into specialties depending on the mode of ritual curing. For example the Rarámuri have herbalist *curanderos*, massage *curanderos*, and pediatric *curanderos* (Mellado Campos et al. 1994:707). *Curandero* shamans exist where native cultures have undergone more European influence, primarily in the center of Mexico. In these cultures, midwives, herbalists, bonesetters, singers, prayer makers, and massage therapists also do much of the curing. The magical curers, the *curandero* shamans, do not have a strong connection to an original native worldview.

The myths that lie at the foundation of traditional shamanic curing are not dead literature but are ongoing beliefs that are modified daily through visions and logical prescientific philosophy. Shamans exert only a provisional, contested control over their patients' understanding (Brown 1988).

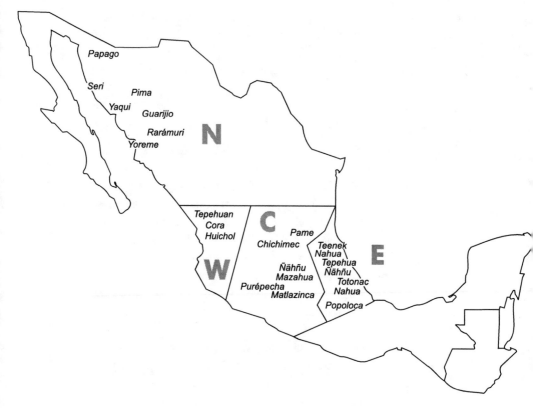

FIGURE 4.1: Locations of native cultures whose shamans are described in this chapter. The regions are north (**N**), west (**W**), central (**C**), and east (**E**).

Each cure provides an opportunity to remake and expand the mythic basis for shamanic healing.

Traditional shamanism is found primarily among the groups that were changed the least by the haciendas of the eighteenth and nineteenth centuries. These cultures are generally in the mountainous areas to the east and west of central Mexico, shown in Figure 4.1.

The cultures that support traditional shamans are the Nahua, Sierra Ñähñu (Sierra Otomí), Totonac, Teenek (Huastec), Tepehua, Cora, and Huichol. All these shamanic traditions have ancient roots in pre-Columbian cultures.

Conceptual Models of Illness

A model of how the world is constructed lies behind shamanic healing. Shamanism is simply based on the laws of nature as Native Americans see them. This traditional worldview is fundamentally animistic. People believe that an animating force is contained within all living things and moving objects. Animating forces are the essence of life. An animating force is usually called a soul or *alma* in European languages, but this translation distorts its meaning by adding irrelevant Christian connotations. Anthropologists have sometimes conceptualized the idea of animating forces as a visit by the shaman to another spirit world. My interpretation of the philosophy is that the forces are part of the present world and that the average person is just insensitive to them. Thus the traditional shaman seeks greater awareness of what is in this world, not awareness of another world. As Eger Valdez notes (1996:300), the philosophy is profoundly ecological and most appropriate to cultures that depend on foraging and agriculture instead of science and industry.

Uncontaminated animistic philosophy is relatively simple. All things move and act because their animating forces give them the power to do so. In the native worldview, no distinction is made between symbolic and physical effects or between psychological and medicinal causality. All significant actions are the result of animating forces at work. The forces exist in a hierarchy of power with the sun and moon at the top and stones on the bottom. The animating forces of humans are in between these two extremes. Humans have total power over stones, which have no animating force, but no power to change the motion of the sun or stars, which have powerful animating forces. Humans dominate animals. Beings that are more powerful dominate humans.

Traditional shamans are able to see and manipulate the animating forces. Although this concept also lies behind the work of *curandero* shamans, traditional shamans seek knowledge of the forces. The traditional shaman's quest for knowledge has its own spiritual rewards beyond being simply a practical means of curing. The community is drawn into the quest and supports it as a religious calling. The traditional shaman returns this support by leading rituals for the community. The traditional shaman is also a religious leader.

Shamanic magic is consistent with Malinowski's (1948:30) observation that magic in general is an extension of human effort beyond the point where ordinary technology fails. When herbalists and shamans exist in the same community, the herbalists are enlisted for routine medical problems where sorcery is not suspected and where a positive outcome is likely. When the illness proves to be more intractable, a shaman is called in to deal with the underlying animating forces. The difference between herbalists and shamans is that the herbalists confine themselves to prescribing botanical treatments and avoid dealing with the animating forces. The shaman, on the other hand, confronts the underlying animating forces.

Traditional shamans use visions and trances to see and deal with the animating forces. In the western region, shamans go on vision quests; for example, some Huichol shamans go to the forests to commune with wolves and receive wolf power (Eger Valdez 1996:273–274). In the east shamans enter trances during rituals. Hallucinogenic plants such as peyote (Furst 1972), datura, and cannabis (Emboden 1972:229) aid these visions and are regarded as spiritual beings in their own right. The most noteworthy hallucinogenic plant in the west and north is peyote (Furst 1972). The first non-Indian to investigate the vision quests of the Huichol was Fernando Benítez (1968). The peyote visions carry a divine message using the symbols of Huichol myth (Benzi 1969). In the east, the Sierra Ñähñu and the Tepehua use cannabis (Williams García 1963:215–221). Cannabis has also been used in the west. Lumholtz reported it among the Tepehuan as early as 1902 (Emboden 1972:229). It was called *rosa maría* there. In the east it is called *santa rosa*. In general, cannabis, an Old World plant, seems to have been substituted in some places for New World plants such as peyote, datura, morning glory, and hallucinogenic mushrooms because of its superior effects or because there was a lack of the original hallucinogen.

As a spiritual leader, the traditional shaman can lead pilgrimages to places of spiritual power. With such leadership the average person can become aware of the animating forces without becoming a shaman himself. Huichol shamans lead groups of devotees on pilgrimages to the place where they gather peyote plants. Through prayers and rituals, the landscape is reconstructed as a Huichol mythical place called Wirikúta (Furst 1972; Myerhoff 1974). The Cora also believe in Wirikúta, and their shamans see it while in trance (Mellado Campos et al. 1994:80).

In the eastern part of central Mexico, Sierra Ñähñu go on pilgrimages to a mythic place called "México Chiquito," or "Mayonikha" (Galinier 1990:313). In fact, there are a number of cave shrines in the sacred mountains of this area that can serve as the mythic locus. The difference between a pilgrimage and a trip to a mountain shrine is simply in the length of the preparation and the length of the journey. Mayonikha refers to the place of an ancient church or a dual church (Galinier 1990:313). Since the original Tenochtitlán (México) contained the main Aztec dual temple, the idea of México Chiquito (Little México) as a place of pilgrimage recapitulates a pilgrimage to the Aztec dual temple at Tenochtitlán. The memory of ancient Mexico City as a place of pilgrimage still lingers on in the Sierra Ñähñu vocabulary. Today Mexico City is called Mändä (Middle), a shortened form of Ra Mändä Zäna (The Middle of the Moon), which recalls the ancient name of the lake in which Tenochtitlán was built, the Lake of the Moon. Another legendary place of pilgrimage for the Sierra Ñähñu is La Laguna (The Lake), where the goddess of the fresh waters, Maka Xumpɸ Dehe, resides.

The Sierra Ñähñu and Nahua believe that companion spirit animals (*tonales*) guard a person's animating force. The companion spirit animals are born at the same time as the person. They are seldom seen but aid the individual supernaturally to overcome hardships along his or her life journey. Shamans can see the companion spirit animals and are able to work with them. The power to manipulate the animating forces implies the power to manipulate them for evil as well as good. Therefore, the belief in sorcery is widespread in Mexican subcultures. Even if a subculture has many Catholic beliefs, it often retains a concept of sorcery. For example, the Purépecha magical curers deal with the evil eye, cleanse patients of "evils" (*maleficios*), and get rid of "disgusting things" (*cochinadas*) that may have been planted in their houses by enemies (Mellado Campos et al. 1994:668), yet most Purépecha consider themselves to be Catholics.

Perhaps stimulated by the success of modern biomedicine, Mexican natives often distinguish between "good" illnesses curable by medicines and "bad" illnesses curable only by shamanic ritual. For example, the Sierra Ñähñu say that "good" illnesses are sent by God, who has also placed on earth the means—herbs and medicines—by which they can be cured (Dow 1986a:9). However, when it is determined that an illness was sent by evil beings or by evil persons and not by God, shamans must intervene because such illnesses will not yield to simple treatments. The Cora believe that sorcery cannot be cured by medicine, although the symptoms may be the same as those of an ordinary illness (Mellado Campos et al. 1994:73). Shamans treat persistent diseases that have resisted common treatments and that people have come to believe are the result of some hidden evil.

A patient's moral transgressions can lead to illness. The native cultures of central and north Mexico have many rules for polite, civil behavior. In a number of cultures, people believe that the violation of these rules can lead to illness. The extent to which immorality is blamed for illness varies. The Teenek and the Cora are particularly concerned with illness caused by improper behavior. The Teenek believe that breaking the rules either deliberately by sorcery or accidentally by mistake eventually leads to illness (Alcorn 1984:21).

Evil Beings

Malevolent beings exist in the native worldview and can be generally classified as

1. evil godlings
2. airs
3. evil companion spirit animals
4. transforming witches

The evil godlings vary from place to place. People believe that they are quite willing to offer their services to sorcerers. Among the Teenek they are referred to as "punishers" (Alcorn 1984:231). They are often able to command airs, a type of rabid immaterial being that attacks anyone. The Sierra Ñähñu cut paper figures of evil beings, such as Lord of the Jews, Queen of the Earth, Lightning, and Rainbow (Sandstrom and Sandstrom 1986:152).

The companion spirit animals of sorcerers are evil. For example, Huichol myth names the owl and the fox as minions of sorcerers. The Sierra Ñähñu also point to these two evil companion spirit animals. Other animals exist in a more hideous realm. Some people believe in nightmarish bloodsucking beings, usually animals such as vultures or owls that may or may not take human form (Nutini 1993). It is sometimes difficult to distinguish these nightmare creatures from the spirit animals of sorcerers in the folklore of a particular culture.

Attacks

ATTACKS BY IMMATERIAL BEINGS

Airs or winds are evil beings that attack people who get too close to them. Although there is much evidence that a belief in airs is widespread, the belief is phrased in so many different ways that it is not always easy to recognize. The Sierra Ñähñu call them dähi, winds, and believe they live in canyons. They attack suddenly and painfully like rabid dogs (Dow 1986a:92). The Matlazinca believe that airs live in canyons or around springs (Mellado Campos et al. 1994:372). Airs are associated with dead persons. They could be hanging around where someone has died. They can be found where lightning has struck. The Matlazinca distinguish between various types of airs: lightning airs, thunder airs, airs of fright (*espanto*), river-source airs, and airs sent by curses (Mellado Campos et al. 1994:368). In general airs are found in dark, damp, drafty places and places where someone has died. They are like the dark cold wind that sweeps across the land just before a thunderstorm. Some Purépecha in the remote mountainous zones like Charapan still believe in a being called Miríngu or Miringua, "the trickster," an air that appears as a light wind which dries up plants (Mellado Campos et al. 1994:667). The Totonac shamans symbolize airs with humanoid figures (Ichon 1973:271). The Sierra Ñähñu use paper figures (Dow 1986a:32). Among the Sierra Ñähñu, Thunder and Lightning are evil godlings who command airs.

The Totonac, like other natives, believe that airs are basically evil, but they also say that some good things, such as the wooden horse used in the dance of the Santiagueros, is loaded with air. For this reason dancers who have been in contact with the horse must be purified. The Totonac recognize two strengths of airs. Certain individuals such as shamans, certain animals such as the *cojolite* (the bird species *Penelope purpuracens*), and certain objects have a strong air and are particularly dangerous. Other airs are weaker. Contact with the dead and participation in religious ceremonies can also cause seizure by airs (Ichon 1973:249). This accords with the idea that airs are powerful, dangerous, and without conscience. They are evil in the sense that contact with them causes sickness, not in the sense that they intend harm.

In the native worldview, airs are a category of evil being associated with storm gods. The syncretism of this concept with European humoral medical theories about air has obscured the underlying indigenous concept, which can be seen in the cultures where traditional shamans still practice. For example, Nahua beliefs in the Valley of Mexico have led to the following very concrete description of airs.

> The *enanitos* [dwarves], also known as *"los aires"* [the airs], are described in Tecospa as little men and women who stand about one and one-half feet high, wear long hair, dress and live like the Indians of Tecospa, and speak the Otomí tongue. They live in caves in the hills and mountains where they store big barrels containing clouds, rain, lightning, and thunder. When the *enanitos* are angry with a human being, they blow their breath at him, causing him to fall ill with the common disease known as *"aire de cuevas"* [cave air]. This disease usually is inflicted on bad persons who offend the *enanitos* by trespassing in their caves, by carrying food near their caves without giving them any of it, and by pointing or calling to a rainbow. *"Aire de cuevas"* is rarely fatal if the sick person is treated by a curer specializing in treatment of this disease. (W. Madsen 1955:49–50)

Airs have been called "among the most elusive of illness concepts" (Adams and Rubel 1967:338), but there is a clear focus on water, dampness, and storms. Putting these beliefs together, one is led to the conclusion that the concept of airs originated in a folk belief that people who died in storms or drowned went to live with water gods and could return to molest the living.

In the west central region, the Huichol believe in "bewitchment" (*tkiguo re* or *hechizos*) that is similar to airs. They believe that their ancestors send bewitchment to plague persons who have not been living a good life. The idea of airs is not prominent in accounts of Huichol curing, but airlike ideas appear in Huichol myth. The mythic founder of sorcery Kiéri Téwiyári is also called the "Tree of Winds" and can appear as an air (Furst and Myerhoff 1972:73).

ATTACKS UTILIZING MATERIAL OBJECTS

Among the native peoples of central and northern Mexico there is a widespread belief that physical objects implanted in the body or sorcery objects in and around one's house can cause illness. Objects believed to be inside the body are invisible to the average person. Only shamans can see and withdraw them. The nature of a hidden object is revealed when the shaman withdraws it. For example, Popoloca shamans find nails, maguey spines, and stones in the bodies of their patients (Jäcklein 1974:262). Sierra Ñähñu shamans find pieces of rotten blood and flesh (Dow 1986a:108). Tepehua shamans find small bones, coffee beans, corn, or money (Bower 1946:682). The objects are small, definitely foreign to the human body, and some-times disgusting. They define and explain the pain the patient suffers. Bower (1946:682) found an ironic twist in Tepehua belief. A rich man may suffer terribly from money lodged in his body. A man grown wealthy from trade in coffee may suffer from internal coffee beans. It could be said that the Tepehua believe in the supernatural leveling of wealth. They believe that the rich pay a painful price for their wealth.

Sorcery objects, on the other hand, are not in the body. They cause ill-ness by being close to their intended victim. Natives believe that sorcerers create these objects to attack their victims. They act something like radio-active land mines. The sorcery object symbolizes the insult to the victim. For example, among the Sierra Ñähñu, it may be a set of mutilated paper figures.

Diagnosis

Shamanic curing in central and north Mexico begins with a consultation (*consulta*). The consultation has several important dimensions. First, the same Spanish word is used to describe a visit to a biomedical doctor; there-fore, the consultation is a visit to a person with special professional knowl-edge. Second, by means of visions the shaman may also consult other more powerful beings. The consultation is a linking between levels in the hierar-chy of living beings. It is a necessary first step in a cure that links the patient to beings that can help him or her. For this reason, the consultation practi-cally always includes prayers and offerings. Gifts of rum, candles, incense, and other ritual paraphernalia are usually brought by the patient, or his or her family, to the consultation to offer to the superhuman powers that will assist in the cure. Nahua shamans in the Sierra Norte de Puebla use corn kernel divination to discover the identities of saints who will help the patient (Huber 1990b:161). The linking of the patient and shaman to higher pow-ers is almost a reflexive act in these cultures, in which the presence of the supernatural is constantly brought to mind though hundreds of small altars in houses, on the roadside, and in public transportation.

The consultation may put extra emphasis on the shaman's communication with higher beings, as with the Cora. Cora shamans will ask their clients for offerings of *pinole* (toasted corn flour and sugar), money, and cotton. Cotton is a significant symbol and tool for the Cora shamans. It is considered sacred because it is made of fine threads that if unwound would reach to heaven (Mellado Campos et al. 1994:80). Cotton links the levels of the hierarchy of living beings and absorbs illness in cleaning ceremonies. In most shamanic rituals, clients provide the necessary materials, because the clients are the supplicants and because the materials are regarded as gifts.

Diagnosis depends on the knowledge of how different illnesses manifest themselves. A shaman acquires such knowledge from study, visions, and experience. Each type of disease manifests itself in a different way. Each culture has developed different diagnostic traditions. For example, the Matlazinca examine the eyes to see if an air has attacked the person. If an air has attacked, the eyes appear "sad," and the patient appears *aventado,* a syndrome including indigestion, nausea, anorexia, and tiredness (Mellado Campos et al. 1994:372). The symptom of an air among the Sierra Ñähñu is a sudden severe pain (Dow 1986a:93). The Papago shaman simply looks at the patient to tell if an illness has been caused by witchcraft. How this is done has not yet been explained to ethnographers (Mellado Campos et al. 1994:609).

Weakness and depression can be interpreted as symptoms of a loss of animating force. The loss of animating force, soul loss, is a serious illness treated by practically all shamans. In many ways, soul loss is the essence of illness. If the animating force cannot be returned, the patient will die. Don Floriberto, a Popoloca shaman informant, puts it as follows:

> An ill person is simply one who has lost part of his soul, which you can imagine is something like an air, and it is up to you [the shaman] to find the spirit animal that has carried it off. In order to do this the shaman runs though the mountain after the four-legged creature, bird, reptile, or insect which he feels is the soul of the patient, to capture it and return it to the patient.

A preliminary cleaning may reveal the nature of the illness. For example, during the consultation a Cora shaman passes cotton over the body of the patient and then places it in a white napkin on the altar. He blows smoke from his pipe on the patient and, waving his eagle feathers, recites the following prayer.

God who is my father, God who is my brother, God who is my mother, that, through your wisdom, we wish to know the origin of this illness. We entreat you to do us this favor and discover that tiny place from which this evil came. You are the one for certain who casts out the spirits of the earth, and we do not know if they have caused this misfortune.

The cotton is then examined to make the diagnosis. If the fiber, for example, has a dirty spot in the center, it means that the sick person is in danger of dying; if the mark is not very big, there is still hope that the sick person will recover.

Nahua shamans in Morelos use a similar technique with an egg. The egg is passed around the body without touching the body and then pressed or touched lightly to the skin in spots, particularly where the patient feels pain. The shaman shakes the egg near his ear to hear any air that may have been taken up from the body of the patient. Air will sound like water inside the egg. Then the egg is broken in a glass half full of water. It is studied, and the nature of the illness is deduced from what is seen. A foamlike appearance indicates a heart problem. Internal wounds may be seen in the yoke. The white of the egg reveals different types of airs that have attacked the patient. "Airs of the dead" appear as lighted candles, long stones, or a dead body lying in the street. "Canyon airs" appear as places in a field, a canyon, or a hillside spring. Another important conclusion that can be drawn is whether the illness is "hot" or "cold" (Álvarez Heydenreich 1987 : 147–151).

Nahua shamans in the east feel the pulse of the patient (pulsing) to determine the illness. They state that the blood of the patient accuses the sorcerer who has caused the illness. Sierra Ñähñu, Totonac, and Huastec shamans often use crystals to diagnose illness. They say the crystals, made of quartz or colored glass, arrive magically and have the power to reveal an illness inside the body. In actuality, the crystals are found in the ground or are gifts of devoted followers. Typically, a crystal is held up to a candle near the patient. Transmitted through the crystal, the lights of the candle reveal the location and nature of the illness. Totonac crystals are kept in a napkin or in a painted gourd on the altar. Before using a crystal, the Totonac shaman passes it through the smoke of the censer, and, after he or she has finished with it, dips it in white rum to "give it a drink" (Ichon 1973 : 267).

The visions of the shaman are always important. There are often times in the diagnostic process when the shaman will retire to receive visions. Shamans speak of certain symbols that they look for in their dreams. For example, the following dream symbols indicate sorcery to a Rarámuri shaman: the victim's hair being burned in a cross, a sick cow reviving, or the person's clothes being washed away by a river (Mellado Campos et al. 1994:715). Airs appear to Sierra Ñähñu shamans as thin pigs, masked dancers, or black cows (Dow 1986a:94). The vision symbols vary from shaman to shaman and from culture to culture.

Treatment

Shamanic diagnosis and treatment go together. The shaman starts treatment as soon as the illness reveals itself. As more is learned, new treatments may be started or prescribed. Treatments are logically related to the way that an illness is conceptualized. Illnesses seldom are simple, so treatment can be complex. The patient and the patient's family provide the materials for the treatment. The shaman tells them what to buy and when the rituals will be held, and the shaman receives a fee for his or her work. Fees among the Sierra Ñähñu are charged according to the value of the cure to the patient (Dow 1986a:41).

REGIONAL VARIATIONS IN TECHNIQUES AND BELIEFS

Throughout central and north Mexico, as in other parts of Mesoamerica, there are innumerable outdoor shrines where native superhuman beings exert their powers. In the east, caves, mountains, and lakes are especially propitious locations for shrines. The Ñähñu and Nahua worship the sun god on mountaintops. Caves are the abodes of the rain, earth, and mountain gods. Lakes and springs can be the home of the goddess of the fresh waters. Ñähñu and Nahua shamans cooperate in their pilgrimages to sacred shrines (Sandstrom 1991:300, personal communication). Traditional shamans and their followers leave offerings at these shrines, and the shaman says prayers. In the mountains of the west there are shrines to tutelary beings such as wolves (Eger Valdez 1996:275). A Papago shaman of the north has said:

> I cannot speak of this goddess because I don't have the permission of my elders. If the elders would permit it I could tell you about her. I can only say that she is a very beautiful girl dressed in blue with long

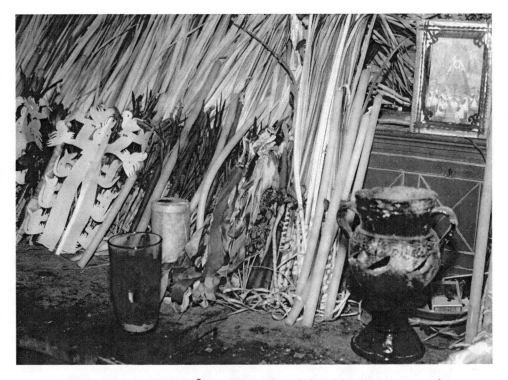

FIGURE 4.2: Altar of a Sierra Ñähñu Shaman. From left to right one can see paper figures representing the animating force of the patient, stacks of flower offerings, ribbons and paper figures covering the shaman's two wands, long candles, an image of a Catholic saint, a chest containing images of the shaman's tutelary beings, and the shaman's censer.

> bead necklaces and that she appears in the cave of La Petaca, where there was a stone found in her likeness. My prayers are songs in the O'otam language and I say them in the mountains. The desert and the hills are my altars. (Mellado Campos et al. 1994:609)

Curing usually takes place in the patient's house or in a special part of the shaman's house devoted to this work. Every place where curing is practiced should have an altar (see Figure 4.2).

Traditional shamans also lead rituals in oratories or special temples that serve a local kinship group, a larger neighborhood, or the entire village. They may also utilize Catholic churches for their rituals. Altars are complex.

As in Christian churches, they are places where superhuman beings are addressed. Images of tutelary beings can be found on the altar of a shaman. Shamanic utensils such as wands, arrows, crystals, paper, tubes, feathers, and so on, are used. Other objects such as stones and eggs may take on a symbolic significance. Tobacco is usually present in some form during a cure. White rum (*aguardiente*) is often used as a purifying agent.

The ritual objects used by shamans vary from culture to culture. More ritual objects are used in the east, west, and central regions than in the north, possibly because central Mexico has always been more technologically sophisticated. In central Mexico there are east-west variations in paraphernalia. In the east, the Totonac, Tepehua, Sierra Ñähñu, Teenek, and Nahua use small humanoid figures to represent animating forces. Crystals are used in diagnosis. The Sierra Ñähñu, northern Nahua, and Tepehua use paper humanoid figures. The Totonac shamans use solid figures. The Sierra Ñähñu still manufacture the bark paper used for some of the figures. In the center region, ritual paraphernalia is not as elaborate. For example, the Purépecha use playing cards for divination.

In the mountains of the west, the Cora and Huichol shamans use votive arrows, eagle feathers, yarn paintings, and cotton in their ceremonies. The Cora make amulets from the bodies of chameleons to ward off the effects of sorcery (Mellado Campos et al. 1994:609). The Huichol ceremonial arrow has a bundle of hawk, eagle, or turkey feathers tied to it. Power objects such as rattles from rattlesnakes or miniature deer snares may also be attached to the feathers (Myerhoff 1974:110).

There are also east–west variations in belief. In the east, there is a greater belief in companion spirit animals. These are believed to help the patient and the shaman. In the west, there is a greater emphasis on prayer to the gods. Animals such as the wolf and the deer act as tutelary beings in the west. The Cora place great emphasis on the relationship between the patient and their gods. The most powerful Huichol curers are their *mara'akáte* (plural of *mara'akáme*), shamans who have shown themselves to be closest to the gods. In the central and north regions, Catholic beliefs are very important.

Loss of Animating Force (Soul Loss)

Restoration of the animating force of a patient depends on how it was lost in the first place. The animating force can be lost by natural accident, or it can be stolen. It is widely believed that a sudden fright (*espanto* or *susto*) can cause animating force loss. In this case, where the desire to live is intimidated, the animating force must be restored as soon as possible. The Teenek believe that such losses are not caused by transgressions, deviations from the path of goodness, but are natural occurrences that are to be expected as an ordinary part of life. Other natural illnesses for the Teenek are wounds, measles, attacks by evil winds, and colds (Alcorn 1984:217).

If the animating force of the patient has been diminished by fright or has been lost without cause, treatment must restore it. It is widely believed that force loss can result in death if not treated. Companion spirit animals of the shaman may be sent out to look for the lost force. Restoration ceremonies comfort and reassure the patient. Cora shamans sit alone with their seriously ill patients chanting for hours in an effort to contact gods "above their heads" and below the earth in an effort to restore the animating force. The shaman enters a trance and is able to journey to Virikuta, the Cora mythic world, to bring back the animating force of the patient (Mellado Campos et al. 1994:80).

If the animating force has been stolen, a confrontation between the thief and the curer is necessary. Stealing an animating force is a dastardly act of sorcery. Sierra Ñähñu shamans send their powerful companion spirit animals to do battle with the companion spirit animals of the sorcerer in order to recapture the animating force of the patient (Dow 1986a:63).

Since the restoration of the animating force of the patient is a fundamental object of shamanic curing, a ritual to restore it is often woven into other larger ritual complexes. For example, the Totonac cure has four phases: cleaning, the reinforcement of the animating force, the washing, and the herbal refreshment (Ichon 1973:251). The Sierra Ñähñu shamans can restore the animating force within any ritual by preparing a white paper figure that represents the animating force surrounded by the patient's companion spirit animals (see Figure 4.3).

The Cleaning Ritual (*Limpia*)

A cleaning ritual (*limpia*) removes an intrusive disease or invisible sorcery. A sucking ritual removes a solid object. Table 4.1 compares the cleaning with the sucking treatment.

The cleaning ritual is without a doubt the most common magical healing

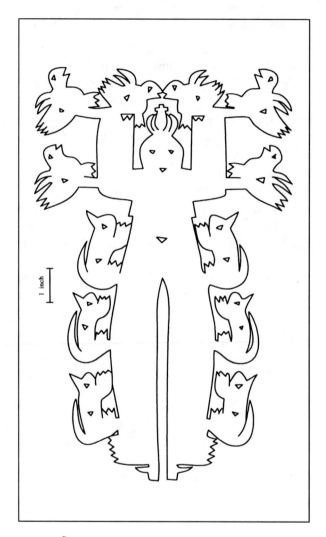

1 inch

FIGURE 4.3: Sierra Ñähñu paper figure representing the animating force of the patient with companion spirit animals.

ritual in Mexico. It is often named in the native languages by words that connote cleaning up, sweeping out, or fixing up. Cleanings are aimed primarily at withdrawing airs, the most common invisible beings that invade the body. The ritual exists in a variety of forms ranging from those based on purely native belief to those based on a great deal of Christian belief. The central act of the cleaning is to pass a ritual object, an attractor, around the body of the patient to attract and absorb the animate illness within. The ritual object varies from culture to culture. In the native eastern escarpment and the Huasteca, it is usually a collection of anthropomorphic figures. In the central region and among the Nahua of the Sierra de Puebla, it is often a chicken egg. In the west, it is usually eagle feathers or votive arrows. Christian forms of the *limpia* found widely in the center region make use of objects blessed by a priest or votive candles that were lit before the image of a saint.

The cleaning ritual is usually part of a more elaborate curing complex that often includes the restoration of the animating force and various other subrituals that depend on the culture and the shaman's particular sense of what is needed. Cleaning rituals can also be part of a diagnosis. The Cora method of observing the cotton used in a cleaning and the Nahua method of observing an egg used in cleaning are examples of how cleaning contributes to diagnosis. Magical treatment is never delayed and can become part of diagnosis.

In the east among the Nahua of the Huasteca, Ñähñu, and Tepehua, paper figures are used in cleanings. The figures are cut to represent the animating forces of airs and the evil godlings that control them. The Sierra Ñähñu perform two levels of cleanings, the small and the large. The small

TABLE 4.1: FEATURES OF CLEANING AND SUCKING TREATMENTS

	Cleaning	Sucking
Goal	To extract illness from the body	To extract illness from the body
Physical nature of illness extracted	Invisible, airlike, air or wind	Visible, solid
Moral quality of illness extracted	Evil	Evil
Animate status of extract	Animate and more powerful than ordinary human, requires shaman to dominate	Inanimate but buried in the body, requires magic to remove
Method of arrival of the extract in patient	Arrives under own volition or led by a more powerful being, can be sent by sorcery	Appears accidentally or can be shot or implanted by sorcery

one is simpler, requires less paraphernalia, and costs less. The large one requires a full layout of figures representing the evil godlings, such as Rainbow, Thunder, the Lord of the Jews, and Santa Catarina. One should note that the figures represent the animating forces of the beings, not the beings themselves, and they give the shaman magical power over them. In the large cleaning, a live black pullet is bundled with the papers. The pullet conveniently dies after the airs have been swept out of the patient into the bundle, lending further credence to the belief that a potentially lethal illness has been withdrawn. The Totonac also use a live chicken in their cleaning. The Totonac attractor is herbs or an altar candle.

The typical practice in the eastern region is to take the bundle of attractors that have swept up the airs far from the house of the patient. It can be thrown into a canyon; airs are believed to live in canyons. It can be hung in the forest on the west side of a mountain so that the sun god will take the airs on his journey to the underworld. It should not be placed anywhere near where people will travel, unless the patient demands vengeance against persons who he or she believes have sent the illness. In that case, after serious consultation with the shaman, the bundle may be placed near the enemy's house.

In the center region, the goal of Matlazinca cleaning is to remove airs, which are typically considered to have a cold temperature. Several types of cleanings are performed. The most common utilizes an egg together with *chile ancho, chilaca,* or both. Another, called the sweeping (*barrida*), makes use of herb and flower branches of perch, *romero,* and *cempoalxuchitl,* or *santamaría* and *ruda.* Similar herbs are sometimes incorporated into the large cleaning of the Sierra Ñähñu (Dow 1986a: 102). Branches symbolize cleaning, since branches of other plants are used daily to sweep the houses and to clean the skin in a sweat bath.

In the western region, Cora therapeutic cleaning makes use of sacred hawk or eagle feathers. Extensive prayers are offered to their gods during the cleaning. The Huichol cleaning ritual is also complex. The diagnostic phase makes use of a mirror around 4 cm in diameter, a wand to which eight eagle feathers are attached, a candle, an arrow, and a crucifix. The mirror is placed on the chest of the patient. The collection of other things is passed over the body of the patient and placed next to the mirror. The shaman then waits for a vision that will reveal the nature of the sickness. If "bewitchment" is revealed, the shaman cleans the patient with his eagle feathers and the arrow. The shaman throws the money and the candle offerings in the sea, and the patient takes the arrow to offer later to the gods who have been responsible for the cure (Mellado Campos et al. 1994:291).

Sucking

Sucking is a shamanic treatment for object intrusion. The object is first manipulated inside the body and brought toward the surface. Then, the shaman puts his or her lips on the skin and sucks the object out. A tube of some sort may also be used for this purpose. In Totonac culture, female shamans use the lips or fist to suck, whereas male shamans use a reed. Only male shamans can use a reed because the reed is associated with the Sun god, a male deity of maximal importance (Ichon 1973:283). Sleight of hand may also be used to produce a visible object, but the belief in the withdrawal of an unseen evil is often enough to produce relief from pain.

The Teenek shaman passes a crystal over the body. The shaman peers through the crystal at the patient's body, illuminated by a candle or pine-stick flame, and sucks the illness out through a reed. In the center region in the Valley of Mexico, Nahua curers combine an egg attractor with suction. The shaman fills his mouth with water and places one end of an egg on top of the patient's head and sucks on the other end. This is repeated on other parts of the body such as the temples, the elbows, the palms of the hands, and anywhere pain is felt. The air passes through the egg into the water in the curer's mouth, which is spit onto the floor after the sucking (Madsen 1955:53). The egg, like the chicken, a living thing, symbolizes the animate food-seeking nature of the air.

Sorcery

In central and north Mexico, a belief in sorcery is practically universal. It represents a breakdown in good social relations; it focuses blame on another member of the community. Envy is a common motivation for sorcery. For example, the Rarámuri believe that envy can drive a person to put an evil object (*mal puesto*) in the path of his or her victim. They believe it will cause the victim to suffer an illness that can lead to death if not treated immediately. They say that the sorcery is like a black moth that flies into the heart of the victim; only a shaman can remove it (Mellado Campos et al. 1994:

714). The Papago believe that the desire to seduce the spouse of another person is a cause of sorcery.

In general, native Mexicans usually believe that a person who suffers and wastes away is a victim of sorcery. In spite of these widely held beliefs, one meets very few sorcerers, if any at all. So who and where are they? Most of them apparently exist only in the minds of their supposed victims and the shamans who treat the victims. Very little has been recorded in the ethnographic literature about actual acts of sorcery. There are two possible reasons for this: (1) that very few real acts of sorcery actually occur and (2) that all such acts are carefully hidden to avoid retaliation. Possibly, aggrieved parties who are not recognized as shamans perform most real acts of sorcery. They may enlist the help of a shaman, but that shaman is likely to be a novice or to be from a different area where he or she is protected from retaliation. The best evidence that real acts of sorcery exist are shamans who admit that they occasionally practice it and material evidence that is found from time to time. For example, one day I was walking behind a Sierra Ñähñu graveyard and came across a group of paper figures that were partially burned and mutilated (see Figure 4.4). The cuttings were not as well executed as those done by the shamans I knew. Although the craftsmanship seemed amateurish, the intent was clear. The airs of the dead were being called on to harm some hapless victim.

The power to heal implies the power to harm, so shamans have professional ethics as doctors do. The issue of vengeance against an attacking neighbor or other human enemy is separate from curing and marked by ethical considerations. It may be practiced if the patient insists on it, but it is not a necessary part of a cure. Most shamans discourage vengeance sorcery. It can lead to blood feuds and much community distress. The communities in which shamans work have precarious economies in which people have little material wealth. They are small, rural, and often overpopulated. People spy on each other. Face-to-face contact over generations leads to friction and envy. People are suspicious of neighbors who are not perfectly helpful; resentments can fester. Neighbors and kinsmen may try to take small bits of land from each other. The work of the shaman is to calm people's anger and to heal psychic distress. Thus, in general, shamans are not eager to involve themselves in disputes by sending disease. They have to work with a widespread belief in sorcery, but only under extraordinary circumstances do they actually seem to practice it.

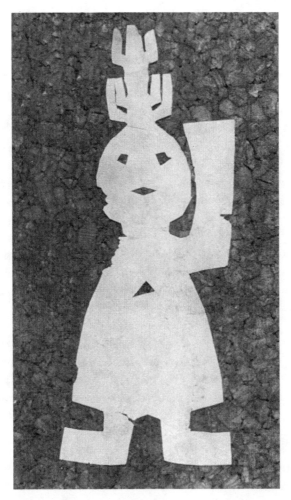

FIGURE 4.4: Mutilated paper figure found beside the graveyard in Tenango de Doria.

Don Floriberto, a Popoloca shaman in the east region, admitted to sorcery but only as a mail order business. He would perform it for distant persons sending him the details in the mail along with a money order (Jäcklein 1974:208). In the Highland Ñähñu village of Xuchitlán in the Mezquital, people believe in sorcery, but there are no practicing shamans or sorcerers anywhere near the village. To find a shaman or sorcerer the residents have to travel hours by bus to the Huasteca (Tranfo 1974:236). There are no shamans in Xuchitlán, either. Where rapid cultural change creates stresses in places like this, people become nervous about the possibility of sorcery, and, as a consequence, curers cannot practice safely for fear of being accused of sorcery. The growth of capitalist modes of production can create stresses that result in sorcery accusations. Isaac (1996) recounts a case where conflicts among Purépecha producers in a growing tourist handicraft industry resulted in accusations of sorcery.

The Sierra Ñähñu treatment for sorcery is to magically bring the sorcery deposit to the shaman, where it is neutralized. The deposit is usually a set of mutilated paper figures causing damage to the animating force of the patient. The retrieval ceremony lasts all night. It may be part of a native flower ritual called the *costumbre*. In the middle of the night, the shaman will send his powerful companion spirit animals out to fly over the land and track down the sorcery. All participants are told to stay inside the shaman's *oratorio*, because evil lurks outside. A knocking is heard at the door. The shaman opens it and reveals a foul-smelling wad of mashed papers. This is brought inside and neutralized by blowing white rum on it.

A very common type of sorcery attack is one in which airs are sent against the victim. In that case, the treatment is a cleaning to get rid of the airs. The Papago have shamans who specialize in the treatment of sorcery. They ask the victim to wear an amulet made from the head of a chameleon and pray to the goddess Quiva (Mellado Campos et al. 1994:609).

Other Shamanic Services

The traditional shaman is a specialist in manipulating the unseen, living animating forces. Many troubling things in the animated world besides illness can be brought to him or her. Sierra Ñähñu and Totonac shamans use their powers to discover thieves. Some Totonac shamans specialize in theft. They attach a cord to an image of San Antonio, who tracks down the thief. The thief can also be made to suffer until he returns the stolen objects. If the shaman burns oil before the image, the thief will die (Ichon 1973:283).

Much of the work of shamans as healers includes the religious counseling of families and individuals. There is a great deal of comforting and ego building in the healing ceremonies. The patient is reassured that all the forces of nature are mobilized to deal with his or her illness. Prayers may be said to the native gods for days on end.

Broken love relationships in the home may be healed by magic. The Sierra Ñähñu believe that shamans can make people love, or lust for, each other by manipulating their animating forces. Clients go to the Sierra Ñähñu shamans with the hope that a wayward spouse can be influenced to return. This is done in a ritual in which paper figures are cut to represent the animating forces of the couple. In the ceremony, the two paper figures are brought together. Love magic that does not reunite a once loving couple is handled carefully because of its potential for causing jealous rages and adultery.

In public religious ceremonies, shamans often act as magico-religious specialists. Traditional shamans in central and north Mexico are the equivalent of native priests. In the west region the most respected Huichol shamans, the *mara'akáte*, study to achieve spiritual enlightenment and are graded in a hierarchy of spiritual attainment. About the east region, Alan Sandstrom (1991:300) writes that nearly twenty-five Nahua and Ñähñu shamans gathered together to organize a pilgrimage to the sacred lake. They cut over twenty-five thousand paper figures in preparation for the journey. This was a major religious event in both cultures.

Shamans usually have a group of followers for whom they lead worship ceremonies. The context of these ceremonies depends on the extent of competition from Christian religions. Ceremonies led by shamans may involve an entire village or just one or two families within it. Where there is little competition, traditional shamans lead large community rituals. Practically always, other persons, not the shamans, sponsor the rituals. The entire community may sponsor the ritual, or a single household may sponsor it. The ritual will bring the sponsor recognition and prestige and provide an opportunity for the conspicuous redistribution of wealth. A traditional shaman as the person with the greatest knowledge of the beings being worshiped will direct the ceremony. For example, Sierra Ñähñu shamans conduct worship ceremonies for local deities called *antiguas* and for their principal gods: the Goddess of the Fresh Water, Grandfather Fire, the Intercessor God, the Earth God, and the Sun Cross. The *antiguas* are represented by small family images. Among the Nahua of the southern Huasteca, for example, shamans lead the major midwinter festival to Tonantsij, the mother goddess, and the blessing of the seeds festival at the end of the dry season (Sandstrom 1991: 279–296). The Huichol *mara'akáme* officiates and teaches traditional Huichol beliefs in the *tuki*, the Huichol community temple (Myerhoff 1974:95).

Competing Christian religions, such as Roman Catholicism and various forms of Evangelical Protestantism, reduce the participation of shamans in public ceremonies. These imported religions have considerable political impact. Roman Catholicism is the religion of the dominant Euro-Mexican culture and enjoys much prestige because of its association with wealth and political power. There is often a native form of Catholicism that introduces Catholic images into a local fiesta system. The extent to which Christian ideas and forms have penetrated native Mexican culture varies widely even in the same cultural region. This penetration has resulted in some interesting combinations of Christian and native religious rituals. For example, in Tenango de Doria, before a Sierra Ñähñu *mayordomo* can dress the image of his saint in the church, he must take the clothes to a mountain stream to be washed in the sacred water of the Goddess of Fresh Water. Shamans appear in public rituals whenever their knowledge of the native gods and the animating forces is needed and whenever the influence of Christian churches is weak.

The Social Status of the Shaman

The participation of women in the shamanic profession varies from culture to culture in central Mexico. There are only a few female shamans among the Huichol. Mellado Campos et al. (1994:279) believe it is a masculine profession there; however, Myerhoff (1974:96) mentions the existence of a female shaman. She notes that the profession is open to women, as it is in practically all native cultures. Since the Huichol have grades of shamanic excellence, it is difficult to say who is a certified shaman and who is not. Apparently the female shamans do not have the same status as the male shamans. Since Huichol shamans have many priestly functions, their culture is consistent with Huber's (1990:170) observation, made for the Nahua, that male shamans tend to function as priests, whereas female shamans only cure and do not officiate at public ceremonies.

Female shamans predominate among the Nahua of the Sierra de Puebla (Huber 1990b:160). Native people sometimes see the male shaman as a stronger warrior against evil; however, female shamans can be the majority of successful practitioners at the same time. Bower (1946:680) writes that female Tepehua midwives are assistants to a male shaman. Don Antonio, a Sierra Ñähñu shaman, expresses a masculine bias by saying that shamanism is hard and dangerous work and that women are sometimes not strong enough (have weaker blood) for the work (Dow 1986a:131). Nevertheless, there are many successful female shamans among the Sierra Ñähñu. Many curers and most midwives, shamans or not, are female in central and north Mexican native cultures.

The core of belief that supports shamanic healing is supported by myth. Each shaman has a personal myth that explains how he or she began to cure and how that power was acquired. This personal myth needs to be conceptually separated from the actual learning process that shamans go though to acquire their skills. Mendelson (1965:217) writes of Mesoamerican shamans: "In actual fact, short of believing in shamanism ourselves, we must agree that all shamans in some way or another do learn from living teachers." The personal myth usually tells of a dramatic trial in which the person almost dies and is forced into recognizing that he or she is destined to be a curer. To turn away from this path that the tutelary beings have set for one would bring their wrath down on the person and probably result in his or her death. The myth is widely told and serves to explain and enhance the shaman's power to cure. For example, Don Soltero, a Nahua traditional shaman, was attacked by rain dwarves. They agreed to release him from a deadly sickness only when he agreed to become a curer (W. Madsen 1955:50).

The myth is developed during a period of initiation in which the novice commits him- or herself to the profession. New Nahua shamans of the Northern Sierra de Puebla enter a quasi-liminal period during which they decide for or against becoming a curer. The *tamatinime*, wise powerful spirits who live in caves and frequent streams, waterfalls, forests, and the ocean, play a part in helping them to decide (Huber 1990b:159). When a Teenek person is stricken by illness, such as insanity or loss of consciousness, a curer may find that he or she must become a curer in order to have his or her spirit put back in order. A chicken is sacrificed and its stomach is examined. If thorns appear, the person is destined to become a sorcerer. If quartz crystals are found, the person is destined to be a curer (Alcorn 1984:241–243). Among the Tepehua, a sickly state and mystical dreams are indications that a person wants to be a shaman (Williams García 1963:142).

The actual learning process starts with participating in curing ceremonies, often in the context of one's family. Many children of shamans become shamans themselves. Later one may become an assistant to a shaman. Alcorn (1984:239) writes of "loose apprenticeship" among the Teenek. The Cora novice shaman accepts the gift of healing from God. Then he learns from another experienced healer or begins to learn on his own (Mellado Campos et al. 1994:69). Finally, the novice starts to cure on his or her own. If successful, his or her reputation grows and he or she is recognized in the community. Some communities have a number of failed and unrecognized shamans who are unable to garner reputations. Such persons need to get out of the business before they are accused of sorcery.

CHAPTER 5

A Comparative Analysis of Southern Mexican and Guatemalan Shamans

Frank J. Lipp

Introduction

In Mexico it is estimated that fifteen to twenty million of the inhabitants utilize traditional medicine and the services of its 180,000 practitioners (Lagarriga 1978a:56; Schendel 1968:144). Although homeopathy, herbalism, hydrotherapy, and other forms of alternative medicine are an integral part of health behavior in Mesoamerican urban centers, traditional medicine, having its syncretic roots in pre-Hispanic and Spanish colonial culture, is more prevalent in the rural hinterlands (Barba de Piña Chan 1980).

In order to arrive at a better understanding of traditional medicine in Mesoamerica, this chapter analyzes and compares the traditional medical practitioners working among the indigenous populations of Oaxaca and the Mayan-speaking region of Mexico and Guatemala. The discussion is subdivided into eight main sections: (1) sociodemographic and economic characteristics, (2) therapeutic specializations, (3) social organization, (4) signs and instruments, (5) recruitment, (6) training and initiation, (7) dreams and spirits, and (8) etiology, diagnosis, and treatment of illnesses.

Since the days of the Spanish Conquest, indigenous *curanderos* or curers have been the target of persecution and ridicule. Since indigenous medicine was closely linked to the native religions, Indian curers were considered to be agents of the devil, and even the use and administration of medicinal plants were legally prosecuted during the colonial period (Aguirre Beltrán 1963; Quezada 1976:57). The banning of hygienic and medicinal procedures such as daily bathing, circumcision, and the native vapor bath, which killed syphilitic spirochetes and other microbes, greatly contributed to the spread of disease and epidemic infections (Krumbach 1977:147; Schendel 1968:87). The opposition to native curers took on a different form when, during the 1930s, the village *curandera* was portrayed in national campaigns as impeding the life-saving work of government health workers and thereby causing needless deaths (Schendel 1968:155; Steinbeck 1941). Until recently, campaigns of harassment against traditional medical practitioners were instituted in many parts of Mexico and Guatemala (Redfield 1941:316). The general attitude of physicians toward folk medicine in Oaxaca today is that of condescending indifference, if not outright contempt. Because they are so frequently regarded as quacks, *curanderos* are highly secretive, and do their best to appear inconspicuous.

There are 6 million Mayan speakers and approximately 1.2 million speakers of indigenous languages living in Oaxaca. In view of these numbers, the ethnographic literature dealing with these groups must be considered sporadic at best. Given the marked intervillage variability and known lacunae in the ethnographic record for many sections of southern Mesoamerica, any general conclusions must be approached with a word of caution. A bloody civil war, expanded government health services, increased education, and Protestant conversion have also left a marked impact on the region. Many of the ethnographic reports upon which this study is based are decades old and only cover three or four villages at best for entire linguistic groups. Hence, many of the facts reported for a particular village will no longer hold true but may still be the case for other undescribed communities within the same language group. In certain instances, however, striking continuities were noted between older and more contemporary descriptions.

Indigenous traditional medical practitioners have been variously described as witch doctors, shamans, or as hybrid shaman-priests, sorcerer-priests, shaman-diviners, priest-healers, doctor-priests, shaman-healers, and priest-shamans. Replacing these terms with new labels would lead to only more semantic confusion and conceptual ambiguity. The terms utilized in this paper have, in general, been those used in the studies cited.

Sociodemographic and Economic Characteristics

The number of traditional medical practitioners working in Mayan and Oaxacan communities is highly variable and is dependent upon population size, culture change, and other factors. The ratio of curers to total population ranges from 1 to 27 in some Zinacantan hamlets to 1 curer for 300 individuals in a Cakchiquel community (Fabrega and Silver 1973:30; Tenzel 1970:373). Available sources yield a median ratio of 1 curer for every 47 inhabitants, although a ratio of 1 to 282 is reported for the highland Maya of Chiapas (Freyermuth Enciso 1993:89). Some communities may have no curing specialist, such as the Lacandón, where the function of curer is part of the social role of the male head of the household (Freyermuth Enciso 1993:70; Mellado Campos et al. 1994:333). The drastic reduction of the number of curers in Tzeltal Tenejapa—1 to 25 to 1 to 98—during a twenty-year period is perhaps better explained by religious conversion and modernization, rather than sampling error (Fabrega and Silver 1973:29; Freyermuth Enciso 1993:89).

The ages of curers range from 13 to 85 years of age, with a median age of 55 years. Although Mazatec and Tzotzil curers are reported to begin their careers as young as 13, most begin working after 30 years of age (Favre 1973:251; Gillin 1948:397; Holland 1963:176, 204; Johnson 1939a:132; Mellado Campos et al. 1994:86, 300, 488; Valladares 1957:220; Vogt 1970: 1151; Wagley 1949:68). In a survey of curers in twelve highland Mayan communities in Chiapas, 4 percent were under 20, 29 percent were 20 to 39, 33 percent were 40 to 59, and 33 percent were 60 and over (Freyermuth Enciso 1993:133).

In terms of gender, Oaxacan curers are described as being mostly females, including the Zapotec, Mixtec (55 percent), Chocho (80 percent), Chontal, Ixcatec (75 percent), Mazatec (60 percent), Mixe (70 percent), and Zoque (70 percent) (De la Fuente 1949:321; Mellado Campos et al. 1994: 160, 197, 300, 471, 488, 502, 913; Romney and Romney 1966:77). Freyermuth Enciso (1993:133) reported the percentage of female highland Chiapan curers to be 64 percent, which is much higher than previously reported estimates (Fabrega and Silver 1973:30; Vogt 1969b:416, 1970:1151). This discrepancy is undoubtedly due to the primary concern of the Harvard Chiapas Project with shamanistic curing rituals and public ceremonies, in which female curers did not participate (Fabrega and Silver 1973:30; Vogt

1966:363). Among the Atitlán Tz'utujil, Quetzaltenango K'iche', and other highland Maya groups, male curers outnumber female curers, with approximately 37 percent being women (Bunzel 1952:79; Carlsen and Prechtel 1994:91; Oakes 1969:21; Rodríguez Rouanet 1969:71). In Yucatan, the number of female curers was found to be more balanced, with 52 percent of the total (Mellado Campos et al. 1994:383).

The majority of Mazatec female curers and midwives are widows or "abandoned" wives (Boege 1988:172). The curing role provides them with a means of income, social status and power, and a sacral aura which disinterests potential suitors (Benítez 1964:50).[1]

Attending to the sick is for most curers (70 to 90 percent) a part-time specialty, which supplements agricultural, household, and artisan labor (Freyermuth Enciso 1993:136; Mellado Campos et al. 1994:142, 263, 488). Practitioners become full-time specialists when their practice thrives and becomes highly successful, at which time working their land may be requested in lieu of a monetary fee (Holland 1963:202; Shaw and Neuenswander 1966:23n).

Although some are described as making considerable sums in curing the sick, the majority of Mesoamerican curers are not in a favored economic position and are little differentiated, in terms of wealth, from their neighbors. Social status, prestige, and consequent authority and influence in the community, rather than monetary remuneration, is commonly considered a more important motive for taking on a curing role (Favre 1973:252; Ruz 1983:180).

Due to fluctuating exchange rates over time, it is difficult to arrive at exact figures for curing fees. Fees may vary according to the reputation and competence of the curer, the severity of the illness, or the patient's ability to pay (Carlsen and Prechtel 1994:91; Lipp 1991:149; Ruz 1983:180). Since they are entrusted to serve the community, some curers do not charge a fee, or it may be voluntary and left up to the discretion of the client (Bunzel 1952:78; Rodríguez Rouanet 1969:61, 67–68; Tedlock 1992a:71). Mixe curers are forbidden by the deities to demand high fees; their curing power would be taken away and they would suffer a misfortune if they did so (Lipp 1991:149). If a seriously ill patient is cured, some families will wish to give a substantial sum or cattle to the curer. Not all curers, however, will accept such aggrandized payments.

Fees for curing *susto* and other culture-bound illnesses are modest or

consist of food, liquor, or labor services (Bunzel 1952:299; Cheney 1979:
88; Hermitte 1970:65; Holland 1963:171, 185; La Farge and Byers 1931:
150; Mak 1959:141; Oakes 1969:92; Thompson 1930:68). At times, small
gifts of eggs, maize, or beans may be presented to the curer at each curing
session. Complex curing rituals, which require a substantial fee as well as the
purchase of fowl, large amounts of candles, incense, and other ritual paraphernalia, are a considerable financial burden on the villagers (Gillin 1948:
389). Curers also receive high fees for community-wide rituals during epidemics or intervillage land disputes (Lipp 1991:149; Ruz 1983:181). If fowl
are sacrificed, the curer normally gets a goodly portion of the cooked meat
(Lipp 1991:149; Villa Rojas 1945:74).

Therapeutic Specializations

Medical specialists such as midwives, diviners, bonesetters, massagers, individuals treating snakebites, as well as general practitioners, or *curanderos*, are
present in practically all Mesoamerican communities. Many native healers,
however, practice a combination of two or three specialties (De la Fuente
1949:321; Freyermuth Enciso 1993:70; Tedlock 1992a:57, 74; Wisdom
1940:343). Some bonesetters attend other physical illnesses, such as tooth-
aches, intestinal worms, diarrhea, and "female disorders," while other bonesetters can perform a full range of shamanic curing and ritual procedures
(Fabrega and Silver 1973:41; Rodríguez Rouanet 1969:64). Similarly, midwives frequently have a specialized knowledge of medicinal plants, with
which they treat rheumatism, snake bites, vomiting, female disorders, and
other emotional and physical ailments (Mellado Campos et al. 1994:87,
107, 214; Rodríguez Rouanet 1969:57; Romney and Romney 1966:77;
Wisdom 1940:354). Some midwives are also diviners or prayer sayers, remove object intrusions by sucking, or are ritual calendar specialists (Oakes
1969:184; Parsons 1931:60). The Huave have midwives, bonesetters, and
three other kinds of traditional curers with overlapping roles. Although
they also treat minor illnesses, the most common type are primarily diag-
nosticians of illness (*neandüy*). On the basis of a diagnostic interview and
examination, the *neandüy* directs the patient to a specialist or, in difficult
cases, to another diagnostician to verify the initial finding[2] (Signorini 1979:
221–222). Although they neither examine the sick nor prescribe treatment,
the most prestigious category of specialists are the incensors (*neasomüy*). In-

censors specialize in treating grave emotional illnesses caused by shame, anger, fright, despondency, or the dead by means of confession, prayer, and ritual offerings (Cheney 1979:66–68). Another kind of curer (*neashaing*) specializes in treating illnesses due to injured, lost, or captured guardian spirits by means of a shamanic trance journey acted out with dramatic gestures and postures (Signorini 1979:253–254).

Social Organization

Although Chinantec and Mazatec curers form part of the council of elders, Oaxacan curers are not organized in any formal corporate group (Barabas 1973:8; Boege 1988:168). Rather, competition, professional jealousy, and a tendency to deprecate the abilities of fellow healers mark their relationships (Boege 1988:176; Lipp 1991:149; Parsons 1931:60; Signorini 1979:221). During an epidemic or other crisis, village shaman-curers may convene in order to put together the most effective countermeasures possible. At times, elderly curers of the Loxicha Zapotec region will meet to discuss important matters and resolve difficult problems (Ravicz 1960:84).

Oaxacan village curers are informally ranked in terms of their competency and the range of illnesses they can treat. As in Yucatan, more prestige is accorded to male curers who are able to divine unresolved issues, family problems, and carry out complex rituals pertaining to illness, life crises, and subsistence activities, as opposed to female practitioners involved solely with curing physically and culturally bound syndromes, such as fright illness (Redfield 1941:314–315).

In Tzotzil Larraínzar there is an informal tripartite hierarchy of prestige, whereby curers of flesh and bone with little ritual knowledge are accorded less status than those who cure spiritual illnesses by means of complex rituals (Holland 1963:173–175). Although this situation may now be reversed, as in Chimaltenango, Coloteca Mam *chimanes* who cure illnesses primarily due to transgressions and sin by exclusively ritual means also have greater prestige than curers (*k'anal*) utilizing medicinal plants and patent drugs (Valladares 1957:217–218). Similarly, Pinola Tzeltal and Tojolabal curers of external diseases with medicinal plants are accorded less prestige than diviners of internal, spiritual illnesses (Hermitte 1970:149; Ruz 1983: 179). In Quetzaltenango minor ailments are also treated with medicinal plants, whereas acute, dangerous illnesses, which are due to moral trans-gression, must be drawn from the soul by confession and ritual offerings (Bunzel 1952:150). The Chorti' extend this distinction to accord greater prestige to all diviners and curers who possess spiritual power, unlike mid-wives, massagers, and herbalists, who lack this power (Wisdom 1940:343).

In Tzotzil Zinacantan all shamans (*H?iloletik*) are in strict rank order on the lineage, waterhole group, hamlet, and community level, depending upon the time of service (Vogt 1966:362, 1969b:418–420). A small group of se-nior *H?iloletik* exercise authority over the rest, and plan and supervise ham-let ceremonies (Fabrega and Silver 1973:36). The most senior *h'ilol* directs the ceremonies, levies public funds, and assigns groups of shamans to visit various shrines. Since his position is permanent, it is analogous to the Ixil *b'o•q'ol b'a•lwaҫti•sh*, Q'anjob'al *aqom be kalap*, K'iche' *aj cum*, and the Mam *chmaan tnam*. These are the one or two principal priest-shamans of the community, whose functions include the training and initiation of novice shaman-priests, the selection by divinatory means of village officials, setting the dates for and directing important community rituals, and serving as ritual consultants to senior cargo officials (La Farge 1947:134; Oakes 1969: 56; Wagley 1957:217; Watanabe 1992:107). As the most powerful shaman-diviner in the community, the *aj cum* once possessed absolute power over the other shaman-priests (Sapper 1924:395). Previously inherited from fa-ther to son, the position of municipal shaman-diviner is received today through nomination by senior officials (Valladares 1957:212).

A similar hierarchical organization of priest-shamans on the lineage, ward, canton, and community level occurs in K'iche' Momostenango (Ted-lock 1992a:35). Termed *chuchkajaw*, or mother-father, these calendrical di-viners and ritual specialists are drawn from a large number of day keepers. In Chichicastenango only the *chuchkajaw* may carry out rituals at certain hillside shrines (Tedlock 1992a:84–85).

Among the Chuj, Jakalteko, Q'anjob'al, and other Maya groups, shaman-priests are accorded ranked positions and considerable influence within the religious cargo system and sodalities (Bunzel 1952:324; Carlsen and Prech-tel 1994:86; Siegel 1941:67n; Termer 1930:431; Valladares 1957:209, 214). In Momostenango members of the society of shaman-priests proceed through different grades or levels by which the most intelligent and re-spected enter the select group of elders (Tedlock 1992a:37, 41). In this

K'iche' town, also, the position of mayor in the civil hierarchy is held by a priest-shaman and every other year by a medium "bearer of the table" (Tedlock 1992a: 74).

Signs and Instruments

At birth, some Chinantec, Tojolabal, and Tzotzil infants display peculiar configurations of the cranium, teeth, and umbilical cord or are said to be born with caps, horns, or shoulder bags, foretelling their adult curing role (Barabas 1973:13; Favre 1973:251; Paul and Paul 1975:708; Ruz 1983: 174). These physical signs rapidly disappear after birth, unlike the powerful animal guardian spirits with which Tzotzil and Tojolabal shamans are born (Holland 1963:303; Nash 1970:139; Ruz 1983:175; Vogt 1970:1157).

Insignia of their sacred office are the staffs and black tunics worn by Jakalteko and Tzotzil shamans (La Farge and Byers 1931:143; Vogt 1966: 362). Although the bamboo staffs are usually presented at a formal initiation ceremony, this is not the case with Mixe shamans, some of whom also carry a wooden staff or carry a special shoulder bag (Lipp 1991:150). In K'iche' Momostenango the staff is a shamanic instrument, much like the divining crystal or *sastun* widely used by Yucatecan *h'men* or seers (Hanks 1990:246; Redfield and Redfield 1940:72; Tedlock 1992b:456; Villa Rojas 1945:74, 137). For Mopan Maya curers, receiving a divining crystal from the spirits is the final step of training, preceded by several petitionary ceremonies. In a dream a shaman-spirit wearing jaguar pelts informs the novitiate of the crystal's use (Arvigo 1993:26).

At the end of their training Cakchiquel, Mochó, Mam, and Ixil shaman-priests receive an altar-like table, used for divining, from their mentor, a senior diviner, at a formal ceremony (Betts 1993:56; Carlsen and Prechtel 1994:102; Colby and Colby 1981:67, 142; García-Ruiz 1984:331; Oakes 1969:90; Valladares 1957:214). Similarly, the *ki'ijbal* (day instrument), a sacred bundle containing divinatory seeds and crystals, and identifying K'iche' calendar priests, is transmitted at a formal ceremony (Bunzel 1952: 287; Tedlock 1992a:59). Chorti', Mam, and K'iche' shaman-priests are also said to possess a special divinatory soul or spirit, which manifests as sensations in the calf muscle or blood, enabling them to correctly divine illnesses (Bunzel 1952:148, 290; Oakes 1969:183; Tedlock 1992a:53, 1992b:466; Wagley 1949:72, 1957:214; Wisdom 1940:343).

Recruitment

People become curers as a result of divine election, hereditary transmission, or as a personal quest. These should not be viewed as discrete, separate entities but typically occur concurrently. Upon receiving the power and techniques to cure from a higher spiritual being in a vivid dream, the individual undergoes a lengthy period of self-learning or apprenticeship at the side of an experienced family member or older shaman.

A significant number (19 to 37 percent) of curers learn to heal on their own initiative with no superhuman or familial aid (Freyermuth Enciso 1993:135; Rodríguez Rouanet 1969:73). By inquiring in the community for remedies for certain illnesses, they gradually acquire the knowledge and practice to cure minor ailments, utilizing herbal remedies and ritual cleansings (Heinrich 1994:74). Some curers utilize patent medicines, injections, cauterization, dextrose infusions, and minor surgery, which they learn to use from missionary staff or by working in hospitals or the army. Some of these medical practitioners only utilize Western medicine, while others combine this with prayers and ritual cleansings.

Although 59 to 69 percent of highland Maya curers reported other *curanderas* as family members, and 26 to 33 percent reported being taught by their family, 63 percent acquired the capacity to cure in revelatory dreams (Freyermuth Enciso 1993:134–136; Rodríguez Rouanet 1969:72–73). The number of Yucatecan Maya and Zapotec curers stemming from families of healers is even higher; 98 percent and 88 percent, respectively (Mellado Campos et al. 1994:384, 878). In some cases, however, an individual stemming from a long family line of curers may not be taught by them and only begins to cure at midlife, subsequent to a life crisis.

Divine election occurs within a context of some physical or emotional crisis: economic hardship, a severe, chronic, or life-threatening sickness, or death(s) in the family or vicinity (Arvigo 1993:21; Benítez 1964:46,78; Favre 1973:252; Gillin 1956:132; La Farge and Byers 1931:140; Munn 1973:102; Oakes 1969:152; Tenzel 1970:373). In a vivid dream, the individual is informed by a spirit being—saint, angel, Keeper of the Game, Sun and Moon, ancestral curer—that she or he will receive the divine gift to cure illnesses (Betts 1993:51, 53; Mak 1959:140). Although the person may resist the calling, refusal results in worsening sickness or death (Gillin 1948: 397; Lincoln 1942:121; Siegel 1941:70; Wagley 1949:73, 1957:215–217).

In Zinacantan the individual's soul is summoned, in a dream, before the council of ancestral deities inside a sacred mountain. In a series of three dreams, the acolyte is instructed in how to carry out curing ceremonies and is shown a number of patients, who he must successfully diagnose and cure (Holland 1963:172; Vogt 1966:361–362, 1969b:416–418).

During the initiatory dream vision the individual may experience temporary insanity or unconsciousness, and a death experience whereupon he or she is reborn as a person with shamanic power and knowledge (Boege 1988:174–175, 180; Mak 1959:140; Mellado Campos et al. 1994:815; Sharon 1976:76). In Tzotzil Chamula, the ability to cure illnesses of increasing severity is dependent upon the number of times the shaman has lost consciousness in a trance (Pozas 1959:194).

Invariably, the illness disappears when the individual begins initiatory training or curing (Oakes 1969:91; Paul 1976:79; Rodríguez Rouanet 1969: 57, 67; Tedlock 1992a:54; Wagley 1957:215). Among the Jakalteko, Mam, and other Maya groups, a diviner informs the sick person that the illness or even death of a family member is a sign that he or she should become a curer (Bunzel 1952:322–323; La Farge and Byers 1931:141; Tedlock 1992a:49; Valladares 1957:214, 220; Wagley 1949:75).

Initially, the fledgling curer heals a sick family member, then neighbors, friends, and ritual kin. At first only able to cure a few minor illnesses, with spiritual help and practice, the curer is able to deal with more severe illnesses (Fabrega and Silver 1973:33; Holland 1963:180). People start to call on the healer to ameliorate the sick, and as cures progress, so does the curer's reputation.

Training and Initiation

The nature of nonfamilial apprenticeship and formal initiation is related to the presence or absence of a lineage-based social organization and a concomitant community-wide hierarchy of shamans. The various ethnic groups in Oaxaca and several Maya-speaking groups follow a bilateral and generational kinship pattern and lack an ancestor-based vertical arrangement (Elliott 1977:261; Merrifield 1981; Romney 1967:224–228). Among these groups formal recognition and initiation by a lineage-based priest-shaman, as found in the highland Mayan area, is not required.

The length of apprenticeship depends upon the amount of knowledge the pupil wishes to acquire and may last for years (Follér 1996:2; Wagley 1957:207). Although the individual may have been taught as a child by his or her grandfather or another relative, and later on by the deities and spirits in a series of dreams, many shamans will seek further short-term apprenticeships with different master shamans in order to develop further skills and specialized knowledge. In addition to establishing ritual kin relationships, paying for training or exchanging ritual information, the instructor will have the pupil at his beck and call, collecting and chopping firewood, cleaning the yard, and doing sundry other onerous chores (Arvigo 1993:22).

Under the tutelage of his or her teacher, the aspiring Mazatec shaman repeatedly ingests morning glory (*Ipomoea violacea*) seeds or *Psilocybe spp.* mushrooms in increasing dosages. In a vision the neophyte is transported to the Cave of the East at the end of the world, where the Principal Beings, deceased curers and relatives, teach him or her how to cure with plants and rituals (Villa Rojas 1955:118). A similar process is present in the Chatino-speaking region, except that here there is no teacher-guide. Having an incurable illness, the individual ingests the vision-inducing mushrooms, which inform him or her how to cure the illness. Later, he or she cures a sick family member and then learns how to cure other illnesses using the same procedure (Bartolomé and Barabas 1996:133). Some Mixe curers also receive a call from Earth under the influence of *Psilocybe* mushrooms to become shamans by undertaking a vision quest on a mountain (Lipp 1991:150–151).

Among the Mopan Maya, the pupil takes a series of nine herbal baths before his or her teacher performs an initiation ceremony, petitioning the nine Mayan spirits to accept the individual as an apprentice (Arvigo 1993:23–24). In Q'eqchi' San Antonio, the instructor teaches the initiate the prayers and procedures for curing in an isolated area away from the village. At the end of the training period, a boa appears to the acolyte, who is in an altered state of awareness, and puts its tongue in the initiate's mouth, or licks and swallows him, imparting occult knowledge (Thompson 1930:68). A similar initiation is believed to occur among Nebaj Ixil and Chinantec shamans, who are said to understand the language of serpents and receive the knowledge and power to cure from them (Basauri 1940:560–561; Thompson 1941:104). Formal initiation among the snake bite healers of Popoluca Sayula consists of a revelatory dream and ritual. In the initiatory test, several serpents are set to twine about the initiate's body to ascertain whether he is able to surmount his fear (Guiteras Holmes 1970:120; Módena 1990:167).

Apprenticeship and formal initiation follow a different pattern among societies with lineage-based land ownership and formal and informal hierarchies of shaman-curers. In Zinacantan the aspiring shaman informs his senior hamlet *h'ilol* of his premonitory dream and then asks a senior shaman to perform a ritual circuit of sacred localities with him. Or, to avoid service in unrewarding public ceremonies, the *h'ilol* practices surreptitiously until he is reported to the authorities, whereupon he is forced to publicly declare his status by partaking in community-wide ceremonies (Fabrega and Silver 1973:33–34).

In Momostenango aspiring novices are evaluated by other priest-shamans on the basis of auspicious birth dates, culture-specific initiatory illnesses, and dream experiences. Interlaced with training in the use of the sacred calendar and divinatory bundle, the novice carries out with his teacher nine consecutive ceremonies, forty and twenty days apart. Determined by the 260-day calendar, these rituals, consisting largely of offerings of prayers, candles, and incense at lineage shrines and other sacred localities, serve to present the novice to the deities and to petition for his acceptability (Tedlock 1992a:66). At the more important last and fifth, or midpoint, rituals, the pupil, teacher, assistants, and their wives, as well as their parents, all interact as married couples (Bunzel 1952:332–334). The ninth ceremony, a complex, public initiation and presentation, may last for several days, involving a series of feasts and meals interspersed by offerings of prayers, candles, incense, and fowl at hillside altars. To publicly announce the novice's debut to the community, a feast, accompanied by a marimba band and fireworks, is attended by a large number of neighbors and friends (Bunzel 1952:332; Valladares 1957:221). Prior to their arrival, the novice and his wife formally receive their divining bundle and altar cross. Subsequent to the formal initiation ceremony, the new priest-shaman carries out a series of ceremonies at mountain shrines and receives further instruction in calendrical divination and the performance of rituals (Bunzel 1952:34; Schultze-Jena 1933:175–179). The shaman-priest may then seek further training and initiation in midwifery, bonesetting, and other specialties, under the tutelage of the appropriate peer group (Tedlock 1992a:71–74). Nebaj Ixil day keepers receive instruction in the use of the sacred calendar and bundle primarily in dreams and by participating in ceremonies (Colby and Colby 1981:63).

At their initiation ceremony K'iche' "bearers of the table" (*aj'mes*) receive the spirits which will be summoned in future séances (Earle 1984: 399; Valladares 1957:221). Similarly, Mazatec novitiates receive an altar-like table with which they conduct divinations and "masses," the sacred objects on the table representing powers interceding for or against the client (Johnson 1939a:132; Munn 1973:104).

In order to commence curing, the Mochó novitiate must be recognized by a veteran curer. Following a ritual sacrifice on a mountain, the shaman brings a wooden cross to the house of the novitiate to be installed as his personal defense. Upon receiving the cross, the novitiate may begin to work as a "defender" of the community (García-Ruiz 1984:338).

Dreams and Spirits

The interaction of the shaman with helping spirits in dreams is continuous throughout his or her curing career. In a series of dreams the curer is taught the culturally specific modalities of diagnosis and healing (Gillin 1948:397, 1956:134; Hermitte 1970:68–74; Holland 1963:172–173; Paul 1976:80; Tedlock 1992b:456). After praying for the sick client, the curer goes to sleep under his or her altar to contact the spirit world, or prays to the spirits for a revelatory dream, which appears the following night (Arvigo 1993:24; Münch Galindo 1984:440–441). Dream visions may occur unsolicited; or, in cases of recalcitrant or poorly understood illnesses, the curer prays to his or her helping spirits, who then, in dream form, reveal the nature and etiology of the illness and the means to cure it (Paul and Paul 1975:712; Rodríguez Rouanet 1969:69).

Although there is tremendous variability in shamanic dream narratives of visitations to deities' houses, journeys with spirit helpers to chthonic and celestial realms, and mortal combat with monsters and sorcerers, accounts of shaman visitations, journeys, and combat are patterned in Mesoamerica (Grambo 1973:425; Lincoln 1935:326).

Some Mixe curers have a continuous and intimate relationship with one or more helping spirits. Considered as the curer's defender or "attorney," the tutelary spirit may take the form of a woman, young girl, or snake. In the guise of the wind or a girl-child, the tutelary spirit appears during the curer's diagnosis to inform him or her whether the individual will live and how to cure the patient (Lipp 1991:171). If no spirit appears spontaneously in a dream or vision, she may be secured by means of an initiatory, nocturnal ceremony. Wearing white clothing, the petitionary prays and offers fowl at an altar table constructed on a mountaintop.

Over time, the shaman-curer obtains additional secondary guardian spirits, which are under the control of the main helper spirit (Gillin 1956: 135; Lipp 1991: 150). The tutelary and secondary helper spirits accompany the shaman in dream journeys to various realms and in combating spirits sent by sorcerers. In cases of serious illness, Zapotec, Mixe, and Tzotzil shaman-curers descend into the underworld or upper world to rescue souls or replace their faltering or damaged soul-candles (Eber 1995: 153; Gossen 1975: 450, 455; Laughlin 1988: 91; Lipp 1991: 152; Radin 1945: 93–94).

Lucid and regular dream states of increasing intensity are developed by fasting, social isolation, and by cultivating the intention for lucidity. Lucid dreams are typically triggered by thunder and lightning, and a degree of control is maintained over them by prayer and a special oration. The dream's subjective power, felt meaning, and portent is enhanced by the increased sensory clarity, sense of body presence, vividness, and exhilaration exhibited by lucid dreams (Varela 1997: 104). Lucid dreams are referred to by Mixe shamans as "clear vision" and "illumination," which have a close metaphorical semblance to Momostecan notions of "clear light" and "white light" (Tedlock 1983: 117, 1992b: 470).

Some Mesoamerican shamans are endowed with extremely rich, imaginal creativity. As a parallel reality, experiences in the realm of the spirit world are woven seamlessly into the discourse of everyday life (Guiteras Holmes 1961: 297; Hermitte 1970: 131; Lipp 1991: 153; Ruz 1983: 171).

Some Oaxacan shamans ingest a psychotropic plant in order to communicate with Earth and the owners of nature for diagnosing and ascertaining an adequate cure (Bartolomé and Barabas 1996: 133; Cortés 1976: 351; Ravicz 1960: 84; Rubel and Gettelfinger-Krejci 1976: 238).

In terms of the hierarchy of resort, the sick in Mam society initially consult female herbal curers (*xhbo'ol*). If the person is not healed, the family then consults a calendrical diviner (*aj qi'i*), and as the last resort a "bearer of the table" (*aj'mes*) (Watanabe 1992: 190). These shaman-diviners disclose the etiology of illnesses, extract confessions, interpret dreams, and prescribe healing procedures and medicines during nocturnal seances, in which Maximón, the Sacred World, or an ancestral shade possesses and speaks through the shaman's body (Oakes 1969: 111–113, 147, 203; Saler 1962: 107). Maya "bearers of the table" exhibit a variety of possession experiences, including total memory loss and lucid and simultaneous dual personality possession, where the subject may or may not be controlled by a possessing agent but retains memory of consciousness and encounters the other entity in the same dreamlike dimension (Earle 1984:399; Peck and Peck 1966:176). In possessing the greatest prestige and highest office, and being closely associated with sorcery, K'iche' and Mam *aj'mes* are analogous to the Tzotzil "talking saints" (*me'santo*) (Fabrega and Silver 1973:35, 43; Holland 1963: 199; Tedlock 1992a:74, 111).

Etiology, Diagnosis, and Treatment

In Mesoamerican traditional medicine, illnesses are signs of natural disequilibrium or disorder, and therapeutic treatment is fundamentally concerned with restoring harmonious relations between internal bodily processes and the physical, social, and cosmological order (Adams 1952:20; Colby and Colby 1981:50; Freyermuth Enciso 1993:74; Holland and Tharp 1964: 44–45; Hurtado 1973:16–17; Mellado Campos et al. 1994:106; Nash 1970:137; Ruz 1973:167; Vogt 1976:88).[3]

Illnesses may be caused by imbalances in somatic harmony brought on by disturbed emotional states (i.e., fear, anger, envy, intense desires), excessive amounts of certain foods, overwork, and sudden shifts in body temperature (Campos 1983:211; Mellado Campos et al. 1994:93, 206, 225, 267, 403; Méndez Domínguez 1983:272; Redfield and Villa Rojas 1934:161). Drinking or bathing in cold water in an overheated condition, drinking hot coffee in the cold air, going out into the cold air when one is warm, or eating cold food when the body is hot weakens the body or results in cramps, stomachaches, and other illnesses (Adams 1952:18, 25; Mellado Campos et al. 1994:92, 207; Méndez Domínguez 1983:276–277; Nash 1967:139). Rheumatism is gradually brought on by continuously working in cold, wet conditions (Mellado Campos et al. 1994:100). Rather than being solely expressions of a symbolic hot-cold complex, these preventive rules serve as empirical adaptations to certain climatic conditions (McCullough 1973).

Infants which have weak resistance may become ill as a result of contact with persons with strong blood, emotions, or desires (Adams 1952:33; Simeon 1973:437; Wisdom 1940:310). Emotional upsets such as anger in infants may result in stomachaches, diarrhea, and fever (Mellado Campos et al. 1994:153, 274, 323; Romney and Romney 1966:77). Eating in a state of anger or fear results in a swollen stomach and diarrhea (Lipp 1988:436). In the aforementioned examples, illness is always a result of a temporal imbalance of internal and external conditions (Adams 1952:17).

In adults, anger and aggression make the body susceptible to illnesses sent by the deities. Postpartum tranquility disturbed by quarreling sickens the infant and weakens the mother (Hurtado 1973:18; Lipp 1992:21). Illnesses brought about by social conflict in the community or family are cured by ritual means (Boege 1988:207; Lipp 1991:175; Nash 1967:140; Vogt 1966:365).

Sudden stress caused by thunder, a poisonous snake, falling into a river, or some other emotional shock debilitates the body or dislocates one of the free souls, which is then captured by a malign spirit (Klein 1978; Lipp 1988; Rubel, O'Nell, and Collado 1985; Tousignant 1979). Folk illnesses caused by sudden fright, evil winds, and the evil eye are generally treated by "cleansing" the body by rubbing or passing an egg, aromatic plants, or a fowl over it; blowing breath on or spraying the body with liquids and incensing with strong fumes (Campos 1983:214; Gillin 1950, 1951:112; Hermitte 1970:101; Mellado Campos et al. 1994:92, 96, 101, 110, 150, 200, 205, 207, 476; Redfield and Villa Rojas 1934:173; Wisdom 1940:347–350, 1952:133). Colds, headaches, skin and pulmonary infections, diarrhea, and other digestive disorders are treated with combinations of medicinal plants in the form of teas, baths, and poultices, accompanied by dietary restrictions (Browner 1985; Comerford 1996; Girard 1947; Lipp 1996:113; Rätsch 1994:46–52; Steggerda 1943). The use of medicinal plants by curers is always accompanied by prayers which invest them with therapeutic efficacy (Arvigo 1993:24; Fabrega and Silver 1973:211; Mellen 1967:109; Metzger and Williams 1972:400).

When a family member becomes ill, household remedies are initially used, particularly if the illness is relatively benign. These include the use of patent medicines, medicinal plants, fright-illness rituals, massage, and sweat baths (Bunzel 1952:144–145; Fabrega and Silver 1973:144; León 1911:215). If no relief is obtained from regular therapy, the illness is considered serious and recourse is made to a shaman-curer (Hermitte 1970:112; Metzger and Williams 1972:405; Villa Rojas 1945:137). The illness is then treated as the result of an imbalance between the individual and superhuman entities resulting from sorcery, soul loss, or moral transgressions, such as aggression and violation of family or ritual obligations (Bunzel 1952:78,

146, 291; Fabrega and Silver 1973:92, 231–232; Favre 1973:253; Hermitte 1970:64, 66, 163; Holland 1963:121–123; Redfield 1941:329; Redfield and Villa Rojas 1934:177).

The diagnosis of illness is carried out primarily by maize divination and taking the pulse (Bunzel 1952:286–292; Fabrega and Silver 1973:151–152; Holland 1963:191; Hermitte 1970:113; Metzger and Williams 1972:399; Nash 1970:147; Vogt 1976:62). Pulse indications are based upon binomial discriminations of hot/cold, rapid/slow, strong/weak, and regular/erratic, with eighteen kinds of pulses known to some curers (Arvigo 1993:18; Favre 1973:252; Lipp 1991:166). Mazatec and Poqomchi' shaman-curers enter an alternate state of consciousness before divining (Johnson 1939b:143; Sapper and Narciso 1904:411).

Central to Mesoamerican ritual curing is the concept of the innate and animal companion soul. During dreams the soul ventures dangerously from the body; extreme fright may dislodge the soul. The soul may be stolen by angels or ancestral spirits. The animal companion soul may be imprisoned, injured, or abandoned by the deities, or the individual's personal guardian spirit may be devoured by the animal companion soul of a witch (Alcorn 1984:225; Fabrega and Silver 1973:149, 231; Hermitte 1970:4, 51–52, 55, 74–76, 98, 105; Holland 1963:143, 165; Holland and Tharp 1964:44; Hurtado 1973:19; Schwartz 1974:18; Vogt 1969b:372, 1976:18–19; Wasson et al. 1974:71, 73).

The curing rite is related to the regulation of human conduct and the process of social control (Fabrega and Silver 1973:373; Hermitte 1970: 142–143; Vogt 1969b:373, 1976:19). Sorcery-induced illness is viewed and treated as the effect of direct or mediated punishment for social conduct not in accord with community norms, such as refusing to share wealth or not fulfilling promises made (Hermitte 1970:64, 66). The state of the body is identified with the fundamental principles on which the social life of the group is based (Boege 1988:168; Nash 1967:139). In Chichicastenango, if the sick person does not improve despite medical treatment, family members publicly confess and forgive their mutual wrongdoings at a meeting (Bunzel 1952:292, 325).

The family and relatives, as well as the shaman and patient, are actively involved in curing ceremonies, consisting of a complex assemblage of prayers, sacrificial offerings, pilgrimages to mountain shrines, and ritual meals (Bunzel 1952:299–320, 347–365; Fabrega and Silver 1973:166–196, 256–

269; Hanks 1984, 1993; Lipp 1991:171–180; Köhler 1977; Vogt 1969b: 421–446, 1976:61–96). Nonorganic, belief-inspired healing practices are usually regarded as irrational by outsiders, but often contribute to recovery by helping to unconsciously mobilize the inherent mechanisms for spontaneous healing. The effectiveness of spiritual healing lies in the expectant faith and positive confidence of the patient in the curer and his or her treatment—the powers of suggestion, empathy, and charismatic personality of the healer, and the dynamic rapport of the doctor-patient relationship (Benson 1996:32; Frank 1979:250–252; Holland and Tharp 1964:50–51).

Discussion

To what extent, if any, are Mesoamerican native curers related to Asian shamans, with their emotionally charged, dramatic performances and elaborate use of voice, dialogue, and body pantomime (Atkinson 1989; Laderman 1991)? Although this question has been addressed before, it requires a more exact and extended treatment (Köhler 1990; Madsen 1955; Tedlock 1992a: 48–52). Because attempts to define shamanism—a study in itself—yielded the categories of "true," "derivative," and "impure" shamans, some writers, under the sway of anti-essentialism, have called for the deconstruction of the category "shaman" as a subject of inquiry (Holmberg 1993:174; Rouse 1978; Thomas and Humphrey 1994:2–6; Voigt 1984:16). Indeed, when the term is generalized, it collapses a diversity of ritual roles into one category. For analytic utility in cross-cultural comparisons of continuities and differences, terms must have definitive and precise properties associated with them. Although definitions are necessary for rational discussion, problems arise when these definitions are then applied wholesale to the complex diversity of specific historical and cultural phenomena. Definitions cease to be legitimate when the definer forgets that people existed before and independent of any schemes.

Mircea Eliade (1974:5) regarded shamans as masters of the technique of ecstasy and explained the latter concept in emic, experiential terms as a journey of the soul to the spirit world. "Ecstasy," however, is a rather diffuse concept, used to describe a wide range of extraordinary experiences among poets, early Greek and Coptic seers, and Pentecostal and medieval Christian monks (Laski 1961; MacDermot 1971). The terms "trance," "ecstasy," and "altered state of consciousness," present in all definitions of shamanism, pose a problem since they are often vague and used indiscriminately. The psychiatric definition of "trance," for example, as a mental state in which a person is not reflectively conscious of mental contents or salient features of the environment is one incongruous with the word's usage in much of the ethnographic literature. Alfred Schutz (1962:232, 343) even suggests that we experience multiple states of consciousness each day, each with its own "specific accent of reality," incompatible with other finite provinces of meaning.

Bourguignon (1989:141) and others differentiate the native theory of the physical presence of an alien spirit in a human body (possession trance) from a residual category, referred to as "visionary trance," which encompasses the shamanic state of awareness. A variety of levels and intermediate states of consciousness occur in possession trance even within a single culture, and amnesia, part of the ideology of possession practitioners, may not be present (Cardeña 1990; Frigerio 1989; Leacock and Leacock 1975:208; Mischel and Mischel 1958:253). Along with the presence of different kinds of shamans, a number of cultures evidence the coexistence of soul journeys, possession, and other trance states in the same culture and individuals even during a single séance (Heinze 1988:22; Hughes 1991:181; Kloos 1968; Krippner 1989:384; Laderman 1991:88–89; Lewis 1981:31; Nishimura 1987:s59–s60; Peters 1982:25–26; Shi 1996:7; Vitebsky 1995:25).

Shirokogoroff (1935:269) claims that shamans control and possess mastery of spirits and can induce spirits into their body and expel them at will. However, the shaman's mastery over the spirits is never a secure attainment. Among the Chukchi and other groups, slight disobedience of the helping-spirits is severely punished and the insatiable spirits may overpower the shaman, dominate his actions against his will, or drain him of strength (Durrenberger 1975:9; Findeisen 1960:195; Hines 1993:27; Lot-Falck 1970:126). Rather than mastery over spirits, Peters and Price-Williams (1980:399) posit control of the trance as the crucial element in shamanic states of consciousness. In possession trance religions, however, practitioners, much like developing shamans, learn to control their trance states and master the highly specialized behavioral mannerisms of their possessing spirits (Leacock and Leacock 1975:173).

Some writers have suggested that the term "shaman" be restricted to religious practitioners of ecstasy in hunting and gathering societies (Shaara and Strathern 1992; Winkelman 1990). The dynamic development of urban shamanism in South America, various types of Chinese shamans operating a stone's throw from Wall Street, Japanese shaman-queens, and Kangly, Kypchak, Naiman, and Uyghur shaman-kings run counter to confining shamans to any socioeconomic formation, however (Chaumeil 1992; Dienes 1981; Goodrich 1951; Pelliot 1913:466; Roux 1959:422). Studying the neurophysiological correlates of physical trance and possession states may alleviate the definitional imprecision, which several workers have attempted to do (Goodman 1989; Winkelman 1986; Wright 1989, 1994). These studies, though, are largely based on electroencephalographic activity, which varies depending upon the experience evoked during the trance (AvRuskin 1988:295). The history of neurophysiology, moreover, is rife with misidentifications of functional specializations of regions of the brain, prior to the advent of positron emission tomography (PET) and similar neuroimaging techniques (Zeki 1993:131–132).

In the sense of the term utilized here, a shaman is a religious practitioner who enters an alternate state of awareness in order to contact the supernatural world with the help of spirits on behalf of his or her community (Harner 1973:xi; Hultkrantz 1973:34; Reinhard 1976:16). More specifically, the tutelary or helper spirit constitutes the active component of the shaman, and without the tutelary spirit, there can be no shaman. For it is the guardian spirit which gives a shaman the ability to cure and helps him or her to directly expel illnesses from the patient's body.

Unlike shamans, who are arrant individualists, priests do not receive their presumptive powers in dreams or visions but through their association with a highly structured religious corporation. Power is vested in the religious office itself and priests are usually in charge of an established calendar of rituals for a particular religion. The priestly nature of K'iche' mother-fathers, for example, can be seen in their notion that the office of *chuchkajaw* belongs to Christ and the ancestors, and is merely held in trust by those who presently exercise it (Bunzel 1952:76). Priests and shamans should not, however, be thought of as mutually exclusive, in that many north Asiatic shamans have priestly functions and perform religious ceremonies for the benefit of the community (Findeisen 1957:200; Schröder 1955:880). Although all shamans are curers, not all Mesoamerican curers are shamans (Campos-Navarro 1997:11). Nevertheless, the relationship between Mesoamerican curers and their guardian spirits over time has never been the subject of sustained, focused ethnographic inquiry, and has too often been subordinate to securing data of a cosmological and ritual nature. The dearth of data on the existence of close, interpersonal relationships between curers and their guardian spirits limits our comprehension of the distribution and extent of shamanic healing in Mesoamerica.

Among the traditional medical practitioners of southern Mesoamerica, shamanic themes or traits are most clearly present in their recruitment, training, and initiation. The shamanic curing séances conducted with community participation in southeast and northern Asia occur only sporadically among the Huave, Mixe, and probably other Mesoamerican groups. Unlike in Asia and South America, the I-thou relationship between the Mesoamerican curer-shaman and his or her helping spirits is a closely guarded, private affair, and not publically proclaimed in the healing situation. Although the retrieval of the patient's soul by means of a visionary journey is, as we have seen, present in southern Mesoamerica, it is, except for Mayan spirit mediums (*aj'mes*), a private, not public, act. Far more prevalent in Mesoamerica is the restitution of the patient's lost or captured soul by ritual, rather than visionary, means.

The functional roles commonly attributed to shamans—healer, priest, seer, sorcerer, political leader, judge, keeper and preserver of myths and tradition—typically coexist in each individual, albeit in unequal proportions, and take on greater or lesser prominence in developmental phases of the individual's career. When Mayan shaman-priests become lineage heads or assume the roles of elected prayer sayers and civil-religious officials, the curing role becomes subordinate to more priestly and secular ones. Tedlock's (1992a) mother-fathers, for example, are diviners having both shamanistic and priestly attributes with no medical roles to speak of, although we know from other sources that the K'iche' *chuchkajawib* do have decided curing functions.

There are Mesoamerican shamans who cure solely by ritual means and lack any particular knowledge of medicinal plants. There are also other shamans who do possess specialized plant knowledge, which they receive in dreams and plant-induced visions. There are, at the same time, Mesoamerican curers primarily utilizing plants who have no intimate communication with the spirit world. Nevertheless, they all incorporate prayers and some ritual in their practice, since the most important, common denominator present in all Mesoamerican healers is a sentiment of fervent religiosity in their vocation.

Notes

1. In Yucatan Redfield (1941:314–315) noted a general shift from male *h-men* to female curers and related this to a breakdown in family life, freeing women of family ties and obliging them to support themselves.
2. Individuals who primarily divine the cause of an illness and then advise the patient as to the best curer to see also occur among the Chorti' and Jakalteko (La Farge and Byers 1931:141; Wisdom 1940:343).
3. Claude Bernard noted long ago that the function of the physiological organ systems and metabolic processes was to maintain homeostasis between the internal and external environment. Recent research into the areas of stress and psychoneuroimmunology indicates that there is an interactive system linking cellular respiration, nervous, endocrine, and other organ system functions with the external psychosocial and physical environment (Glaser et al. 1987; Pelletier and Herzing 1988:46).

CHAPTER 6

Mistress of *Lo Espiritual*

Kaja Finkler

Introduction

There was a time when it was believed that as biomedical knowledge advanced and became more and more successful in treating human ills, alternative healers would disappear. Biomedicine has indeed acquired an exquisite understanding of anatomy and physiology. It has developed spectacular techniques in organ transplantation, in saving human life under numerous emergencies, and in various forms of in vitro fertilization, as well as demonstrating many other achievements at which we unceasingly marvel. Yet paradoxically, alternative healing systems, with their simple technologies and in many instances religious underpinnings, have flourished, rather than disappeared. Moreover, whereas traditional healers used to be regarded as charlatans and quacks, currently there is great interest in and respect for alternative healing systems, both sacred and secular. In fact, the last decade of the twentieth century witnessed a significant turnabout regarding alternative healing. The U.S. Department of Health and Human Services has opened a department dedicated to the study of alternative healing systems, and in the January 28, 1993 issue of the *New England Journal of Medicine* (Eisenberg et al. 1993:246), there was an article entitled "Unconventional Medicine in the United States" in which the authors reported, with some surprise, that 34 percent of Americans have used what they called "unconventional medicine." Significantly, and to the surprise of another group led by Eisenberg (1998) whose findings were reported in the *Journal of the American Medical Association,* that percentage had increased to 42.1 by 1997.

Alternative healers in Mexico come in many different guises, but they can be classified into at least two broad categories: sacred and secular. Secular healers include herbalists, bonesetters, naturopaths, acupuncturists, homeopaths, yoga practitioners, chiropractors, injection specialists, and specialists in treating *cintura* (lower back). Sacred healers include *curanderas,* who may also treat, among many other complaints, cases of witchcraft, and who usually work within a sacred context, such as a temple or church.

Generally speaking sacred healers include many different types of shamans and religious healers, all of whom are embedded in religious ideology and practices. This chapter focuses on Spiritualism, one type of sacred healing system in Mexico that I studied as a participant and observer for two years and subsequently followed for more than twenty years. Unlike secular healers, sacred healers, such as the Spiritualists, are usually legitimated by their contact with the divine and mobilize the spirit world by entering an altered state of consciousness.

When I first described my project to Mexican physicians, they invariably responded that because people initially went to quacks such as Spiritualist healers, it was too late for them to treat the patients by the time they arrived in their offices. And when I began attending Spiritualist healing sessions, the Spiritualist healers told me that they could not always heal patients successfully because, by the time people came to them to seek their treatment, it was too late. Interestingly, during the course of my two-year research in a Spiritualist temple, I discovered that of the four hundred patients I studied who visited the temple for the *first* time, every one of them had sought treatment from more than one physician *before* seeking treatment from the Spiritualists. I thus posed the question: How do Spiritualist healers heal and how effective are they from the *patients'* perspective?

In this chapter I will (1) describe the people who seek treatment from Spiritualist healers, (2) examine the healing practices of the Spiritualist healers and recruitment into the healing role; (3) discuss how Spiritualist healers heal from the patients' perspectives, (4) compare the Spiritualists' knowledge with that of their patients, (5) discuss the status of the healers and the role of women in Mexican Spiritualism, and (6) note a few differences between Spiritualist healing and biomedicine. The comparison suggests why Spiritualist healing in Mexico has been continually growing in numbers of followers and healers. In fact, in 1998 on my last visit to a Spiritualist temple situated in a rural area of Mexico that I had initially studied from 1977 to 1979, the number of healers had grown from about eight to thirty-five, ministering in three shifts to hundreds of people a week. I will conclude with a few suggestions for further study of Spiritualism in Mexico.

People Who Seek Treatment from Spiritualist Healers

The people who seek treatment from Spiritualist healers are of all ages and usually, but not exclusively, originate from the poor strata of Mexican society. With some exceptions, they usually seek treatment for what are commonly described as non-life-threatening chronic illnesses, the kinds of afflictions which biomedicine frequently fails to alleviate.

I observed twelve hundred people who comprised at least three categories of patients. *First comers* had seen numerous physicians for gastrointestinal, musculoskeletal, and respiratory distress; skin eruptions; gynecological problems; headaches; and personal problems that were associated with bodily discomforts before seeking treatment at the temple. A second category was what I call the *habitual temple users*. These people had usually been successfully treated by temple healers before, but may have had a recurring episode, returning to seek treatment for disorders such as mild diarrhea, catarrh, "nerves," throat pain, back pain, and general discomfort.

The third category of patients were the *regulars*. These people's afflictions were not alleviated by routine temple treatments and they were recruited into the movement as healers or other functionaries. It is important to separate patients into these three categories because we often regard people seeking treatment from alternative healers as an undifferentiated mass, all following the same healing-seeking strategies with the same expectations.

Healing Practices and Recruitment

Mexican Spiritualism is both a religious movement and a healing system. As a religion, it is rigidly organized on a national level and recognized by the Mexican government as a legitimate religion. The head temple and its affiliates are formally registered with one of the Mexican government ministries and thus have official and formal recognition as a minority religion, along with a variety of Protestant sects. Unlike Protestants and members of other minority religious groups in Mexico, however, Spiritualists may be regarded by many as witches. This reputation no doubt stems from an implicit assumption that anyone who can control good spirits must possess the power to call upon evil spirits as well. When the movement arose in the nineteenth century, it was a small community of dissidents. It later gained momentum, however, and the head temple was established in Mexico City in 1923, signaling the emergence of a formal, hierarchical organizational structure. Many temples are formally affiliated with at least one other Spiritualist temple of a higher rank in the hierarchy. First in importance is the head temple in Mexico City, which is referred to as the "womb" and which has founded branch temples through Mexico and other parts of Latin America, as well as the United States. The second most important temple is situated several blocks from the head temple, and the third-ranking temple is located in the city of Puebla. Heads of branch temples are expected to come once a month both to the head temple and to the second Mexico City temple for instructions. Visits to the Puebla temple need to be made once a year. Each branch temple has a head (usually the branch founder), various functionaries that officiate during religious rituals, and healers. The head temple sets down the rituals and healing procedures that branch temples are expected to follow. These are often reinforced by individuals from the head temple who come to officiate at religious ceremonies at a branch temple. Branch temples seek affiliation with the head temple in Mexico City because official affiliation confers societal legitimacy which they otherwise may lack. Heads of branch temples may travel to participate in each other's anniversary celebrations. In this manner branch temple heads and some accompanying members maintain contact and exchange information about ritual practices. As a result, the ideological beliefs and practices of the movement tend to retain a degree of uniformity.

A branch temple may disintegrate with the death of its head, who in most cases is also its founder. The branch temple's existence is tied to its head's ability to maintain her flock and to groom a successor, usually a member of her family, as was the case in the temple that I originally studied. Temples may also disintegrate owing to dissension between various functionaries. However, no matter what the fate of an individual temple, Spiritualism as a religious structure endures, in great part because of its hierarchical nature.[1]

Healing practices and recruitment into Spiritualism are closely intertwined. Mexican Spiritualist healers are primarily women, including the head of the "mother" temple in Mexico City. This is significant, and I will return to this point later.

Mexican Spiritualists tame the spirits of the dead that roam the universe and harness them for the good of humankind, that is, for healing the sick. Healers minister to the sick gratis through spirit protectors who possess their bodies when they enter into a trance. Each healer possesses one spirit protector throughout her career. This spirit initially identifies himself to her during the course of training, or what Spiritualists refer to as "development" (*desarollo*), which may last from six months to ten years or more, depending on the individual and her readiness to receive the protector. These spirit protectors manifest themselves on healing days after the healer has arrived in the temple, put on a white robe, approached the altar to listen to a brief prayer recited by the temple head, and entered the healing room. To summon the protector the healer sits down, closes her eyes, and mildly shakes the upper half of her body. The healer ceases to shake when the spirit protector has temporarily settled in her body, identified himself by name, and greeted everyone present. Following this proceeding, which may take just a minute or two, the healer is prepared to receive patients.

Spiritualist healers usually heal in a room designated for healing within or adjacent to a Spiritualist temple, where religious rituals are conducted on Sundays and other specially designated days.[2] The healing room may vary in size, depending on the temple head's financial possibilities. In the temple where I conducted my original study, the healing room was a small bare room with a broken window, painted in blue, containing chairs for the healers and a little bench on which various liquids were set that some healers used during healing. Healers sit side by side in trance. As each patient comes up to a healer and gives a special salute, the healer declares that she has heard the patient, and the patient then reports his or her disturbances.

Variation exists among the individual healers' forms of ministration. Some may use liquids (usually ammonia) or a rosemary branch during the cleansing a patient receives, whereas others use no props whatsoever. Those healers who do not use any props during their ministrations are considered more spiritual. But generally speaking all healers resort to a wide variety of healing techniques that include the use of an extensive pharmacopoeia. Patients are instructed to purchase or to search for a variety of botanicals in the surrounding fields. These items may be used to make teas or for massages or baths (using a combination of herbs dipped in alcohol), as well as for ritual cleansings. Purgative treatments often include a prescription for Phillips Milk of Magnesia. Other treatments include spiritual surgeries that symbolically extract the sickness from the patient's body; attendance at weekly, monthly, and specially designated days of religious rituals; pharmaceuticals, including Dramamine and occasionally antibiotics and anti-diarrhea medications; and what I call "passive catharsis." Passive catharsis refers to a process in which a patient experiences a sense of release and relief without having to say anything. In these instances, the healer tells the patient what he or she is experiencing and the patient gratefully shakes his or her head in agreement.

Healers usually hold the patient's hands as the patient stands facing the healer, and the healer moves her hands up and down the patient's body. Part of this practice includes a ritual cleansing that is especially important from the patient's perspective, as I will discuss shortly. When there is a particularly difficult case, such as, for example, paralysis, the healer, while she is giving the patient a cleansing, falls backward in her seat. As she does so, a voice is heard inquiring, "Where am I? What am I doing here in this sacred place?" This suggests immediately that the evil spirit possessing the patient has been transferred to the healer and has captured the healer's spirit protector. The two spirits engage in combat. During the course of a few minutes a powerful struggle takes place within the healer's body between the patient's evil spirit and the healer's spirit protector. At that moment, the head of the temple or another functionary runs over to the healer and addresses the evil spirit that has taken over the healer's body. The evil spirit is told to leave this sacred place immediately, and after a few minutes the evil spirit does. The spirit protector returns triumphantly into the body of the healer, salutes all present, and announces that he is back to minister to mankind. This mesmerizing scene is especially effective from the patient's perspective in removing the evil that had enveloped her.

Besides attributing sickness to attacks by spirits that must be tamed and transformed into healing spirits, Spiritualists share traditional folk beliefs regarding sickness causality that include environmental hazards such as inclement weather, or *aire*,[3] nutritional deficits, and emotional discharges, especially anger and fright (*susto*). However, in day-to-day practice, Spiritualist healers are not concerned with etiological explanations. Such etiologies as they do offer, however, are relatively limited and unchanging compared to those of biomedicine. Spiritualist healers confer a coherent system of explanations, which in the final analysis is usually reduced to assaults by evil spirits. Spiritualists believe that afflictions that stubbornly resist both biomedical and Spiritualist ministrations, including baths, massages, and teas, have been caused by the intrusion of a bad spirit that requires removal from the body. These causal explanations are comforting to patients, who are frequently confused by the lack of certainty and the different etiologies physicians may have given them.

On the whole, Spiritualist healers fail to provide the patient with a definitive diagnosis. When they do, it usually consists of informing the person either that he or she is possessed by an obscure spirit that requires extrication or that he or she possesses a gift (*don*) that requires cultivation.[4] Normally, people whose illnesses are not readily alleviated by standard Spiritualist procedures are given a diagnosis that they possess a special gift, and they are instructed to enter training to develop the gift for healing or to expel the evil spirit. The declaration that the patient possesses the gift of healing or is possessed by an evil spirit is a sure way of recruiting the patient into the ranks of Spiritualism. In fact, a patient's failure to respond to routine Spiritualist treatment frequently triggers recruitment. Thus the patient and the healing role are intricately related in Mexican Spiritualism. In fact, according to Spiritualist doctrine, all human beings have a capacity to heal as long as the spirit protector has identified him- or herself to the individual.[5] In the words of the head of one temple, "protectors give us power." Once the individual agrees to enter development and attend the religious rituals as part of Spiritualist therapy, she forms part of the Spiritualist community.

A typical example of how Spiritualists recruit individuals into the healing role and into the movement is Lupita: Lupita was a forty-eight-year-old mother of eight living children when I met her. For much of her life she worked as a vegetable vendor, buying her merchandise in Mexico City, returning with it on her back, and selling it in the countryside.

She initially came to the temple as a patient when she was fifteen years old, two years after her marriage. At that time she was experiencing a feeling of her tongue becoming inflamed, she could not talk, and she suffered from severe diarrhea and vomiting. She was very fearful of everything. Her vision was blurred. At first she attributed her disorder to eating food and drinking pulque,[6] which her mother-in-law gave her. Later she ascribed her condition to nerves resulting from the difficult life she had with her husband and her mother-in-law. Her husband beat her incessantly. Her first sickness episode coincided with the death of her first-born infant at four months of age. She held herself responsible for its death.

Lupita sought treatment from various physicians who diagnosed her condition as a liver dysfunction; another doctor told her she had a cerebral infarction due to an embolism. Lupita herself continued to ascribe her dysfunction to nerves. Her sickness was not relieved by any of the physicians from whom she sought treatment, and a friend suggested that she go to a Spiritualist temple. After some treatment there she was told that she possessed a gift and she must enter development. The Spiritualist healer diagnosed her condition as an "open *cerebro*,"[7] which made her susceptible to attacks by perturbed spirits who were causing her sickness.

During a Spiritualist religious ritual, Lupita was ordered by God to stand before Him. He told her that the baby's death was not her fault but rather that it was His will, that she was being tested, and that it was her duty to serve Him in His house, meaning the Spiritualist temple. He designated her to work as a healer and clairvoyant during temple rituals. Subsequently, she recovered from her sickness.

Lupita's case represents the majority of people that I studied—persons that tended to suffer from disorders not readily amenable to treatment either by biophysicians or by standard Spiritualist treatment procedures. Of course, not all patients ordered by healers to participate in rituals and in development do so, as Lupita did. Some attend only once or twice, but those who become incorporated into the temple community, either as functionaries or simply as adherents to Spiritualism by attending regularly religious ceremonies, identify their religion as Spiritualism and become "regulars." These individuals will often, but not uniformly, recruit members of their own families to enter development and be marked by God for a special functionary role. Functionaries, who comprise the core membership in a temple, enter the movement after having been "marked" by God for a specific position during a special ceremony. Novices marked for the healing role are eased into their task as soon as their spirit protectors have identified themselves.

What is most remarkable about this form of recruitment—and I must emphasize that this is not unique to Mexican Spiritualism but may be common to sacred healing in general—is that a sick person is converted into a health provider. In fact, the different ways in which Spiritualist healers and physicians are recruited into their respective roles have different effects on patients. Whereas those recruited into the medical profession are usually healthy individuals, those recruited into Spiritualist healing usually have experienced an affliction themselves before becoming healers. As formerly sick people who have become health providers, Spiritualist healers are themselves examples of the potential for recovery through Spiritualist ministrations. Importantly, they convey to the patient that they have grasped the patient's anguish through their personal experience. They experienced the pain in the past in the same way the patient is experiencing it in the present. Spiritualist healers proudly announce that their therapies induce a transformation in the person from having been sick to healing others. Significantly, whereas the conversion of a patient to health practitioner, or to a functionary serving God and the spirit world, forms part of the Spiritualist therapeutic repertoire, it also makes the person's health dependent on her participation in healing and in the religious movement.

How Spiritualist Healers Heal from the Patients' Perspectives

When I questioned patients about the pains that had been alleviated by Spiritualist healing and the aspects of the treatment that had relieved their condition, all responded first and foremost that it was the cleansing they had received. Some also added the massages and baths. Cleansings may be regarded from our perspective as a form of symbolic healing. Symbols are of course intrinsic to all healing systems and cannot be disentangled from "real remedies." When, for example, we take an aspirin, which undoubtedly contains properties that alleviate our headaches, the aspirin possesses symbolic power as well, because we think of it as a medicine for headaches. Similarly, whether cleansing has symbolic or "real" effects owing to the therapeutic touch (Finkler 1994b) is arguably less relevant than the fact that patients recognize it as a powerful healing mechanism. Symbols developed in a particular culture speak to the most profound concerns of the individual in that culture. Cleansings represent a form of purification cross-culturally by removing evil and thereby restoring order into the patient's existence. By way of illustrating the ways in which Spiritualist symbols become transmitted during treatment, consider one patient who subsequently became a healer after having suffered from heart palpitations. The healer linked these heart palpitations to crystalline drops falling into an empty glass, with the drops symbolizing God's words transmitted during Spiritualist rituals, and the patient representing the empty glass. The patient constantly referred to these metaphors when she spoke about having recovered from her chest pains and headaches.

Additionally, on an existential level, those who become regulars and adherents in the movement embody a spirit through trance and in so doing experience their bodies in a new and sacred way. Uniformly, all healers and functionaries who entered a trance to fulfill their healing tasks reported that they experienced a tingling effect in their bodies, a heightening of the senses, and a vision of extraordinary colors. This new transcendent experience may in and of itself be healing.

Spiritualist Healers' Knowledge as Compared with Their Patients'

As mentioned earlier, Spiritualists, like Mexicans from the same social strata, believe in the same causes of illness. However, there are differences as well. Whereas generally speaking people believe in witchcraft (Finkler 1991, 1994b), the Spiritualists I studied do not. Further, Spiritualists do not believe in the traditional unified, holistic view of body, spirit, and mind, but rather, firmly believe in a dualism based upon the division of spirit and body. Spiritualists clearly separate suffering of the body—*lo material*—from spiritual suffering. This is not commonly done in traditional Mexican culture.

Whereas the people who came to seek treatment from the Spiritualists for the first time believed that their affliction was due to malfeasance *because* biophysicians had failed to heal them, the Spiritualists healers vigorously denied that possibility. Also, healers possess a larger store of information than their patients about traditional remedies in general (Finkler 1984). They have greater knowledge of the local botanical plants and commercially sold herbal remedies than the average patient who seeks their ministrations (Finkler 1984). Thus the healers are set apart by their superior knowledge of medicinal plants and the ways in which such plants are to be used. The healers have also developed a separate vocabulary from that of their patients, even though they emerge from the same sociocultural strata, with the same level of education (generally confined to primary school). For example, whereas people use the term *"médicos"* when referring to doctors,

Spiritualists healers refer to them as *lo material*. Healers use the word "*desa-lojo*" to refer to a dislodgment, a healing technique that removes evil spirits, whereas their patients use "*limpia*," to the consternation of the healers. By sharing the same experiences, the healers develop a similar fund of knowledge which differentiates them from their patients. The shared knowledge among healers derives from their extensive experience with illnesses. Their widespread knowledge of medicinal plants is not linked to any professional training; it is, however, related to their intense interest in the native pharmacopoeia, probably nurtured by lengthy exposure to illness. While there is a strong cultural commitment to herbal medicines among Mexicans from all social strata, the patients I studied would claim that they knew little about a particular plant's specific applications respecting dosage, mode of preparation, or the part of the plant to use. By the time people become Spiritualist healers, almost all have had extensive experience with afflictions unsuccessfully managed biomedically, as we saw previously, and these earlier experiences form the basis of their recruitment into Spiritualism and the healing role.

Moreover, the healers can manipulate supernatural forces that their patients cannot. In the final analysis these forces give them legitimacy to heal that is recognized by the people who seek their treatment. However, the control of these forces fails to give them status outside their immediate temples. Given the healers' powers to manipulate supernatural forces, one might ask from an analytical perspective about their emotional and psychological health, or how they differ in this respect from the population at large. Spiritualists tend to restore patients to health by imbuing them with beliefs that human beings communicate with spirits. How do persons with such beliefs fit into Mexican society? To what degree do these people stand apart from other Mexicans of the same social strata? It is true that, although an ideology of the existence of spirits is not alien to Mexican traditional thinking (witness, for example the belief in *aire*), Mexicans do not ordinarily believe, as Spiritualists do, that humans can communicate with spirits. Nevertheless my data suggest that Spiritualist healers are psychologically as sound as ordinary Mexicans. In fact, a comparison of regulars and a control group of healthy individuals who had never attended a Spiritualist temple revealed no psychological differences on a standardized measure of mental health (Finkler 1994b). Indeed, Spiritualists who become temple heads are not only psychologically sound, but also display exceptional abilities. Directing a temple, whether large or small, requires an enterprising spirit and the ability to manipulate the social environment. Mariana, the head of one temple, is a case in point. When I first met her she was in her mid-fifties. She was literate, intelligent, energetic, and self-sustaining (Finkler 1981). She was remarkably active and alert, as was reflected in her penetrating gaze.

My work did reveal behavioral differences between male regulars and the larger male population, however. Male regulars tend to relinquish their machismo, which is defined by heavy drinking, womanizing, and wife beating. Men who were recruited and who chose to become regulars usually had a history of heavy drinking. Although Spiritualists are not teetotalers, they prohibit drunkenness, and when a man joins the temple, he is taught to give up his drinking. This sets him apart from the majority of Mexican macho men, whose drinking patterns (and womanizing) define them as men. In fact, whereas Spiritualists reinforce traditional female behaviors in women, they attempt to remodel male conduct by deemphasizing masculine behavioral traits associated with machismo.[8]

Status of the Healers and the
Role of Women in Mexican Spiritualism

Spiritualist healers are not accorded special privileges, prestige, or status within Mexican society at large, within the communities in which they reside, or even within the temple hierarchy, despite their superior knowledge of healing and botanicals, and despite their ability to control supernatural forces. That Spiritualist healers lack social status in the society at large is, of course, not surprising. By and large Spiritualists form part of Mexico's lower and marginal socioeconomic sector. Moreover, the Spiritualists' power to manipulate the spirits is a double-edged sword. Whereas it confers on them the legitimacy to be healers, it is also considered threatening to the society at large, since those who can control the spirits for benevolent purposes might, as Spiritualists are sometimes falsely accused, also do so for malevolent reasons. In fact, some clergy often call Spiritualists *brujas* or sorcerers, and they may similarly be viewed by practicing Catholics.

With the exception of the temple head (Finkler 1981), Spiritualist healers also fail to attain high status or prestige within the community of patients whom they serve. The fact that they lack prestige and status within Spiritualism itself is created by an interesting contradiction intrinsic to Spiritualism. In order to gain legitimacy, Spiritualist healers must disclaim their healing abilities as human beings by deferring to the spirit protectors that they summon during an altered state of consciousness. The healers incessantly stress to everyone that any healing powers they possess flow from their protectors, not from them. Their favorite metaphor is that they are just "radio transmitters" for the spirits. In fact, healers dissociate themselves completely from the spirit protectors during normal consciousness to the extent that some even repudiate any knowledge of healing or medicinal plants.

Consider this. I attempted to query four healers about specific medicinal properties, preparations, and uses of plants that I had observed them routinely prescribe to patients.[9] During informal interactions—at meals and on other occasions—healers delighted in instructing me about all aspects of illness and its remedies. But when I asked each individual for more formal instructions on these subjects, the healers disclaimed any knowledge of the *materia médica*, or cures, on the grounds that their therapies and knowledge stemmed from their spirit protectors, and they claimed total ignorance of such matters during a normal waking state. With these disclaimers the healers strove to maintain a logical consistency, but they also denied themselves any possibility of attaining prestige in their communities on the basis of having superior knowledge. Additionally, all healing protectors are regarded as having equal powers.

Nor is Spiritualism a vehicle for economic mobility. Healers are, in fact, even penalized economically because they must usually devote at least two days a week to treating patients at the temple, for which they receive no remuneration. The frequency with which healers participate in healing and in temple rituals depends upon their home situation. I have observed them being under extraordinary pressures at home because women healers must also fulfill their household chores. Furthermore, by serving as healers in the temple, both men and women are foreclosed from engaging in economic activities. In fact, participation in temple activities requires considerable expenditures of time and money for travel to the temple and incidental expenses away from home.

Some of the healers were supported by their husbands and were not engaged in financially remunerative enterprises. Others, both men and women, lost potential income on the days they worked as healers. While healers recognized the financial losses, they acknowledged that by ministering to others they were also ministering to themselves. In fact, many claimed that when they were absent from the temple and failed to carry out their assigned tasks, they suffered from various forms of distress as a result of their failure to fulfill their obligations to God. Thus by becoming riveted to the temple, the healers become anchored in a socioeconomic status quo because participation in Spiritualism limits rather than promotes socioeconomic mobility.

Paradoxically, on the level of the individual, then, while Spiritualist healing restores one and gives one healing powers, on the level of the collectivity, Spiritualism tends to lock in its participants economically.

Nevertheless, and significantly, Spiritualism has a particular attraction for women. Over 75 percent of patients seeking treatment from Spiritualist healers were women, and the majority of adherents are women as well. The significant question here is, "Why do many more women than men become Spiritualists and healers?" There are undoubtedly numerous reasons to explain this difference, and several levels of explanation. I will attempt here to provide three explanations.

First, unlike the Catholic Church, Spiritualism opened positions of leadership for women from its inception, when their founder, a recalcitrant priest, allocated twelve sacerdotal positions to men and twelve sacerdotal positions to women in 1861. And the founder's earliest followers and functionaries were indeed women. The movement grew and gained momentum, and in 1923 the head Spiritualist temple, known as the "womb," was founded in Mexico City (Finkler 1983). The headship of this temple is transmitted matrilineally, and the heads have always been women who claim direct descent from the woman who was awarded one of the twelve sacerdotal positions. Indeed, the numerous Spiritualist temples dispersed throughout Mexico are headed almost exclusively by women.[10] Thus one could characterize Mexican Spiritualism as a woman's religion, as for example Starr Sered (1994) has done.

Second and concomitantly it can be argued, as Lewis (1971) has, that dissident religious movements such as Spiritualism, in which spirit possession is central to their creed, are expressions of powerlessness and tend to attract individuals from politically and economically disadvantaged sectors of society. Some women of the Spiritualist movement support this assertion. Lewis' thesis regarding dissident religious movements is still valid: "it is in terms of the exclusion of women from full participation in social and political affairs and their final subjugation to men that we should seek to understand their marked prominence in peripheral possession" (1971:88) such as that practiced by Mexican Spiritualists.

Moreover, Spiritualism emphasizes abstention from alcohol and inter-active male–female relations. A prime motivation for women to become Spiritualists is that they are married to men who drink excessively. If the woman can prevail on the man to join also, he usually abandons his drinking. When a man gives up drinking, the woman is shielded from his acts of vio-lence after a drinking binge, and the resources that are usually diverted for alcohol consumption revert to the household.

As mentioned earlier, Spiritualist healing, in fact, differentially reorders men's and women's lives. It reorders men's lives to the ostensible advantage of women. Spiritualists preach against machismo in men, leading them to cease drinking heavily and womanizing. The men tend to spend their leisure time with their wives and families rather than with their former male friends or women other than their wives. By restructuring men's lives, Spiritualism promotes smoother marital relationships, changes women recognize as salu-tary and healthful. Not surprisingly, more women than men are attracted to such a movement.

Lastly, there is another important dimension to explain why women pre-dominate as healers and participants in Mexican Spiritualism. As we saw earlier, recruitment to Spiritualism occurs mainly through the sick. Signifi-cantly, more women than men experience sickness, for reasons I explore in great depth elsewhere (Finkler 1994c). Here I will only note that more women than men are exposed to what I have termed *life's lesions*, that is, perceived adversities of existence, including inimical social relationships, unresolved contradictions, and moral dilemmas in which a human being is entrenched and which gnaw at the person's being. These lesions become inscribed on the body and fester. They become manifested in anguish, in generalized pain experienced in the entire body, and in non-life-threatening symptomatologies of the kind that patients present to Spiritualist healers.

As I have shown (Finkler 1994c), more women than men are exposed to existential conditions and moral contradictions that lead them to experience life's lesions. The contradictions and moral dilemmas that women encoun-ter are often rooted in their relationships with their mates. In fact, the very acts that make men feel macho, drinking and womanizing, are the same acts that produce life's lesions in women. Moreover, women's health in Mexico is greatly influenced by their relations with their mates, resulting in lesions that are produced by such aspects of the relationship as domestic violence (Finkler 1997). It is therefore not surprising that more women than men seek treatment from Spiritualists healers and consequently, more women than men become recruited into Spiritualism in general and Spiritualist healing in particular.

Comparison of Spiritualist Healers and Biophysicians

To conclude the discussion of Mexican Spiritualism I will compare Spiritualist healers and biophysicians. This brings into bold relief the attraction that Spiritualist healing has for patients.[11] This comparison is informed by an outsider's (etic) analysis rather than analyses that patients themselves have made. It is important to emphasize that Mexicans usually do not distinguish between different types of healers. Their preoccupation is pragmatic. Their concern is with who gives the best medicine rather than how a particular practitioner is trained and legitimized—by spirits, or by a medical education and diploma.

There are various differences between Spiritualist healing and biomedicine, and also some similarities that I discuss elsewhere (Finkler 1991, 1994a). I will point out a few here. For example, a major attraction for patients seeking Spiritualist treatment is the fact that Spiritualists are certain of their diagnoses, while physicians, in order to practice good medicine, must usually present their diagnoses as provisional. Spiritualists draw on a limited diagnostic repertoire and eschew multiple diagnoses, unlike biophysicians. There is usually a consistency among different Spiritualist healers regarding the cause of the person's affliction, as well as diagnosis and treatment. From the patient's perspective, consistency and certainty are a relief, especially after a patient has seen numerous physicians and been given a variety of diagnoses. Getting several diagnoses for the same pains and symptomatologies is puzzling and often disturbing to patients.

Most important, there are significant differences in the patient–healer relationship that merit attention. It is usually held that traditional healers, including Spiritualist healers, display greater understanding, more empathy, and more compassion for patients than physicians do. They are presumably more attentive to patients than physicians; this is often measured in terms of healers having more eye contact with patients and spending more time with them. However, this view may represent an idealization of traditional healers. My observations of traditional healers revealed that unlike physicians, Spiritualist healers lack eye contact with their patients and do not recognize the individual standing before them. The healers sit in trance with expressionless faces, eyes closed, holding or stroking the patient. The trance state precludes them from displaying any kind of affect for their patients. By contrast physicians sit facing the patient, who is given a physical examination, and physicians often show a great deal of affect during the encounter.

I found that physicians spent about twenty-one minutes on average with a first-time patient, whereas Spiritualists healers usually spent half that time. Moreover, the physician–patient interaction can be characterized as a drama featuring tension and conflict between the patient and the physician—a component lacking in the Spiritualist–patient interaction (Finkler 1991). In both Spiritualist healing and biomedical practice the meeting between the health provider and patient is *not* like an ordinary encounter between two strangers. However, the conditions that bring the patient and health provider together are *extra ordinary:* one is in pain and under duress and the other is expected to eliminate or transform the condition. In contrast to the Spiritualist healer–patient encounter, the drama in the medical consultation is revealed when the two actors stand in opposition to one another. The encounter scripted by the biomedical model brings two players into conflict. Moved by a crisis, the patient arrives on the stage to seek advice from an expert who presumably knows more about how bodies work than the patient does. The physician claims to have a monopoly on the knowledge of disease. He is the authority on what went wrong. The patient comes laden with personal knowledge encoded by cultural understandings about the working of his or her own body and the authority of experience with the specific condition. The patient is *certain* of his or her individualized experience of pain, whereas the physician is often *uncertain* of the diagnosis. One of the doctors I studied said, "I must sometimes invent a diagnosis."

The drama that exists in the doctor–patient relationship is minimized in the Spiritualist healer–patient association. While a physician's clinical judgment entails uncertainty and is grounded in a process of exclusion, Spiritualist healers treat patients with great certainty. Spiritualist healers are as sure of their diagnoses and course of treatment as patients are certain of their pain. Spiritualist healers do not doubt that the spirits possessing their bodies "in the service of mankind" are omniscient and that they know the person's pain and the required cure.

Significantly, too, while the physician must cast the patient's sickness in a temporal frame and localize the pain in a specific part of the body, the omniscient spirits transcend time and space in the same way that the patient's sickness transcends temporal and spatial dimensions. The patient cannot confine the onset of the afflictions to a specific time because the patient usually experiences the pain as timeless. In contrast, the biomedical diagnostic process incorporates a temporal and topographic dimension. As a result, the physician is often frustrated by the patient's inability to compartmentalize symptoms to a particular anatomical region to conform to the medical history format or to locate the symptoms within a specific time frame.[12] When the patient confronts a Spiritualist healer, he or she need not tell the healer very much for the healer to know everything. In fact, the spirit situated in the body of the healer constantly reminds the patient, "I know everything." The patient is experiencing the passive catharsis that I noted earlier. In this way, the healer reassures the patient and also establishes legitimacy in the healing role. Of course, patients are also assured that the Spiritualist healer knows their pain because they know that Spiritualist healers too have suffered afflictions before becoming healers.

To summarize this brief comparison, Spiritualist healers' diagnoses are relatively simple. However, their treatment repertoires are relatively complex. By contrast, the physician's diagnoses are complex but their curing repertoire is limited. Thus, a comparison of treatment techniques reveals that the physician's treatments include chiefly medications, or in extreme cases, surgery or replacement of body parts. On the other hand, the Spiritualist healer's treatment kit contains a large array of treatment options which also involves patients' participation in various treatment activities. These include the use of pharmaceuticals or herbs and other botanicals that people are required to find in the fields, grow at home, or purchase; massages; baths that require preparation by the patient; and participation in Spiritualist rituals. These activities effectively engage patients in their recovery. In keeping with this point, the physician takes full responsibility for the patient's successful cure, if not for the failure to heal, whereas the Spiritualist healer assigns responsibility to the patient for the cure by constantly reminding her that she must have unrelenting faith in the Spiritualist God and His benevolence, further involving her in her own therapy.[13]

Lastly, physicians do not address the contradictions in which patients are enmeshed. Physicians may blame impersonal pathogens that attack the body or the patients themselves for their poor habits. Biomedicine requires patients to alter their behavior such as diet, work, and drinking habits, but it does not attempt to transform the circumstances of the patients' lives in the way Spiritualists do for those who become regulars. Spiritualist healing can gradually transform the person's existence by incorporating him or her, and in some instances, his or her entire family, into a religious community, a family in which members refer to one another as siblings. Over the long term, Spiritualist healing provides new interpersonal networks and also places the person in a new and transcendent relationship with God. In the latter instance, relationships with other human beings become submerged with interactions with God. Spiritualist healing progressively reorders the existence of the regulars by incorporating them into a community of sufferers who share a satisfying religious reality and symbolic meanings, by God appointing them as functionaries in the movement, and by His having chosen them to become healers because they possess a gift. As I have emphasized elsewhere (Finkler 1994b), Spiritualist healers do not produce miraculous cures. All transformations are achieved gradually, and some patients even experience great pain in the process of recovery.

To the degree that Spiritualist healers succeed in easing marital strain and changing the person's existence, they are also promoting health. Clearly, biomedicine does not address the existential dilemmas that produce life's lesions, or reinterpret these dilemmas and give them new meanings, or change the social relationships in which a patient is embedded, including those between husband and wife.

Spiritualist healing encompasses the lives of patients that it succeeds in converting into participants and believers. The bodies of regulars become an extension of the Spiritualist congregation, upon which they become totally dependent, and this also forms part of their cure. While Spiritualist healers may not succeed in eradicating life's lesions, participation in the Spiritualist movement exerts power over the patients' existence because, as many patients readily admit, if they failed to attend to various rituals and to heal others, they would revert to their morbid states.

In the final analysis, Spiritualist healers, like physicians, fall short of healing their patients when they fail to attend to their patient's lived world. To succeed in resolving non-life-threatening subacute conditions, a healing system must address its patients' life's lesions and concurrently transform their perceived existence. Biomedicine fails to do this, whereas Spiritualist healing succeeds mainly with the regulars in transforming their lives.

By way of conclusion, I will note, as I have earlier, that during the course of twenty-five years of contact with Spiritualist healers in Mexico, I have watched Mexican Spiritualism grow immensely. This growth is probably associated with many factors. To cite but two, as globalization comes into full force, people tend to reemphasize their own cultural practices, including their healing traditions, in response to the perceived or actual forces of homogenization associated with the globalization process.

But more important, as modern medicine advances and people's expectations are heightened by its success, its failures become less explicable and more frustrating. People will therefore turn more and more to alternative healing of the secular and sacred kind, as they have in the United States, for conditions that biomedicine fails to heal, including those that are produced by life's lesions. The non-life-threatening symptomatologies produced by life's lesions cannot be healed unless their causes are addressed and the person's life is transformed. For this reason I anticipate that traditional healing of the Spiritualist kind will continue to grow and thrive in Mexico and elsewhere.

To conclude this discussion, I will call attention to several avenues of further research that could be carried out to expand our understanding of sacred healing (see also Csordas 1994).

First, the experiential aspects of sacred healing require further exploration. How does the interaction between *lo espiritual* and *lo material* influence the healer's experience of her body? How does the dualism of the body and spirit in Spiritualism differ experientially from the dualism of body and mind in biomedicine?

Second, very little research has been done on the iatrogenic effects of sacred healing practices such as Spiritualism. As I note elsewhere (Finkler 1994b), to become a Spiritualist entails negative as well as positive aspects. To join the Spiritualist movement creates numerous conflicts for the individual, and these conflicts, some of which impede the healing process, need to be explored.

Third, Spiritualism has to some degree incorporated pharmacological treatments. What are the various influences of biomedicine on beliefs and practices of sacred healing such as Spiritualism?

Fourth, how do Spiritualist healers integrate their religious doctrines into their daily practice? For example, the Spiritualist healers that I studied vehemently denounced beliefs in witchcraft in accordance with the twenty-two laws Spiritualists are expected to obey and repeat at every religious ritual (Finkler 1985). Do Spiritualists throughout Mexico adhere to this injunction, which has important consequences for the healing process and for day-to-day social relations?

Fifth, Spiritualism and its practices in the United States need to be explored from sociological and phenomenological perspectives.

Spiritualist healing is a vibrant and growing movement in Mexico at the beginning of the twenty-first century that exists side by side with the advances made in biomedicine. Its study must be continued.

Notes

1. For a more detailed discussion of Spiritualism as a religion, see the *Diccionario enciclopédico de la medicina tradicional mexicana* (Mata Pinzón et al. 1994; see also Finkler 1994b; Ortiz Echáriz 1977).
2. Spiritualists conduct services on the first, seventh, thirteenth, and twenty-first of each month in addition to Christmas, New Years, November 2, Easter, and the founding day of the temple, which is celebrated annually.
3. "Bad air" refers to a traditional type of illness produced by a tormented spirit roaming around and possessing the body of an individual, especially one who passes a cemetery. The predominant symptom is a crooked mouth, or Bell's Palsy.
4. While I reported no illnesses to the healers, they nevertheless regarded me as possessing a gift for healing and I was placed into training to become a healer.
5. While the majority of healers are women, their spirit protectors are usually male, suggesting that the power acquired through possession trance is reinforced by the spirit guide's gender.
6. *Pulque* is an alcoholic beverage that is extracted from the agave plant.
7. *Cerebro* refers to the occipital region of the skull.
8. For further discussion of this point and some vignettes, see Finkler (1994b).
9. I never succeeded in entering an altered state of consciousness or to have a spirit protector descend into my body, but I did spend two years as an assistant to the healers. Each healer had an assistant who recorded the prescriptions on a slip of paper to give to the patient.
10. While the Spiritualist movement discussed here originated in Mexico, it is widespread in other countries in Latin America (for Guatemala, see Cosminsky 1987) and in the United States. Spiritualists meet annually in Mexico City, at which time each representative from a temple carries a banner indicating where he or she is living and worshiping. When I attended these annual meetings I saw banners from Houston, San Antonio, and other cities in the United States. For a complete history of Spiritualism, see Ortiz Echáriz (1977). Lagarriga (1975, 1978a, 1978b) has also written about Mexican Spiritualism.

11. After having studied Spiritualist healers, I spent two years studying Mexican physicians because I wished to understand patients' responses to biomedicine (Finkler 1991).

12. In my study of Mexican physicians (Finkler 1991) I often observed how physicians would say to a patient, "Tell me where it hurts," and the patient would point to many different areas of the body, or the physician would ask when the pain began, and to their frustration the patient would respond with different time periods.

13. Similarly, I have found that patients' participation in the physician–patient encounter significantly influences recovery (see Finkler 1996).

CHAPTER 7

Recruitment, Training, and Practice of Indigenous Midwives

From the Mexico–United States Border to the Isthmus of Tehuantepec

Brad R. Huber and Alan R. Sandstrom

Introduction

The authors[1] of this chapter undertake a comparative study of indigenous midwives living in seven subregions in Mexico that extend from the United States border to the Isthmus of Tehuantepec. Considerable variability exists in the geographic distribution of midwives, their medical and ritual roles, methods of recruitment and training, and in the manner in which midwives interact with other medical personnel and government organizations. A significant portion of this variability is correlated with ecological and demographic factors.

The most comprehensive publication on indigenous Mexican midwifery is a three-volume book by Mellado Campos et al. (1994). This source and those listed in Table 7.1 were used to collect data on midwives from 1900 to the present. The findings that emerged from this literature review are illustrated with information collected by the first author and three field assistants from fifteen Nahuat-speaking midwives. These midwives live in San Andrés Hueyapan, a rural community of approximately seven thousand people in the Sierra Norte de Puebla, a part of the eastern subregion. Seven midwives were interviewed on one or more occasions during the 1980s and again in 1996. In 1996, eight more were identified and interviewed. Most of Hueyapan's midwives have been practicing for several decades; only four began their practices in the last ten years. Hueyapan currently has one

TABLE 7.1: SOURCES USED FOR REGIONAL COMPARISONS OF INDIGENOUS MIDWIVES FROM THE MEXICO–UNITED STATES BORDER TO THE ISTHMUS OF TEHUANTEPEC

Name	State	First Author	Year of Publication
NORTHWEST REGION			
Kickapoo	Coahuila	Fabila	1945
Kickapoo	Coahuila	Latorre	1976
Kiliwa	Baja California	Ochoa Zazueta	1992
Opata	Sonora	Hrdlička	1904
Seri	Sonora	Felger	1991
Seri	Sonora	Griffen	1959
Seri	Sonora	Kroeber	1964
Seri	Sonora	Moser	1982
Seri	Sonora	Nolasco	1967
Tarahumara	Chihuahua	Bennett	1986
Tarahumara	Chihuahua	Fried	1951
Tarahumara	Chihuahua	Lumholtz	1902
Tarahumara	Chihuahua	Pennington	1963
Yaqui	Sonora	Ochoa Robles	1990
Yaqui	Sonora	Zayas	1992
WEST REGION			
Cora	Nayarit	Dahlgren Jordan	1994
Cora	Nayarit	De la Cerda Silva	1943
Cora	Nayarit	González Ramos	1992
Cora	Nayarit	Grimes	1972
Huichol	Jalisco	Basauri	1990
Huichol	Jalisco	Fabila	1959
Huichol	Jalisco	Grimes	1972
Huichol	Jalisco	Mata Torres	1982
Huichol	Jalisco	Zingg	1982
Tepehuani	Durango	Riley	1972
EAST REGION			
Huastec	Various	Alcorn	1984
Huastec	Veracruz	Bonfil Batalla	1969

TABLE 7.1 (cont.)

Name	State	First Author	Year of Publication
Nahua	Puebla	Huber	1990a, 1990b
Nahua	Puebla	Huber	Forthcoming
Nahua	Hidalgo	Montoya Briones	1964, 1969
Nahua	Veracruz	Münch Galindo	1983
Nahua	Puebla	Sanchez Flores	1982
Nahua	Veracruz	Sandstrom	1975, 1991
Nahua	Veracruz	Sandstrom	1986
Nahua	Puebla	Tuynman-Kret	1982
Nahua	Veracruz	Unidad Regional	1983
Nahua	Veracruz	Vargas Ramírez	1983, 1995
Nahua	Puebla	Vexler	1981
Nahua	Veracruz	Williams García	1957
Otomí	Various	Galinier	1987, 1990
Otomí	Hidalgo	Tranfo	1974
Tepehua	Veracruz	Williams García	1963
Totonac	Veracruz	Francisco Velasco	1985
Totonac	Various	Garma Navarro	1995
Totonac	Various	Ichon	1973
Totonac	Veracruz	Kelly	1953, 1956
Totonac	Puebla	Roldán Q.	1990

CENTRAL REGION

Name	State	First Author	Year of Publication
Chichimec	Guanajuato	Nava L.	1995
Nahua	Morelos	Álvarez Heydenreich	1976, 1987
Nahua	Various	Baytelman	1986
Nahua	Morelos	Lewis	1963
Nahua	Mexico	Madsen	1968
Nahua	Various	Nutini	1968, 1974
Nahua	Morelos	Redfield, M.	1928
Nahua	Morelos	Redfield, R.	1930
Nahua	Tlaxcala	Scheffler	1977
Purépecha	Michoacán	Beals	1973a
Purépecha	Michoacán	Larme	1985
Purépecha	Michoacán	Prado	1984

TABLE 7.1 (cont.)

Name	State	First Author	Year of Publication
Purépecha	Michoacán	Young	1978
Tlahuica	Mexico	Basauri	1990
Tlahuica	Mexico	Vázquez Rojas	1995

NORTH AND CENTRAL OAXACA REGION

Chinantec	Oaxaca	Stebbins	1984
Mazatec	Oaxaca	Incháustegui	1994
Zapotec	Oaxaca	Beltrán Morales	1982
Zapotec	Oaxaca	De la Fuente	1949
Zapotec	Oaxaca	Greene	1988
Zapotec	Oaxaca	Parsons	1936
Zapotec	Oaxaca	Taub	1992

SOUTHERN PACIFIC REGION

Amuzgo	Guerrero	Tapia García	1985
Chatino	Oaxaca	Bartolomé	1996
Mixtec	Oaxaca	Ibach	1981
Mixtec	Oaxaca	Katz	1992
Mixtec	Oaxaca	Mak	1959
Mixtec	Oaxaca	Monaghan	1995
Mixtec	Guerrero	Muñoz	1963
Mixtec	Oaxaca	Romney	1966
Tlapanec	Guerrero	Muñoz	1963
Trique	Oaxaca	García Alcaraz	1997

ISTHMUS OF TEHUANTEPEC REGION

Chontal	Oaxaca	Galante	1980
Chontal	Tabasco	Rubio	1995
Chontal	Oaxaca	Sesia	1992
Chontal	Oaxaca	Turner	1984
Huave	Oaxaca	Cheney	1972
Huave	Oaxaca	Dalton	1992
Huave	Oaxaca	Rita	1979
Huave	Oaxaca	Sesia	1992

TABLE 7.1 (cont.)

Name	State	First Author	Year of Publication
Huave	Oaxaca	Signorini	1979
Mixe	Oaxaca	Alvarado	1991
Mixe	Oaxaca	Beals	1973b
Mixe	Oaxaca	González Villanueva	1989
Mixe	Oaxaca	Kuroda	1993
Mixe	Oaxaca	Nahmad	1965

active male midwife, although other men have served as midwives in the recent past.

Geographic Distribution of Midwives

Table 7.2 shows that midwives are common in most indigenous groups from this part of Mesoamerica with the notable exception of the Kiliwa (and other Baja California groups), the Tarahumara, Cora, Huichol, and Tepehuani. In these western and northwestern groups, indigenous women often give birth alone or are attended by experienced female relatives. Curers may also be routinely present or called in to help when women experience problems. Midwives may be absent or scarce because these groups experienced an especially turbulent history and a once viable midwifery tradition was lost. Or, midwifery never developed as a medical specialty among these groups due to their having a relatively small population, a low population density, and relatively few births per year occurring over a relatively large geographic area. Only "generalist" healers like shamans are found under these circumstances.

The ecological conditions under which these groups live cannot support large, dense, populations. The terrain is often extremely rugged with high mountains cut by deep canyons (Cora, Huichol, Tarahumara). Most groups have access only to lands with poor soils composed of clay or rock (Tarahumara, Tepehuani) or that are subject to extreme variations in temperature, droughts, or prolonged periods of heavy rains (Kiliwa, Huichol, Tarahumara). Their precarious subsistence pattern, often consisting of a

TABLE 7.2: GEOGRAPHIC DISTRIBUTION OF MIDWIVES AND OTHER BIRTH ATTENDANTS FROM THE MEXICO–UNITED STATES BORDER TO THE ISTHMUS OF TEHUANTEPEC

Group	Absence or Scarcity of Midwives	Experienced Woman Present at Birth	Curer Routinely Present at Birth
NORTHWEST REGION			
Kiliwa	XXXX	XXXX	
Guarijío			
Kikapoo			
Mayo			
Opata			
Papago			
Pima			
Seri		XXXX	
Tarahumara	XXXX	XXXX	XXXX
Yaqui		XXXX	
WEST REGION			
Cora	XXXX	XXXX	XXXX
Huichol	XXXX	XXXX	
Tepehuani	XXXX	XXXX	XXXX
EAST REGION			
Huastec			
Nahua		XXXX	
Otomí			
Pame			
Popoloca			XXXX
Tepehua			
Totonac			
CENTRAL REGION			
Chichimec			
Mazahua			
Nahua			
Otomí			
Purépecha			
Tlahuica		XXXX	XXXX

TABLE 7.2 (cont.)

Group	Absence or Scarcity of Midwives	Experienced Woman Present at Birth	Curer Routinely Present at Birth
NORTH AND CENTRAL OAXACA REGION			
Chinantec			
Chocho			
Cuicatec			
Ixcatec			
Mazatec			
Zapotec			
SOUTHERN PACIFIC REGION			
Amuzgo			
Chatino			
Mixtec		XXXX	XXXX
Tlapanec			
Trique			XXXX
ISTHMUS OF TEHUANTEPEC REGION			
Chontal			
Huave			
Mixe		XXXX	XXXX
Popoluca			

mixture of agriculture, animal husbandry, fishing, hunting, or gathering is insufficient to support people unless a considerable number of people migrate to other regions in Mexico or to the United States in search of work in light industries (Kiliwa), the harvesting of tobacco or sugar cane (Cora, Tepehuani), etc. The Huichol and the Tarahumara live in two of the most isolated regions of Mexico, and the latter is classified by the Mexican government as "very highly marginalized" (Mellado Campos et al. 1994:706).

146   **Mesoamerican Healers**

Overview of the Midwife Role

PRENATAL CARE

Massaging pregnant women is an essential part of indigenous Mexican midwifery. Massage makes pregnant women more comfortable and is used to determine the position of the fetus and, when necessary, to change it. See Mellado Campos et al. (1989:94) for a good description of prenatal massage.

A more rigorous kind of massage used to change the position of the fetus is the *manteada*. A blanket (*manta*) is folded to form a thick sash and is placed underneath the pregnant woman's waist while she is lying down. The midwife straddles the woman and pulls firmly on each end of the sash two or three times. A technique related to the *manteada* consists of the midwife partially picking up a pregnant woman by her legs and shaking her in the manner of a bell (*campanear*). Table 7.3 shows that the *manteada* and similar techniques are found mostly in central Mexico and in north and central Oaxaca. The prenatal customs of binding a pregnant woman's abdomen with a sash, entering a *temazcal* (sweat bath), and having a procedure like a *limpia* (cleansing) performed are not as widely reported.

Like other indigenous Mesoamerican midwives, Hueyapan's midwives attach great importance to prenatal care. Natividad[2] claims to make ten to fifteen prenatal visits beginning during the second trimester.[3] The rest of Hueyapan's midwives make between one and four prenatal consultations. Occasionally, women contact a midwife for the first time just prior to birth (see also Lewis 1963:356; Sanchez Flores 1982:23; Vexler 1981:133). It is more common for the midwife to visit the client's home than vice versa.

In Hueyapan, only one midwife employs a *manteada*. However, all massage[4] women during their prenatal visits. The majority are also concerned about preventing and treating *mal aire*. Some, like Felicia and Rafaela, report applying an ointment during a massage,[5] while others perform *limpias*. For example, Natividad passes rue and elder sprigs, and an egg over a woman's entire body, but especially over the woman's abdomen. Medicinal teas prepared with rue, elder, and zapote leaves, aspirin, ribbons, sewing needles, porcupine spines, starfish, and sand dollars are also used (see also Álvarez Heydenreich 1976:94; Lewis 1963:357; Redfield 1930:135). Note the use of sharp, pointed objects to prevent the intrusion of a *mal aire*.[6]

Hueyapan's midwives may enter a *temazcal* with pregnant clients[7] with the goal of warming the body and making the bones, ligaments, and muscles of the pelvis flexible. Some pregnant women dislike entering the *temazcal*, in which case a red hot stone is placed in a bucket of water, and the woman stands over the bucket with a blanket over her head to catch the rising steam. Regardless, Hueyapan's midwives caution that too much heat can harm the unborn child.[8] They also recommend that pregnant women remain as active as possible although they should avoid lifting heavy objects.

CHILDBIRTH

Ana and Pablo generally require that clients come to their homes to give birth, and because of this, Pablo sees a similarity between his practice and that of a doctor's. The other midwives report that women prefer to give birth in their own homes, and if possible, in a room separate from the rest of the house. If the house has just one room, a section is screened off with a hanging blanket.

In general, only the midwife and one other adult woman (e.g., the woman's mother, mother-in-law, or aunt) are present in the birth room. Some midwives, such as Ana and Rafaela, prefer to deliver babies without assistants. In contrast, Mercedes generally brings along her husband to administer an injection to reduce a laboring woman's pain. Pablo typically works with his wife. He recognizes that women feel more comfortable with a woman present when they are giving birth, and when bathing and dressing afterward. Midwives say that some women discourage their husbands from actively assisting in birth while others permit it. Children are made to leave the home altogether, or if it is night, are put to bed.[9]

Prior to the delivery, some of Hueyapan's midwives light a candle on the household altar[10] and say a prayer. As labor proceeds, many routinely administer a medicinal tea to speed delivery. Ana administers injections of oxytocin syntocinon for this purpose.[11] The practice of midwives administering herbal teas is reported for twenty indigenous groups spanning all seven subregions.

The kneeling or squatting birth position is reported for twenty-five indigenous groups and for all seven subregions. The option of lying down while giving birth is reported for eight groups. A semi-erect birth position is reported for the Tarahumara, Cora, and Huichol. Perhaps the rarest birth

TABLE 7.3: PRENATAL ACTIVITIES OF INDIGENOUS MIDWIVES FROM THE MEXICO–UNITED STATES BORDER TO THE ISTHMUS OF TEHUANTEPEC

Group	Manteada or Campanear	Prenatal Use of a Sash	Prenatal Use of Temazcal	Prenatal Ritual
NORTHWEST REGION				
Baja Groups				
Guarijío				
Kikapoo		XXXX		
Mayo				
Opata				
Papago				
Pima	XXXX			
Seri		XXXX		
Tarahumara				XXXX
Yaqui				
WEST REGION				
Cora				
Huichol				
Tepehuani	XXXX			
EAST REGION				
Huastec				
Nahua	XXXX	XXXX	XXXX	XXXX
Otomí				XXXX
Pame				
Popoloca				
Tepehua				
Totonac	XXXX	XXXX		
CENTRAL REGION				
Chichimec				
Mazahua		XXXX		
Nahua	XXXX		XXXX	
Otomí	XXXX			
Purépecha	XXXX			
Tlahuica				

TABLE 7.3 (cont.)

Group	Manteada or Campanear	Prenatal Use of a Sash	Prenatal Use of Temazcal	Prenatal Ritual
NORTH AND CENTRAL OAXACA REGION				
Chinantec				
Chocho	XXXX			
Cuicatec				
Ixcatec	XXXX			
Mazatec	XXXX			XXXX
Zapotec	XXXX		XXXX	
SOUTHERN PACIFIC REGION				
Amuzgo				
Chatino	XXXX			
Mixtec		XXXX		
Tlapanec	XXXX			XXXX
Trique			XXXX	XXXX
ISTHMUS OF TEHUANTEPEC REGION				
Chontal	XXXX			XXXX
Huave				
Mixe			XXXX	
Popoluca				

position is that reported by Seri women in the 1950s. The mother sits in a reclining position in the lap of one midwife who is sitting on the ground with her knees spread and doubled under her. A second midwife sits on the ground facing the parturient with her hands on the ground beneath her skirt, waiting for the baby to be born (Moser 1982 : 225).

Most of Hueyapan's midwives prefer that women kneel or squat when giving birth (see also Sanchez Flores 1982 : 24). Women steady themselves by holding onto a low stool, a rope hung from a rafter, a pole set into the dirt floor, or a wooden crate. Blankets, a sheet, clean rags, or a *petate* (palm mat) are placed underneath the woman.[12] Most midwives position themselves behind the woman and put their arms around the woman's abdomen to squeeze. Sometimes, midwives position themselves at the squatting woman's side or in front of her. When women give birth lying down, midwives stand at the foot of the bed facing the woman. Most of Hueyapan's midwives report applying quite a bit of pressure to the woman's abdomen to facilitate the child's birth. In at least five indigenous groups, including the Nahuas of the eastern region, a woman is tightly bound with a sash while giving birth.

The majority of infants begin breathing on their own shortly after birth. If they do not, Hueyapan's midwives sprinkle alcohol or water on the infant's face, back, or chest, gently pull on the umbilical cord, or make a loud noise near the infant's ear by tapping on a hoe or by having a rooster crow. After the delivery, they clean the newborn's eyes, nose, and mouth, tie the umbilical cord, and cut it with a small knife, scissors, or a sharp piece of cane several finger widths away from the umbilicus.[13] A piece of cotton gauze or cloth is placed around the end of the cord, and the cord itself is wrapped in cloth and held in place by a small belt. The baby's lower body is wrapped with a square piece of cloth or a diaper which is held in place with another belt. Some midwives bathe an infant in warm water about an hour after birth; others wait until the following day. Regardless, the infant is wrapped in warm cloths and placed in a warm blanket.[14]

A sharp piece of cane or bamboo is the most commonly reported tool used to cut the umbilical cord by midwives from these forty-one indigenous groups. Some midwives believe metal cutting tools such as scissors, knives, razor blades, machetes, and sickle blades may harm infants, and conscientiously avoid them. Nevertheless, they are used widely. Rarest of all is the use of stone (e.g., obsidian) blades to cut umbilical cords. Fifty years ago, stone blades were reportedly used by the Huichol and Tarahumara. Midwives from eleven different groups customarily cauterize the end of the cord attached to the newborn child.

After the placenta is expelled, a midwife in Hueyapan helps clean and dress the mother, bind her waist with a sash (*ilpicat*), and place a ball of cloth (*fiador*) underneath the sash to apply abdominal pressure. The postnatal use of the sash is found among eighteen indigenous groups and in all seven subregions. In Hueyapan, a candle is sometimes placed on the household altar as an offering of thanks. With the exception of the mother, Natividad says all of the adults present "drink a shot [of *aguardiente*] and [smoke] a cigarette because everyone is happy about the new being which has just arrived." A woman's husband typically buries the afterbirth and pieces of cloth soiled during birth.[15]

PROLONGED LABOR AND PROBLEMATIC BIRTHS

For prolonged labor, Hueyapan's midwives massage and apply pressure to the woman's stomach, and request that the woman "push" harder. They may also ritually cleanse the woman of *mal aire*.[16] Excessive bleeding is stopped by having women lie down and by administering herbal teas, wines, and patent medicines (see also Baytelman 1986:53; Madsen 1968:102). In cases of a breech birth, several midwives seek the assistance of another midwife (usually Natividad or Ana) or that of a medical doctor (see also Münch Galindo 1983:126; Sanchez Flores 1982:23). If the placenta is slow in coming, midwives place the end of a woman's braided hair in her mouth in an effort to induce gagging and help her "bear down."[17] Midwives stimulating the gag reflex to encourage the birth of the placenta is reported for fourteen indigenous groups. Other methods of dealing with this problem include massage, shaking a woman's abdomen, and having the woman drink an herbal tea.

POSTPARTUM CARE

In Hueyapan, the midwife typically checks up on mother and baby the day after birth. She may bathe the mother with warm water at that time,[18] but most wait two or three days. Hueyapan's midwives are generally expected to return to the mother's house three times after birth to bathe the infant, massage and rebind the woman's abdomen with a sash, and wash soiled blankets and clothing.[19] Midwives report that the latter duty is especially burdensome. There are reports of midwives in six indigenous groups where it is customary for them to wash blankets and clothing.

In the 1950s, it was common for women from Hueyapan to take sweat baths[20] the fourth, eighth, and twelfth day after birth (Nutini and Isaac 1974:188). This is less common now.[21] When Hueyapan's midwives accompany their clients to the sweat bath, they use bunches of herbs referred to as a "*pezma*" to fan and warm the woman's body, especially her vagina.[22] Some midwives also rub *aguardiente* on the woman's body to heat it. After the final sweat bath, the danger of family members becoming ill with *quemadas* is minimized.[23] *Quemadas* are skin rashes thought to be caused by contact with

TABLE 7.4: POSTPARTUM ACTIVITIES IN INDIGENOUS GROUPS FROM THE MEXICO–UNITED STATES BORDER TO THE ISTHMUS OF TEHUANTEPEC

Group	Postpartum Temazcal	Ritual, No Specialist	Ritual with Midwife	Ritual with Curer
NORTHWEST REGION				
Kiliwa	XXXX			
Guarijío				
Kikapoo				
Mayo				
Opata				
Papago				
Pima				
Seri		XXXX		
Tarahumara				XXXX
Yaqui				
WEST REGION				
Cora		XXXX		
Huichol		XXXX	XXXX	XXXX
Tepehuani		XXXX		
EAST REGION				
Huastec			XXXX	
Nahua	XXXX	XXXX	XXXX	XXXX
Otomí	XXXX		XXXX	XXXX
Pame				
Popoloca				
Tepehua	XXXX		XXXX	
Totonac	XXXX		XXXX	XXXX
CENTRAL REGION				
Chichimec				
Mazahua				
Nahua	XXXX	XXXX		
Otomí				
Purépecha				
Tlahuica	XXXX			

TABLE 7.4 (cont.)

Group	Postpartum Temazcal	Ritual, No Specialist	Ritual with Midwife	Ritual with Curer
NORTH AND CENTRAL OAXACA REGION				
Chinantec				
Chocho	XXXX			
Cuicatec				
Ixcatec	XXXX			
Mazatec	XXXX			
Zapotec	XXXX	XXXX		
SOUTHERN PACIFIC REGION				
Amuzgo				
Chatino		XXXX		
Mixtec	XXXX	XXXX	XXXX	XXXX
Tlapanec	XXXX	XXXX		
Trique	XXXX			
ISTHMUS OF TEHUANTEPEC REGION				
Chontal		XXXX		
Huave				
Mixe	XXXX	XXXX	XXXX	XXXX
Popoluca				

a woman shortly after she has given birth. Table 7.4 indicates that the postpartum use of the *temazcal* is found among many indigenous groups, with the notable exception of those from the western and northwestern regions, and other groups from hot, low-lying areas.

In some Nahua communities, *limpias* are performed instead of having the mother enter the *temazcal* (Montoya Briones and Moedano Navarro 1969:282; Nutini 1968:89; Nutini and Isaac 1974). Postpartum *limpias* are reported for six indigenous groups; four are from the eastern region: Huastec, Nahua, Tepehua, and Totonac.

Postpartum Rituals Involving Midwives

Table 7.4 also shows that postpartum rituals involving midwives[24] are generally found in the eastern region. Huastec, Nahua, Otomí, Tepehua, and Totonac midwives (and shamans) show considerable concern about offending supernatural beings with the afterbirth, blood, and amniotic fluid of recently delivered women (Galinier 1987:427; Ichon 1973; Kelly 1953: 180–181; Mellado Campos et al. 1994:802; Roldán 1990:94–95; Sandstrom and Sandstrom 1986:162, 201–202; Williams García 1957:52–54, 1963). For example, Nahua midwives from Ixhuatlán de Madero perform a ritual cleansing of mother and child soon after birth to protect them from supernatural harm, and offer candles, *coyol* palm adornments, *copal* incense, and food to the earth spirit to make recompense[25] (Sandstrom 1991:272, 296; Sandstrom and Sandstrom 1986:72, 78). On the fourth day after birth either the midwife or a special ritual kinswoman (the *axochiteonaj*, or water-flower godmother) ritually cleanses the newborn child by bathing him in water in which herbs have been soaked.[26]

The concern midwives (and shamans) from the eastern region show toward cleansing and returning the earth and people to a state of purity and balanced harmony may very well be due to the fact that the Huasteca was a part of the eastern region dedicated to the worship of Tlazolteotl prior to the Spanish Conquest. Tlazolteotl was the goddess of filth who consumed human sin (see Sandstrom and Sandstrom 1986:282–286; 296–300; 311–317).

In addition to attending birth, providing prenatal and postnatal care, and leading postpartum rituals, Nahua, Tepehua, and Totonac midwives play an important role in healing ill patients who may be under the more general care of shamans. For example, Ichon (1973) reports that the Totonac use the *temazcal* for general curative purposes. Godparents of a sick child may lay him down in a *temazcal* in which a midwife is present. She implores the god of the *temazcal* hearth to restore the child's health.

The role of Nahua midwives in the eastern region is the most extensive of all since they participate in village-wide religious ceremonies. The Xochitlalia is a crop fertility ritual. The Tlacatelilis is a winter solstice ceremony meaning "to cause to be born." On both occasions, the midwife serves as an incense dancer. On the latter occasion, the midwife leads young girls in a procession from house to house (Sandstrom 1991:282–283; Sandstrom and Sandstrom 1986:39, 72–73).

Midwifery Combined with Other Healing Roles

Six of the sixteen individuals who are currently active as midwives in Hue-yapan are also curers. They see patients on a regular basis who are diagnosed with illnesses with supernatural etiologies (e.g., soul loss). There is also one woman who serves as a midwife, curer, and bonesetter.

Mata Pinzón et al. (1994:657) note that midwives do not typically limit themselves to birth and pre- and postnatal care. They are often asked to treat sterility and illnesses that frequently affect pregnant women and new-born infants such as *susto* (fright), *mal de ojo* (evil eye), and *caída de mollera* (fallen fontanelle). Thus, it is not surprising that individuals frequently combine midwifery with other kinds of healing roles. Developing an expertise in two or more healing specialties occurs gradually over time. Clients occasionally ask midwives to recommend an herbal remedy, massage an abdominal complaint or painful joint, or perform a ritual for an illness that is not of a gynecological or obstetrical nature. If these requests become frequent, residents come to recognize them as midwife-curers, midwife-bonesetters, midwife-herbalists, and so on.

Indigenous Mexicans combine midwifery with at least eighteen other kinds of medical specialties. Table 7.5 contains data on the four medical specialties most commonly combined with midwifery.[27] The variability illustrated in Table 7.5 is patterned. Pearson's *r* was calculated to test the hypothesis that the number of healing roles combined with midwifery is positively correlated with population size. Mellado Campos et al. (1994) provide data on population size for thirty-six groups. The five groups in which midwives are scarce or absent are excluded from analysis. Pearson's *r* was found to have a value of .494 with a one-tailed significance level of .002. If the number of healing roles combined with midwifery is used as an indicator of medical specialization in general, then it can be concluded that larger groups tend to support more kinds of medical specialties than smaller ones.

Kinds of Conceptual Models Employed by Midwives

Different kinds of Mesoamerican healers can be placed on a scale according to the type of conceptual model they use to explain and treat illness. Shamans and spiritualists would be found near the sacred end of the scale; physicians, nurses, social workers, herbalists, and bonesetters would fall near the secular end. Indigenous midwives would fall somewhere in the middle since

**TABLE 7.5: THE FOUR MOST COMMON MEDICAL SPECIALTIES COMBINED
WITH MIDWIFERY FROM THE MEXICO–UNITED STATES BORDER TO
THE ISTHMUS OF TEHUANTEPEC**

Group	Curer	Massager	Bonesetter	Herbalist
NORTHWEST REGION				
Baja Groups				
Guarijío		XXXX		
Kikapoo				
Mayo	XXXX	XXXX		
Opata				
Papago				
Pima	XXXX	XXXX		
Seri				
Tarahumara	XXXX	XXXX		
Yaqui	XXXX	XXXX		
WEST REGION				
Cora	XXXX	XXXX	XXXX	XXXX
Huichol				
Tepehuani		XXXX		
EAST REGION				
Huastec	XXXX	XXXX		
Nahua	XXXX		XXXX	
Otomí	XXXX			
Pame				
Popoloca				
Tepehua	XXXX			
Totonac	XXXX	XXXX	XXXX	XXXX
CENTRAL REGION				
Chichimec	XXXX	XXXX		
Mazahua		XXXX		XXXX
Nahua	XXXX	XXXX	XXXX	
Otomí	XXXX	XXXX	XXXX	XXXX
Purépecha	XXXX	XXXX	XXXX	
Tlahuica		XXXX		

TABLE 7.5 (cont.)

Group	Curer	Massager	Bonesetter	Herbalist
NORTH AND CENTRAL OAXACA REGION				
Chinantec	XXXX			
Chocho				
Cuicatec	XXXX			
Ixcatec	XXXX		XXXX	XXXX
Mazatec	XXXX	XXXX	XXXX	XXXX
Zapotec	XXXX	XXXX		
SOUTHERN PACIFIC REGION				
Amuzgo	XXXX	XXXX		
Chatino	XXXX			XXXX
Mixtec	XXXX			XXXX
Tlapanec	XXXX		XXXX	
Trique				
ISTHMUS OF TEHUANTEPEC REGION				
Chontal	XXXX			XXXX
Huave	XXXX			XXXX
Mixe	XXXX	XXXX	XXXX	XXXX
Popoluca	XXXX			XXXX

they combine both supernatural and naturalistic models for understanding pregnancy, childbirth, and gynecological problems.

For example, Hueyapan's midwives employ a variety of mechanical and pharmaceutical "tools" when dealing with pregnancy and childbirth (e.g., massage, herbal teas to stimulate contractions, a sharp piece of cane to cut the umbilical cord, etc.). Observation and experience guide midwives in the use of these tools. On the other hand, when faced with an uncommon or problematic birth outcome, midwives may employ a supernatural explanation. For example, prenatal discomfort is attributed to spirit intrusion, a cleft palate is caused by an eclipse of the moon (a deity), a woman is sterile because she buried one of her dolls when she was a child, and so on. This mixing of supernatural and naturalistic models is also evident in the accounts of midwives being recruited.

Secular Routes to the Midwife Role

Ethnographers report three secular "recruitment paths" to the midwife role. These paths are as follows: (1) being self-taught (e.g., learning from giving birth to one's own children) (eighteen groups), (2) responding to an urgent request for help from an expectant mother (eight groups), and (3) serving an apprenticeship to another midwife (twenty-seven groups).

The distinction among these paths is not always clear. In Hueyapan, women who report being self-taught say that they also responded to an urgent request for help prior to becoming midwives. Recruitment paths 1 and 2 are probably not separate paths but two components of one path. Table 7.6 indicates seven midwives in Hueyapan were pressed into service by a pregnant woman whose birth was imminent. Five served an apprenticeship[28] with a relative such as a mother or sister-in-law. Many had ample opportunity to observe healers at work even though they may not have been directly trained by them. Of thirteen midwives for whom information is available, nine report having one or more relatives who were midwives. Seven also report having relatives who were curers, and two had relatives who were bonesetters. Traditional healing tends to run in families.[29] Mercedes is exceptional in this regard: " . . . my grandmother, grandfather, mother, and father—all of them were midwives. My mother's father was a bonesetter and my grandmothers were curers." Reports of midwives having relatives who are healers are fairly common among other indigenous groups. Twenty-three groups have midwives with relatives who are midwives; six groups have midwives from families with curers; two have midwives with bonesetters as family members.

Sacred Routes to the Midwife Role

Although divine callings are described in some detail by ethnographers of Maya midwifery, they are apparently somewhat uncommon for midwives living between the Isthmus of Tehuantepec and the Mexico–United States border. Divine callings are indicated for Chatino, Cora, Huave, Mazahua, Mazatec, Nahua, Popoloca, Purépecha, and Trique midwives.

Turning again to Table 7.6, the recruitment of a midwife in Hueyapan is seen to combine secular components, sacred ones, or both. Antonia, for example, received a three-component sacred calling, apprenticed herself to a traditional midwife, and responded to an urgent request by a woman who was

TABLE 7.6: SECULAR AND SACRED RECRUITMENT PATHS OF HUEYAPAN'S MIDWIVES

Name	Section	Characteristics of a Secular Calling		Characteristics of a Sacred Calling		
		Apprentice to Midwife	Emergency	Dreams	Illness	Revealed by Curer
GROUP I: NO ASPECTS OF A SACRED CALLING						
Gabriela	I	No	Yes	No	No	No
Francisca	6	Yes	No	No	No	No
Ana	I	No	Yes	No	No	No
Isabel	10	No	Yes	No	No	No
Pablo	7	No	Missing	No	No	No
GROUP II: ONE ASPECT OF A SACRED CALLING						
Ernestina	6	Yes	Yes	Yes	No	No
Margarita	2	Missing	Yes	Yes	No	Missing
Teresa	8	No	No	Yes	No	No
GROUP III: TWO ASPECTS OF A SACRED CALLING						
Natividad	2	Yes	Missing	Yes	Yes	No
Mercedes	10	Yes	No	Yes	Yes	No
Francisca	7	No	Yes	No	Yes	Yes
GROUP IV: THREE ASPECTS OF A SACRED CALLING						
Antonia	6	Yes	Yes	Yes	Yes	Yes
Josefa	3	Missing	Missing	Yes	Yes	Yes
Felicia	3	Missing	Missing	Yes	Yes	Yes
Rafaela	8	No	No	Yes	Yes	Yes
	Total	5	7	9	7	5
		(N = 12)	(N = 11)	(N = 15)	(N = 15)	(N = 14)

about to deliver. Midwives[30] generally experience premonitory dreams and illnesses between the ages of eight and fifteen, although some are well into adulthood when this happens. Their call comes from *tamatinime*, all-knowing supernatural guardians of nature who appear to people in the form of lightning bolts, snakes, little children, and old people in traditional clothing.

Hueyapan's midwives can be ranked by the degree to which their calling is sacred. The top of Table 7.6 shows that five midwives have a purely "secular" calling. None of them report experiencing premonitory dreams, illnesses, or a revelation by a curer that they have a "gift" for midwifery. Four midwives listed at the bottom experienced all three characteristics of a divine calling. This ranking is not recognized by the midwives themselves. However, as an etic construct it is useful in predicting the likelihood that a midwife will collaborate with doctors and nurses. This point is discussed in the following section.

Collaboration with Doctors and Nurses

Collaboration is understood here as regularly assisting, consulting with, or providing childbirth-related data to formally trained health personnel. Five of Hueyapan's traditional midwives report this level of cooperation: Ana, Isabel, Pablo, Ernestina, and Teresa.

For example, Isabel[31] refers pregnant women who are at high risk in Section 10 to the doctor at the head town's Secretaría de Salubridad y Asistencia clinic. She also monitors high-risk births when the doctor is on vacation or otherwise outside of the community, files monthly reports, and requests that parents vaccinate infants. In return, the doctor advises low-risk patients to maintain contact with Isabel.

Teresa[32] reports an even higher level of cooperation. In addition to attending low-risk pregnancies, handling clients when the doctor is on vacation, and referring high-risk women, she vaccinates children, makes home visits with doctors and nurses, and regularly monitors pregnant women from her section. She also advises women to visit the doctor to have their blood pressure monitored and discuss their diet. Prior to a delivery, she consults with the doctor and tells the pregnant woman's family to prepare clean clothing. After delivery, she records birth-related information and takes it to the clinic.

Table 7.7 shows that only midwives with a secular calling collaborate with doctors and nurses. The seven midwives with two or three components of a divine calling do not. Fischer's Exact Test indicates it is very unlikely that this association is due to chance. Evidently, midwives with a sacred calling view midwifery differently than those with a secular calling. We suspect divinely called midwives are reluctant to cooperate with doctors or nurses because

TABLE 7.7: RECRUITMENT (SECULAR VS. SACRED) OF HUEYAPAN'S
MIDWIVES AND REGULAR COLLABORATIONS WITH A DOCTOR, NURSE,
OR CLINIC REGULARLY

Type of Recruitment	Collaborates with Doctor or Nurse on a Regular Basis		Total
	No	Yes	
Secular	3	5	8
Sacred*	7	0	7
TOTALS	10	5	15
Fischer's Exact Test (N = 15)	Exact Significance .026 (Two-Sided)		Exact Significance .019 (One-Sided)

*Midwives with two or three characteristics of a divine calling.

they want to avoid the appearance of being motivated by money, a motivation that they and others may feel is inconsistent with service to a higher power.

Cooperation among Midwives

Midwives from Hueyapan are reluctant to cooperate with each other. In general, competition, envy, and disdain color the way Hueyapan's midwives relate. Midwives avoid cooperation because this might lead to their competing with each other or being blamed for problems for which they are not responsible. However, emergencies do sometimes lead to cooperation. For example, Ana has a reputation for being able to handle problematic births, and the other midwives who reside in the *cabecera* (e.g., Natividad, Ligia, Margarita, Gabriela) consult her when they encounter a life-and-death situation.[33] The only other context in which cooperation takes place is in the training of relatives to become midwives.

The Social-Psychological Impact of Becoming a Midwife

EMOTIONAL REACTIONS

Seven midwives report being fearful and six say they felt ashamed at the time they began their practice. Midwives are initially ashamed because they knew so little about midwifery and because they believe people suspect them of becoming midwives in order to earn money. They are initially afraid of encountering problems during childbirth, especially those that might lead to the death of the infant or mother, and they fear being blamed for these deaths.

These strong emotional reactions are related to the midwife's age: the older the midwife, the more likely she felt ashamed or afraid prior to becoming a midwife. This makes sense since older midwives generally began practicing when a woman's role in Hueyapan was very narrowly defined. In the past, women were strongly discouraged from handling money and working outside of the domestic sphere. Nor were they socialized to take charge in life-and-death situations.

STATUS AMBIGUITY AND ROLE CONFLICT

Lois and Benjamin Paul note that individuals who petition the assistance of midwives from the Zutuhil Maya community of San Pedro la Laguna couch their requests in ceremonial speech, kiss their hands, offer them food and drink, and send them gifts on festive occasions (Paul 1975; Paul and Paul 1975). They are respected for their deep commitment to their profession, technical competence, and special relationship to the supernatural world (e.g., performing rituals designed to ensure the survival of children with special destinies or to protect newborn infants from the destructive spirits of older siblings). Nevertheless, there is "a sharp disjunction between the standards governing the behavior of women in San Pedro and the behavior required of the midwife" (Paul and Paul 1975:139; see also Vexler 1981: 164). Others may criticize her because she is assertive, works outside the domestic sphere, and travels alone at night. In addition, a midwife's husband often resents his wife's unpredictable absences and objects to the taunts of his peers, who insinuate he is living from his wife's money.

In Hueyapan, former clients may greet a midwife in the street using ceremonial speech and respectful terms of address such as "doña," and some even bow slightly. Sometimes, people ask midwives to attend the baptisms of the children they deliver or invite them to a soft drink, beer, or shot of *aguardiente* when they meet in the street. However, ten midwives report they have been criticized; four say their husbands have been criticized too. Husbands may suspect their wives of having extramarital affairs; they may get upset when neighbors greet and bow to their wives; and neighbors may envy and become critical of midwives when they hear of the gifts and cash they receive.

Socioeconomic Status of Midwives

GENDER

Many ethnographers give the impression that Mexican midwives are always women. However, Table 7.8 shows there are many indigenous groups where at least some midwives are male. Based upon our reading of Mellado Campos et al. (1994), we suspect most men who practice midwifery start out as curers and then extend their healing role to include birth and pre- and postnatal care. Male midwives like Pablo, who practices midwifery and no other healing role, are probably rare.

Why male midwives are found in some indigenous groups but not in others is puzzling. We suspect that some parts of Mexico are so lightly populated and remote that pregnant women are forced to seek out the help of men because there are no women in the area willing or able to assist them. Some of these men are curers or the pregnant women's husbands. We have little reason to believe that male midwives tend to be found among groups where the value people place on female modesty is relaxed. The presence of a woman's husband, her children, or a male curer at "normal" (unproblematic) births can be used as indicators of relaxed attitudes toward female modesty. Table 7.8 shows that there is no clear association between male midwives and any of these three indicators.

AGE AND MARITAL STATUS

The average age of indigenous midwives is difficult to compute reliably because (1) midwives may not accurately recall their age or year of birth, and (2) the sample of midwives whose ages an ethnographer reports may not be representative of all of the midwives in the community. Nevertheless, estimates of the mean age of midwives are worth examining since a relatively high mean age may indicate that a midwifery tradition is dying out, with few or no young people being recruited to the role.

Hueyapan's midwives[34] are relatively young compared to midwives from other ethnic groups (Montoya Briones and Moedano Navarro 1969:281; Nutini and Isaac 1974:176; Sandstrom 1975:93, 260; Sandstrom 1991:139;

TABLE 7.8: MALE MIDWIVES, HUSBAND, CHILDREN, AND MALE CURER PRESENT AT BIRTH FROM THE MEXICO–UNITED STATES BORDER TO THE ISTHMUS OF TEHUANTEPEC

Group	Male Midwives	Husband Present	Children Present	Male Curer Routinely Present
NORTHWEST REGION				
Kiliwa		XXXX		
Guarijío		XXXX		
Kikapoo				
Mayo	XXXX			
Opata			XXXX	
Papago				
Pima				
Seri			XXXX	
Tarahumara	XXXX	XXXX		XXXX
Yaqui	XXXX	XXXX	XXXX	
WEST REGION				
Cora	XXXX	XXXX		XXXX
Huichol		XXXX		
Tepehuani	XXXX	XXXX		XXXX
EAST REGION				
Huastec		XXXX		
Nahua	XXXX	XXXX		
Otomí		XXXX	XXXX	
Pame	XXXX			
Popoloca				XXXX
Tepehua	XXXX			
Totonac		XXXX		
CENTRAL REGION				
Chichimec		XXXX		
Mazahua				
Nahua	XXXX	XXXX		
Otomí				
Purépecha	XXXX	XXXX		
Tlahuica				XXXX

TABLE 7.8 (cont.)

Group	Male Midwives	Husband Present	Children Present	Male Curer Routinely Present
NORTH AND CENTRAL OAXACA REGION				
Chinantec	XXXX			
Chocho				
Cuicatec				
Ixcatec		XXXX		
Mazatec	XXXX	XXXX		XXXX
Zapotec	XXXX	XXXX		
SOUTHERN PACIFIC REGION				
Amuzgo	XXXX			
Chatino	XXXX			
Mixtec	XXXX	XXXX		XXXX
Tlapanec	XXXX	XXXX		
Trique		XXXX		XXXX
ISTHMUS OF TEHUANTEPEC REGION				
Chontal	XXXX	XXXX		
Huave	XXXX	XXXX		
Mixe	XXXX	XXXX		XXXX
Popoluca				

Sandstrom and Sandstrom 1986:72; Unidad Regional de Acayucan 1983: 61; Vexler 1981:41, 57). In 1996, Hueyapan's midwives ranged in age from 16 to 88 years old. The mean age was 53 ($N = 16$), a mean similar to that of the Totonacs and groups in central Mexico.[35] (See Table 7.9.)

Somewhat surprisingly, age is unrelated to the likelihood that a midwife cooperates with a doctor or nurse in Hueyapan. However, three of the oldest midwives cooperate with other midwives. None of the midwives under sixty years old do. We hypothesize that older midwives can afford to be more cooperative than younger midwives because older midwives already have an established and relatively large client base. In addition, interview materials suggest that the oldest midwives would actually like to have fewer clients due to declining health or energy.

TABLE 7.9: MEAN AGE OF MIDWIVES IN INDIGENOUS GROUPS FROM THE MEXICO–UNITED STATES BORDER TO THE ISTHMUS OF TEHUANTEPEC

Location of Group	Group	Mean Age
Northwest	Guarijío	56
	Mayo	67
	Tarahumara	66
West	Cora	66
East	Huastec	64
	Nahua	53
	Popoloca	65
	Totonac	50
Central	Mazahua	53
	Nahua	52
	Otomí	54
North and Central Oaxaca	Cuicatec	57
	Ixcatec	68
	Mazatec	59
Southern Pacific	Amuzgo	59
	Mixtec	60
	Tlapanec	51
Isthmus of Tehuantepec	Chontal	58
	Huave	57

COMPENSATION AND ECONOMIC STATUS

In the mid-1980s, Hueyapan's midwives accepted whatever their clients felt was appropriate for their attending births. However, by April of 1996, some midwives charged a fixed fee. Compensation varies between the equivalent of one to fifteen days' wages paid for agricultural work in Hueyapan (approximately $3 to $47 US). They also receive between $0.65 and $1.35 US for a prenatal massage. In addition to cash, midwives may receive small gifts of food, cigarettes, or liquor when clients first come to their homes to request their services, and during subsequent prenatal and postnatal visits. The level at which Hueyapan's midwives are compensated is comparable to that of midwives in other Nahua communities (Lewis 1963:355–356,

361; Montoya Briones 1964:60, 103; Nutini and Isaac 1974; Redfield 1928: 104; Redfield 1930:136; Tuynman-Kret 1982:23, 52; Vexler 1981:117, 135, 137).

In 1996, Hueyapan's midwives varied with respect to their economic status. Five midwives are very poor by local standards. For example, Josefa lives in a small, two-room, wood plank home with a tar paper roof and a packed earth floor. She uses firewood to cook in a ground-level hearth and does not own a bed, table, or chairs. At the other extreme are four midwives who live in households approaching that of Ana's. Ana lives in a four-room cement block home, with plaster walls, a tile roof, and a cement floor. She owns beds, tables, chairs, and a television. Five others have an intermediate status. None of Hueyapan's midwives are wealthy by local standards, although some have improved their standard of living relative to their family of origin.

SOCIOECONOMIC STATUS OF FAMILY OF ORIGIN

All of Hueyapan's midwives report growing up in poor or very poor families. Of the thirteen midwives for whom we have information, six experienced the death of one or both of their parents prior to their marrying. Some were forced to live with a relative, work at an early age, and forego attending school. When Ana was growing up, she lived in poverty in a household headed by her mother. Her father drank heavily, drained the family of resources, and was often absent. Shortly after she married, her husband abandoned her and her two young children. Fortunately, she found work in the *cabecera*'s clinic helping with cleaning chores. She later became a midwife with the encouragement and training of the clinic's doctor.

Caseload

The amount of time indigenous Mexican midwives work is difficult to determine precisely. Although Mellado Campos et al. (1994) report that a few midwives work full time, most work part time with their remaining time spent in childcare, crafts work, agriculture, or animal husbandry. Consider the case of Hueyapan. In 1983, 281 births were recorded at the civil registry. If Hueyapan's ten active midwives had attended all of these births, they would have averaged about twenty-eight deliveries each. However, a 1983 survey of forty-nine women from the head town, ages fifteen to forty-five, revealed that only 71.6 percent reported consulting midwives when they were pregnant.[36] If this is taken into account, each midwife would have a yearly average of approximately twenty deliveries. If it is assumed that midwives visit women three times before and three times after they deliver, then each midwife made 141 house calls in 1983, an average of 2.7 each week. Further adjustments must be made to these estimates because (1) a percentage of births were not recorded at Hueyapan's town hall, (2) some midwives reported treating a few women from other communities, (3) two midwives (Natividad and Ana) were considerably more active than others, and (4) midwives reported that some women request fewer than three prenatal and three postnatal visits.[37]

Training Courses

Mexico has made a major effort to formally train traditional midwives. They participate in training programs sponsored by (1) the Ministry of Health (Secretaría de Salubridad y Asistencia, or SSA), (2) the Mexican Social Security Institute (Instituto Mexicano de Seguro Social, or IMSS), or (3) the National Indian Institute (Instituto Nacional Indigenista, or INI).

Hueyapan's SSA clinic is located in the *cabecera*. It tends to serve people in the immediate vicinity (Sections 1–5) as well as those most distant from Hueyapan's head town (Sections 9 and 10). Four of the seven midwives who received SSA-sponsored training are from these sections. An IMSS clinic is located in Section 6, and generally serves residents from Sections 6, 7, and 8. Two midwives report training by IMSS-Solidaridad, and live in this part of the municipality.[38] Three midwives received training under the auspices of INI, which has established a large number of regional organizations of traditional healers throughout the country. One clinic for midwives, curers, and bonesetters recently opened in Hueyapan's head town. Regional organizations of traditional healers were formed by INI to reinforce the knowledge of traditional healers, legalize their practice, and provide people with an alternative to the formal health sector (Congreso Nacional de Médicos Tradicionales Indígenas 1992).

Table 7.10 shows that traditional medical organizations (TMOs) tend to be absent among very acculturated indigenous groups and groups in the southern Pacific region. The likelihood of INI establishing a TMO is also positively correlated with the size of an indigenous group. Table 7.11 shows the results of a statistical analysis supporting this statement.

Concluding Remarks

The medical ecological perspective can be used to understand the relationship of ecological variables to demographic ones (population size and density), which have, in turn, an important influence on midwifery in the forty-one groups of this region: (1) indigenous groups with large populations are more likely than smaller ones to have one or more INI-sponsored TMOS, and (2) midwives are uncommon or absent in groups with low population densities. We also hypothesize that (3) male midwives are more likely to be found in isolated and sparsely populated hamlets than in more densely populated villages and towns. In addition to these relationships, place of residence affects the type of training indigenous midwives receive. Midwives tend to be trained by representatives from the kind of clinic (SSA, IMSS, INI) closest to their home. Differences in training are related to the direction and rate at which their practice changes.

Over the past twenty-five years, SSA and IMSS clinics and hospitals have become more common in rural communities. Because of their proliferation, Hueyapan's midwives claim they attend fewer births now than in the past. Some pregnant women prefer doctors and nurses because they administer injections to control the pain. Most importantly, women go to rural clinics because they charge relatively little or nothing for their services. Instead of having a quasi-independent, private practice, more and more of Hueyapan's midwives are acting as auxiliary health workers whose primary role is to funnel pregnant women to SSA and IMSS clinics and take orders and training from doctors and nurses.

The SSA and IMSS have also had a significant influence on birthing practice. The use of a sharp piece of cane to cut the umbilical cord, cauterization of the cord end, and the use of the kneeling birth position are declining. Recently incorporated are pincers used while cutting the umbilical cord; a sterile tie, gauze, and tape to wrap the cord; and alcohol to sterilize hands and equipment.

In contrast, INI has had a smaller impact on indigenous midwives. Only a fraction of indigenous Mexican healers actively participate in regional INI clinics for traditional medical practitioners (see also Mellado Campos et al. 1994: 34). Hueyapan's midwives are reluctant to participate because (1) few people go to the clinic, (2) compensation is low, and most importantly, (3) midwives often have to close up their homes during the day or leave some of their children alone at home when they work at the clinic. Even

TABLE 7.10: PRESENCE OF A TRADITIONAL MEDICAL ORGANIZATION AMONG INDIGENOUS GROUPS FROM THE MEXICO–UNITED STATES BORDER TO THE ISTHMUS OF TEHUANTEPEC

Group	Traditional Medical Organization	
	Present	Absent
NORTHWEST REGION		
Baja groups		XXXX
Guarijío		XXXX
Kikapoo		XXXX
Mayo	XXXX	
Opata		XXXX
Papago		XXXX
Pima		XXXX
Seri		XXXX
Tarahumara	XXXX	
Yaqui		XXXX
WEST REGION		
Cora	XXXX	
Huichol	XXXX	
Tepehuani	XXXX	
EAST REGION		
Huastec	XXXX	
Nahua	XXXX	
Otomí	XXXX	
Pame		XXXX
Popoloca		XXXX
Tepehua		XXXX
Totonac	XXXX	
CENTRAL REGION		
Chichimec	XXXX	
Mazahua	XXXX	
Nahua	XXXX	
Otomí	XXXX	
Purépecha	XXXX	
Tlahuica		XXXX

TABLE 7.10 (cont.)

	Traditional Medical Organization	
Group	Present	Absent
NORTH AND CENTRAL OAXACA REGION		
Chinantec	XXXX	
Chocho	XXXX	
Cuicatec	XXXX	
Ixcatec		XXXX
Mazatec	XXXX	
Zapotec	XXXX	
SOUTHERN PACIFIC REGION		
Amuzgo	XXXX	
Chatino		XXXX
Mixtec	XXXX	
Tlapanec		XXXX
Trique		XXXX
ISTHMUS OF TEHUANTEPEC REGION		
Chontal	XXXX	
Huave	XXXX	
Mixe	XXXX	
Popoluca		XXXX

though INI has actively promoted the maintenance of tradition, such as the use of the *temazcal* and local medicinal plants, their influence has been limited.

The overall trend is clear. Indigenous midwives are gradually being incorporated into Mexico's biomedical health care system. Though the future is always difficult to predict, we suspect indigenous Mexican midwifery will soon resemble midwifery in rural Morelos. In Morelos (Mata Pinzón et al. 1994:658–659; Mellado Campos et al. 1989), Nahua midwives play an important role in introducing birth control and participating in public health campaigns. The salience of these roles is evident in the terms people use to refer to them: *parteras pastilleras* (birth-control-pill midwives), *parteras*

TABLE 7.11: TRADITIONAL MEDICAL ORGANIZATION BY SIZE OF POPULATION

		Population[1]		
		High	**Low**	**Total**
Traditional	Absent	61.1%	22.2%	41.7%
Organization	Present	38.9%	77.8%	58.3%
		100%	100%	100%
		$N = 18$	$N = 18$	$N = 36$
		Value	Approximate Significance	
Chi Square		5.600[2]	.01	
Kendall's tau-b		.394	.01	
Gamma		.692	.01	

[1] For purposes of this analysis, groups are divided into those with high and low populations with the median value used as the cutoff point.

[2] 0 cells have expected count less than 5. The minimum expected count is 7.50.

boticarias (patent-medicine midwives), *parteras promotoras* (health-promotion midwives), *parteras adiestradas* or *parteras capacitadas* (trained midwives), and *parteras empíricas diplomadas* (qualified empirical midwives).

Notes

1. Parts of this chapter were presented at the ninety-sixth and ninety-seventh annual meetings of the American Anthropological Association. Huber would like to acknowledge the financial assistance of a Faculty Research Grant from the College of Charleston in spring 1996 and Tinker Research Grants from the University of Pittsburgh in 1986 and 1987. He would also like to thank Antonio Sosa del Carmen, Antonio Toribio Martínez, and their families for their help and many acts of kindness. This chapter benefited from comments made by Marcia Good Maust, Miguel Güémez Pineda, and Robbie Davis-Floyd.
2. Pseudonyms are used to refer to these midwives.
3. Natividad's level of prenatal care is similar to that of Nahua midwives from Tecospa (Madsen 1969:78) and Tepoztlán (Lewis 1963:356).
4. In a massage observed by Huber, Natividad directed the woman to lie on her back with her knees slightly raised. She then lifted her blouse and rubbed and probed her abdomen with her hands and fingers. The massage lasted less than ten minutes, and upon its completion Natividad was offered sweet breads and coffee (see also Lewis 1963:356).

5. In Tatahuicapan, a midwife may apply cooking oil and oil from a zapote fruit during a massage (Unidad Regional de Acayucan 1983:61).

6. I wish to thank Dr. John Rashford (Department of Sociology and Anthropology, College of Charleston) for this insight.

7. It was probably routine for pregnant women from Hueyapan to bathe in the *temazcal* every other day some twenty-five years prior to this study (Nutini and Isaac 1974:188). In general, the use of the *temazcal* has been steadily declining during the last ten years and many have been falling into disrepair.

8. Among Nahuas, prenatal sweat baths vary in frequency from every other day to one per month, with one per week being the most common (Madsen 1969:78; Montoya Briones and Moedano Navarro 1969:279; Nutini and Isaac 1974; Redfield 1928: 102; Redfield 1930:135).

9. In some Nahua communities, the woman's husband, mother, mother-in-law, or adult daughter may actively assist the midwife during childbirth (Madsen 1969:78; Montoya Briones 1964:102; Montoya Briones and Moedano Navarro 1969:281; Nutini 1968:237; Vexler 1981:41–42, 134). In Tepepan and Tecospa as few people as possible attend birth for fear of exposing mother and child to *mal aire*; promiscuous men and women are excluded in particular. If female relatives are present inside the home, they remain outside of the birth room, heating water for the baby's bath, folding diapers, and making coffee (Madsen 1968:130; Madsen 1969:77–78). In Chachahuantla, only the midwife and husband were traditionally allowed to be present during birth. In the late 1970s, male injection givers were tolerated in case of labor complications (Vexler 1981:41–42, 134). In Chiconcuautla, a midwife may assist in birth. However, most births are simply attended by a member of the family or *comadre*. Occasionally, a woman may give birth without any assistance (Tuynman-Kret 1982:71).

10. Pregnant women may light a candle, pray, and put themselves in the hands of the Madre del Buen Parto, the Virgen de Montserrato, or the Virgen de Luz, and midwives may pray to their favorite saint (Madsen 1968:130; Montoya Briones and Moedano Navarro 1969:281).

11. For information about Nahua midwives speeding delivery in other communities see Lewis (1963:163, 357–358), Madsen (1968:130), Montoya Briones and Moedano Navarro (1969:281), Nutini (1968:89), Nutini and Isaac (1974:47), Tuynman-Kret (1982:90), Unidad Regional de Acayucan (1983:62), and Vexler (1981:41, 134).

12. In the Nahua communities of Atla, Chachahuantla, Chiconcuautla, and Tecospa, women kneel or squat during birth. In Tecospa, the midwife sits in front of the woman and a female relative goes behind her to offer support (Madsen 1969:79; Montoya Briones 1964:102; Tuynman-Kret 1982:72; Vexler 1981:134). In Atla, a woman holds on to her husband, mother, or mother-in-law while squatting (Montoya Briones 1964:102). Women from Mecayapan and Xochitlan grasp a rope suspended from the ceiling and alternate between sitting and squatting on the floor (Law 1960:158; Montoya Briones and Moedano Navarro 1969:281). In Contla, a pregnant woman may brace herself by holding onto a ladder (Nutini 1968:89). Both the kneeling and supine positions are reported in Hueyapan (Morelos), Te-

poztlán, and Xochitlan (Álvarez Heydenreich 1976:95; Lewis 1963:358; Montoya Briones and Moedano Navarro 1969:281). Claudia Madsen (1968:130) reports that the traditional kneeling position in Tepepan has been replaced by the supine position due to the influence of Western-trained doctors (see also Unidad Regional de Acayucan 1983:62).

13. Nahua midwives in other communities cauterize and wrap the cord attached to the newborn with a narrow strip of cloth. The cord may also be sealed with tallow, doubled, and held in place with a sash (*fajero*). In Tatahuicapan, alcohol and Merthiolate are applied to the cord so that it dries quickly. The cord is placed on an ear of corn and cut with a knife (Álvarez Heydenreich 1976:95–96; Law 1960:158; Lewis 1963:359–360; Münch Galindo 1983:125; Redfield 1928:102–103; Redfield 1930:134–136; Unidad Regional de Acayucan 1983:62). For other accounts of midwives cutting umbilical cords in Nahua communities, see Lewis (1963:359), Madsen (1968:130), Madsen (1969:79–81), Montoya Briones (1964:102), Nutini and Isaac (1974:222), Redfield (1928:102–103), Redfield (1930:135–136), Sanchez Flores (1982:24), Sandstrom (1991:296), Tuynman-Kret (1982:72), and Unidad Regional de Acayucan (1983:62).

14. For Nahua communities, Madsen (1969:81) reports that Tecospa midwives pick newborns up by their heals, spank them, and blow on their heads to encourage respiration. In addition, their tongue and palate are massaged with lard so that they will suck well. In Tatahuicapan, some midwives incline or wrap a warm cloth around the child's head so that any fluid in the child's mouth or nose is expelled (Unidad Regional de Acayucan 1983:11–12). In Tepoztlán, some midwives drop lemon juice in the baby's eyes and give the newborn a spoonful of castor oil as a purgative (Lewis 1963:360). In Tepoztlán and Hueyapan (Morelos), the newborn child may be cleaned with alcohol and bathed in rose water or water in which rosemary, myrtle, alcohol, or marigold flowers have been soaked (Álvarez Heydenreich 1976:96; Redfield 1928:104).

15. For descriptions of the treatment of the afterbirth in other Nahua communities, see Lewis (1963:360), Madsen (1969:81), Montoya Briones (1964:102), Münch Galindo (1983:126), Redfield (1928:104), Redfield (1930:136), and Unidad Regional de Acayucan (1983:13, 62).

16. In Atla, a man or a second midwife may carefully apply pressure to the woman's abdomen in difficult cases. However, this is resorted to only after a woman drinks a tea made of ground porcupine quills or corn silk and the root of the corn plant (Montoya Briones 1964:102; see also Montoya Briones and Moedano Navarro 1969:281). In Hueyapan (Morelos), the midwife massages the woman's hips and abdomen, applies a plaster made of rosemary and chicken and skunk "oils," and generally tries to keep the woman warm. If she is suffering from very strong labor pains, she may also be rubbed with a deer's hoof and boiled opossum (*tlacuache*) tail (Álvarez Heydenreich 1976:95). In Tepepan, a long oiled turkey feather is used to make a pregnant woman gag. She may also be given an empty bottle to blow on. In Tepoztlán, a chicken feather, an opossum tail, the husband's urine, or dirty, soapy water are used to induce gagging. A pregnant woman from Tepepan and Tepoztlán

who is experiencing a difficult birth is given a drink in which opossum tail has been boiled (Lewis 1963:358; Madsen 1968:131).

17. When the delivery of the placenta is delayed in Hueyapan (Morelos), hips and abdomen are massaged with tobacco mixed with saliva (Álvarez Heydenreich 1976: 96). In Tepoztlán, the delivery of the placenta may be induced by having the mother chew mint leaves, smell salt and onion, or by placing a hot tortilla on the right side of her abdomen (Lewis 1963:359–360). In Tatahuicapan, the midwife gives the mother tea (Münch Galindo 1983:125).

18. In Tepoztlán, a midwife washes the mother's body and hair and then applies a mixture of egg and alcohol or sweet pulque to her body (Lewis 1963:363–364). In Hueyapan (Morelos), the mother's breasts are rubbed with *soapajtle* (*cihuapajtle*) and the nipples are washed with angel herb water and *yolochichi* (Álvarez Heydenreich 1976:96).

19. In other Nahua communities, midwives also return after birth to bathe the mother and infant, massage or bind the mother's abdomen, or wash soiled blankets or clothing (Álvarez Heydenreich 1976:96; Lewis 1963:81; Madsen 1969:81; Redfield 1928:104; Vexler 1981:135). In Tepoztlán, the mother and child are bathed the day after birth because it is felt that they are still too hot immediately after birth. In addition, the midwife massages and rebinds the woman every day for a week. Massage is said to encourage the flow of blood and cleanse the mother internally. The midwife also bathes the baby daily (Lewis 1963:363; Redfield 1930:136). In Cuacuila, midwives bathe the mother and child three times beginning on the first day after birth. Tuynman-Kret (1982:90) also indicates that Chiconcuautla and Cuacuila midwives wash clothes and linens soiled during or after childbirth. In Cuacuila, midwives risk supernatural harm if they wash clothes in a stream on Tuesdays and Fridays (see also Lewis 1963:360).

20. In other Nahua communities, women are given one to twelve postpartum sweat baths which are begun one day to six months after the delivery. Sweat baths may be taken daily, every other day, or every four days, and the midwife, the child, and other female relatives may accompany the mother. If the newborn child accompanies the mother, the child remains inside for a relatively short time, e.g., fifteen minutes or less (Álvarez Heydenreich 1976:96; Baytelman 1986:52; Lewis 1963: 363–364; Montoya Briones 1964:39, 103; Montoya Briones and Moedano Navarro 1969:282; Nutini 1968:89; Nutini and Isaac 1974; Redfield 1928:105; Soustelle 1958:107; Tuynman-Kret 1982:90; Vexler 1981:52, 140–141).

21. Madsen (1968:131–132) reports that Tepepan women had stopped using the sweat bath after parturition entirely some twenty years before she conducted research.

22. In Nahua communities, bunches of banana, cherry, coffee, corn, oak, pine, rosemary, *tlamaca*, *tlazol* (an antiseptic herb), willow, or *xixicastle* leaves are passed over the mother's body or used to fan her.

23. In Chachahuantla, the mother is thought to be dirty and would feel embarrassed if people visited her before she had taken a postpartum sweat bath (Vexler 1981:140–141; see also Montoya Briones 1964:178; Montoya Briones and Moedano Navarro 1969:282).

24. Postpartum rituals involving shamans are often like those involving midwives in that they show concern for purifying areas soiled by women giving birth and include offerings of recompense or of thanks. For example, Totonac shamans perform an evening ceremony that includes a purification of the *temazcal*, a ritual hand washing, a ritual cleansing of the spirits of deceased midwives living in the kitchen hearth, and the removal of all the rubbish (including the birth mat) from the birth room (Kelly 1953:180–181; see also Ichon 1973). Mixtec shamans play a role in making offerings to supernatural beings (Mak 1959:142–143). Tarahumara shamans seem to be most concerned with averting supernaturally caused misfortunes such as lightning strikes and strong winds (Bennett and Zingg 1986:368–369). Huichol shamans reveal a child's name and "baptize" him with water from sacred places (Zingg 1982:246–249). In contrast, postpartum rituals that do not involve healers of any sort often resemble Catholic baptisms in that they involve bathing and blessing the child, bestowing a name, and establishing ritual kinship ties. They are found in northwestern and western groups (Dahlgren Jordan 1994:84; González Ramos 1992:129–131; Griffen 1959:22–23; Grimes and Hinton 1972:95; Mata Torres 1982:257–259; Nolasco 1967:177–179; Riley 1972:135). Other groups that do not involve healers in postpartum rituals are the Tlapanec and Mixtec. They have a ritual whereby offerings of thanks consisting of chickens and flowers are made at the tops of mountains to resident supernaturals (Muñoz 1963:119–120). In some Nahua communities, postpartum activities take on a festive air. For example, the mother is supported by female relatives as she walks to the sweat bath or is carried there on her husband's back or on a board supported by two men. The sweat bath is decorated with flowers and a cross, and an orchestra plays while the mother is inside. The sweat bath may be preceded or followed by a meal. Postpartum activities may also involve dancing and the child's godparents may participate (Álvarez Heydenreich 1976:96; Lewis 1963:363–364; Montoya Briones 1964:102; Montoya Briones and Moedano Navarro 1969:282; Nutini 1968:89; Redfield 1928:105; Redfield 1930:137; see also Madsen 1968:131–132). In Ixhuatlán de Madero, an elaborate ritual cleansing called a *maltisejcone* (the child will bath himself) may be held several days after birth. It creates strong ritual kinship ties, and the new godparents are expected to buy gifts for the baby and may also name him (Sandstrom 1991:296).

25. In San Francisco Xaltepuxtla, the midwife accompanies the mother to the *temazcal* and performs a *limpia*. Then, for each of the next ten days, she bathes the woman in a stream or spring and leaves an offering of flowers and a candle (Nutini and Isaac 1974:238). Sandstrom (1975:260) reports that some curers will perform a ritual cleansing over the buried placenta if the child becomes sick in the future.

26. The *axochiteonaj* also makes a brief offering called a *nacaspitsalistli* (ear blowing) in which kinsmen whisper advice into the baby's ear. At the time Starr (1900:23) did his research in Tlaxcala, a midwife carried an infant outside shortly after it was born. She blew in its ears and held it up to the sun to assure it would be strong. In Tecospa, the midwife baptizes and names the newborn child (Madsen 1969:81; see also Redfield 1928:105).

27. Among a number of groups, the last two specialties are difficult to distinguish in practice and should probably be regarded as the same. There are other healing roles that individuals combine with midwifery. In order of frequency they are midwife-diviner ($N = 7$); midwife-curer of fallen fontanelle ($N = 6$); midwife-spirit exorcist ($N = 5$); midwife-prayer leader ($N = 2$); midwife-curer of "fallen testicles" ($N = 1$); midwife-snake bite healer ($N = 1$); midwife-sucking healer ($N = 1$); midwife-rainmaker ($N = 1$); midwife-curer of soul loss ($N = 1$); midwife-curer of anger ($N = 1$); midwife-injectionist ($N = 1$), midwife-abnormal birth specialist ($N = 1$), midwife-nurse ($N = 1$), and midwife-spiritualist ($N = 1$).

28. This is the most frequently reported method of recruitment for other Nahua communities (Law 1960:158; Nutini and Isaac 1974:176; Sandstrom and Sandstrom 1986:72; Tuynman-Kret 1982:71; Vexler 1981:133).

29. Law (1960:158) and Vexler (1981:133) also report that some Nahua midwives have mothers or other relatives who are midwives.

30. The sacred calling of Hueyapan's midwives shares some basic similarities with the calling of Hueyapan's curers as well as of curers and rainmakers in other Nahua communities (Barrios 1949:65–66; Bonfil Batalla 1968:102; Huber 1990a, 1990b; Madsen 1968:102–104; Madsen 1955:50, 1957:164–165, 1983:114; Montoya Briones 1964:155, Münch Galindo 1983:197, 210; Nutini and Isaac 1974:363–364; Nutini and Nutini 1987:335; Sepúlveda 1973:14; Signorini 1982:322).

31. Isabel has a high level of formal training in midwifery. Prior to her formal training, she helped a pregnant woman who experienced a long and difficult delivery. Residents came to know of her success and were also aware of the fact that her mother "knew a little about midwifery" and her father "knew a little about bonesetting." As a result, she was elected *presidente* of DIF by the residents of Paso Real, a community in Section 10. DIF is part of the national system for the Integral Development of the Family (Desarrollo Integral de la Familia). She then went to Teziutlán where she attended an INI-sponsored course about traditional medicines, and then to Zacapoaxtla for two weeks to learn about patent medicines and procedures for recording birth-related information and referring complicated cases to doctors at hospitals.

32. Like Isabel, Teresa has a relatively high level of formal training. However, she is interesting because she began her healing career with a very traditional three-component sacred calling to become a curer. After curing for about five years she experienced premonitory dreams which led to her developing a strong interest in midwifery. Later she was elected as a member of the Committee on Nutrition in Section 8. This led to her being recommended to two IMSS-Solidaridad training courses by the local health inspector and elementary school teachers. After she received two health auxiliary diplomas and a midwifery certificate, Tanamacoya's IMSS-Solidaridad doctor held a meeting at a school in Section 8 where he told residents Teresa was trained to help pregnant women and that she would be referring clients to Tanamacoya's clinic.

33. Ana and Gabriela are *comadres* (co-mothers). This is the only known instance of midwives in Hueyapan establishing ritual kinship ties among themselves.

34. Three of fifteen are widowed, eight are married, and four are separated or divorced.

35. Hueyapan's midwives are like those from Atla. In this community, a midwife can be a young, middle-aged, or older woman (Montoya Briones 1964: 103).

36. The remainder gave birth without the help of a midwife or were assisted by a doctor or nurse (see also Law 1960: 158–159; Lewis 1963: 357–358; Sanchez Flores 1982: 24).

37. The caseload of midwives in other Nahua communities is even more difficult to estimate. Researchers rarely report the number of midwives serving a community, the birth rate, a community's population, etc. Vexler states three or four midwives serve the 1,730 residents of Chachahuantla and notes that some women give birth in Huauchinango's clinic, though this is the exception rather than the rule (1981: 26, 133). At least ten midwives served Tepoztlán's population of approximately 3,000 in 1926 (Lewis 1960: 6; Redfield 1930: 152). Eight midwives had active practices in Chiconcuautla, a community of 8,459 people (Tuynman-Kret 1982: 22, 71). If the annual birth rate in these communities was sixty births per one thousand residents (a high estimate), then a midwife from Chachahuantla, Tepoztlán, and Chiconcuautla attends between eighteen and twenty-six births per year. The annual caseload of Nahua midwives is neither exceptionally heavy nor light when compared to that of midwives in the Maya area. In five Mayan communities, Paul and Paul (1975: 137–138, 147) indicate that annual caseloads of midwives range from four to fifty-nine deliveries. Midwives in the Zutuhil-Maya community of San Pedro are said to make as many as 1,062 house calls per year, an average of nearly three per day.

38. IMSS-Solidaridad is a program founded in 1988. It is administered by COPLAMAR (Co-ordinación General del Plan Nacional de Zonas Deprimidas y Grupos Marginados), which uses the IMSS to provide health care to poor rural residents. IMSS-Solidaridad clinics such as the one found in Hueyapan also encourage improvements in sanitation, nutrition, housing, and health education.

CHAPTER 8

Maya Midwives of Southern Mexico and Guatemala

Sheila Cosminsky

Introduction

Midwives are one of the most important types of healers and specialists in Mesoamerica today. They still deliver the majority of births in most communities in the region (over 95 percent in some villages). The use of the midwife is greater in rural than urban areas and among indigenous than *ladina* or nonindigenous women, yet midwives still serve a substantial number of urban and *ladina* women (Acevedo and Hurtado 1997:271; Freyermuth 1993). This chapter presents a comparative analysis of midwives in southern Mesoamerica, focusing on the indigenous Mayan groups of Guatemala, Chiapas, and the Yucatan. It addresses the following questions: (1) What are the common patterns and the variations in the role of the midwife, and in her knowledge and practices? (2) What is the impact of medicalization?

More than any other type of healer, midwives have been bombarded with pressures of medicalization. Medicalization here refers to the application of the biomedical model of obstetrics, which views pregnancy and birth as disease or abnormal states, thus to be treated by the official medical system. The process of medicalization involves the contestation of midwives' authoritative knowledge by biomedicine, which becomes accepted as the authoritative one. Midwives acquire biomedical knowledge and practices, such as aseptic procedures, the horizontal delivery position, and use of injections, either as additions or as substitutions for indigenous ones. The midwife's role is increasingly secularized while the sacred and ritual aspects are ignored. Medicalization is promoted through state health care policies, such as requiring certification of midwives. In addition, a hierarchical and authoritarian model of social relationships is imposed, placing the midwife in a subordinate relationship to biomedical personnel but in a dominant relationship to her clients.

One of the major mechanisms promoting medicalization is the midwifery training program. Midwives are taught to recognize "risk" factors and make referrals to the hospital. This can lead to increased hospital deliveries, especially caesareans. Although unanticipated outcomes of training programs are important to recognize, the main focus of this chapter is the impact and effectiveness of training programs and the criteria used to evaluate them.

This chapter examines how the midwife has coped with these pressures of change. The midwife is a repository of knowledge and an agent of social control perpetuating values of the community. However, she is also an agent of change communicating new knowledge and adapting her role to pressures from the government, the official health sector, and the community. As a member of the community, she is subject to community pressures that can affect her status and authority. In part, this is due to the ambivalent attitude community members have toward both her supernatural powers and her acquisition of new knowledge and practices.

The midwife and various aspects of birth have been portrayed in pre-Columbian codices and sculpture and described in Aztec, Mayan, and early Spanish documents. However, until the 1970s, little detailed information on midwives per se was available and that was usually subsumed under birth practices as part of a general monograph of a community or a specific indigenous group. In these studies, no observations of midwives or births were made and informants were usually males.

Several of the earlier ethnographic studies in Mexico and Guatemala were reviewed and compared by Cosminsky (1976b, 1977c). This chapter builds on that earlier work, using data from more recent studies of midwives and birth that have been carried out in southern Mesoamerica. Almost all the studies are from rural areas, except for that done by Maust in Mérida (1995). The sources used for this chapter are anthropological studies of birth and midwives, including the author's own fieldwork in Guatemala; community studies, health surveys, and other research projects which

TABLE 8.1: COMMUNITIES, LANGUAGE GROUPS, AND BIBLIOGRAPHIC SOURCES

Yucatan (Yucatecan Maya)

Pustunich	Güémez Pineda (1989)
Chan Kom	Jordan (1993)
Chichimila	Beyene (1989)
Mérida	Maust (1994, 1995, 1997)
Yaxuna	Sargent and Bascope (1996)
Taj (pseudonym) in Campeche	Faust (1988)
Various	Mellado Campos et al. (1994)

Chiapas

Various (Tojobales)	Mellado Campos et al. (1994)
Various (Tzeltal)	Mellado Campos et al. (1994)
Amatenango del Valle (Tzeltal)	Nash (1970)
Aguacatenango (Tzeltal)	Day (1996, 1997)
Various (Tzotzil)	Mellado Campos et al. (1994)
Zinacantan (Tzotzil)	Laughlin (1980), Vogt (1969b)
Various (Choles, Chujes, Cakchikeles, Jacaltecos, Motozintlecos)	Mellado Campos et al. (1994)
Various	Freyermuth (1993)

Guatemala

San Pedro la Laguna (Tzutuhil)	Paul and Paul (1975)
Santa Lucia Utatlán (Kiché)	Cosminsky (1982a, 1982b)
Finca San Felipe, Retalhuleu	Cosminsky (1977a, 1982a, 1982b)
Santa Catarina Ixtahuacan (Kiché)	Marshall (1981)
Nahualá (Kiché)	Hurtado (1998), Wilson (forth.)
Indigenous Village I (Kiché)	Acevedo and Hurtado (1997)
Indigenous Village II (Cakchikel)	Acevedo and Hurtado (1997)
Quetzaltenango (Kiché)	Hurtado (1998), O'Rourke (1995b)
Momostenango (Kiché)	Hurtado (1998)
Comitancillo, San Marcos	Hurtado (1998)
Nebaj, Chajul, and Cotzal (Ixil, Kiché)	Villatoro (1994)
T'oj Nam (Mam) (pseudonym)	Bossen (1984)
Totonicapán (Kiché)	Greenberg (1982)
San Marcos (Mam)	Greenberg (1982)
Santa Maria Cauqúe (Kaqchikel)	Bartlett and Paz de Bocaletti (1991), Mata (1978)
San Pablo la Laguna (Tzutuhil)	Hurtado (1984)
San Juan Comalapa (Kaqchikel)	Hinojosa (1998)

include data on midwives; and reports on governmental and nongovernmental training programs (see Table 8.1 for a listing of communities). Certain areas and groups are well represented (e.g., Kiché speakers), while others are not represented in the literature (e.g., Kekchi speakers and the department of Alta Verapaz).

The unit of analysis varies in these studies, which can make comparisons somewhat problematical. Some studies are based on research in several communities of a linguistic or ethnic group, for example, Tzeltal (Mellado Campos et al. 1994) or of a geographic region or political division (Freyermuth 1993; Greenberg 1982); some are based on surveys of several communities of different ethnic groups (Acevedo and Hurtado 1997; Güémez Pineda 1997; Villatoro 1994); some use the community or town name in which the research was carried out (Day 1996; Paul 1975); and others use pseudonyms for the communities, for example, T'oj Nam (Bossen 1984). In addition to these problems, several studies are based on observations and intensive interviews with one or only a few midwives (Cosminsky 1977a, 1982a, 1982b; Faust 1988; Freyermuth 1988; Jordan 1993). Whereas questions of representation may be raised concerning data obtained from intensive research with a small number of midwives, such studies have given us a better understanding of the context in which the midwives operate; their relationships to the parturients and their families, other midwives, other healers, and the community; their negotiations with the biomedical system, and their responses to the pressures of medicalization. Despite the heterogeneity of sources, it is possible to ascertain several common patterns, their range of variation, and the changes occurring in midwives' recruitment and training, prenatal care, management of labor, and postpartum care.

Recruitment and Training

A person can become a midwife based on a divine calling as revealed through birth signs, birth date in the Maya ritual calendar, dreams, visions, bodily movements, severe illness, and discovery of special objects. For example, Beyene (1989:43) reports that one woman in the town of Chichimila, Yucatan, started working as a midwife when she was twenty-five years old; she said no one taught her. God chose her to do this job and all the techniques she uses were explained to her in her dreams. She had repeated dreams of "Santa María" telling her she should help in labor. On the other hand, another midwife in the same town claims to have learned about midwifery from her own experience, with no mention of supernatural signs, and started by helping women in her own family and neighborhood. Both midwives participated in a training program given by the Instituto Nacional Indigenista (INI). In another study in Yucatan, Jordan (1993:186) mentions that the calling of a midwife is sanctioned by supernatural forces and that midwives are also ritual specialists who know how to guard against supernatural influences during birth. However, in the case of the midwife with whom she primarily worked, Doña Juana, she makes no mention of any supernatural or ritual aspects. Rather, Jordan emphasizes that midwifery is handed down in family lines (1993:188) and that Doña Juana's mother had been a midwife. Doña Juana also cited the authority of a Dr. Sanchez, who provided her with instructions and equipment. In addition, she had participated in a government training course in Mexico City. Jordan reports that in another Yucatecan hamlet where she conducted interviews, all three midwives came from the same family.

In addition to inheritance of the position from one's mother or grandmother, apprenticeship and emergency or necessity may also determine a midwife's career path. An emergency often triggers the start of the midwife's practice. Other studies in the Yucatan (Güémez Pineda 1989; Mellado Campos et al. 1994; Sargent and Bascope 1997) make no mention of supernatural recruitment. Mellado Campos et al. (1994) mentions that the majority of midwives learned though apprenticeship in the family, often from their own mothers or grandmothers. Some were also self-taught, probably from necessity in relation to giving birth themselves or helping relatives or neighbors who had to give birth alone without medical help or traditional therapy. The few male midwives interviewed learned from having attended their wives. Faust (1988) reports the existence of male midwives or *parteros*, one of whom was also a shaman, in the Maya village in Campeche where she worked.

In the city of Mérida, Maust (1995:46) says that supernatural powers is viewed ambivalently. It can make the midwife vulnerable to criticism. Doña Delia, a midwife with whom Maust worked, said she knows of many prayers which she learned from her father, but does not say them because she does not want people to call her a witch. Maust says Doña Delia learned by experience through delivering her first baby by herself and from her mother (1995), and does not mention any "calling," dreams, rituals, or sacred aspects of the midwife's role. What the midwife will mention concerning her background, training, and practice will differ situationally according to the context and to whom she is talking (Maust, personal communication).

The same recruitment pattern exists in Chiapas. Ninety-five percent of the midwives in Chiapas interviewed by Freyermuth (1993:141) reported their knowledge as being self-taught, dreamed, or inherited from their parents, but she does not differentiate among these. Among the Choles in Chiapas, apprenticeship is usually in the family of a relative (mother, father, or grandmother) who is a healer. However, one also has to have elements of predestination in order to carry out this apprenticeship. Apprenticeship may be a misnomer for the type of "situated learning" that occurs in some of these cases. As Marshall (1981) points out, midwives in Santa Catarina Ixtahuacan, Guatemala, do not ordinarily serve apprenticeships since they have practical knowledge of their work from having been attended to by midwives when giving birth to their own children. The beginning of one's actual practice is often determined by one's own or a relative's necessity (Mellado Campos et al. 1994:178). Most studies in Guatemala report similar combinations, although supernatural calling is mentioned more frequently there than elsewhere (Bossen 1984; Cosminsky 1976c, 1982a; Hinojosa 1998; Hurtado 1984; Marshall 1981; Wilson forthcoming). The most detailed analysis of divine election of midwives is from Lois and Ben Paul's study in San Pedro La Laguna (Paul 1975; Paul and Paul 1975). Divine calling is seen as providing protection for the birth. This *don*, or gift, enables the midwife's hands to perform massages and external versions. As one Comalapan midwife says, "The hands already know" (Hinojosa 1998:146). The call to be a midwife is also in part a hereditary office. One woman in T'oj Nam whose mother and grandmother were midwives fell sick and was told that the only way to become well was to become a midwife (Bossen 1984:102). Thus these criteria are not mutually exclusive, but are often combined.

Necessity or mutual aid was the major factor that led Ixil midwives to practice, especially those living in dispersed communities. Twenty-four of thirty-two of these midwives have also received a training course. The necessity of becoming midwives increased in frequency during the period of violence and terror at the end of the 1970s and 1980s, when many Ixil fled to the *montañas*, and mutual aid was a survival mechanism. The second major factor was inheritance and learning from other maternal relatives who are midwives. All of these women have also received at least one training course. Another group of women became midwives because of a divine calling, and a small number of the midwives interviewed chose the profession because of a summons from the health center. They tend to be young, twenty to twenty-five years of age, and do not have the people's confidence (Villatoro 1994).

In Guatemala midwives are required to be licensed in order to practice legally. The most common way of getting a license is to take a midwifery training course. In the three *municipios* in the Ixil area studied by Villatoro (1994), 80.5 percent of eighty-two midwives had had some type of training course. In more isolated parts of the country, a smaller percentage of midwives have received training. Most midwives who take the programs are already practicing. It is unusual for a midwife to have the training program as her only criterion for assuming the midwife role, because women do not have confidence in such a person. These training programs have not become substitutes for more traditional criteria but rather are additional. Generally, programs that have tried to train young women who are not already practicing midwives have been ineffective because people will not use them (Cosminsky 1982a; Pansini 1980). However, in some communities such as San Pedro la Laguna, older midwives who had divine mandates are not being replaced by "born" midwives and women have no choice but to go to those who have received a training course but do not have the mandate or were not supernaturally selected (Rogoff 1999).

Characteristics of Maya Midwives

Although most midwives are postmenopausal, many began practicing at a younger age, sometimes on a limited scale. In some cases, they are required to have had children (Beyene 1989). The average age of the Yucatecan midwives at the time of the Instituto Nacional Indigenista survey was a little over 55 years (Mellado Campos et al. 1994:385). In the Ixil area, out of 82 midwives, 27 were between 40 and 49 years old and 31 were between 50 and 59. The range was 20 to 78 years of age. The midwives in Santa Catarina Ixtahuacan were older women freed from their usual work with children, and with the exception of the youngest woman, all were widows. Midwifery provides them with the opportunity to earn some money and acquire food (Marshall 1981). This opportunity is very important among the Ixil, where, according to Villatoro, most of the midwives live in conditions of extreme poverty and are chronically malnourished. They weave and sell maize, beans, or greens in the market as well. The midwives that live in the more urban areas do not have major problems. Those that live in the more isolated areas face difficult conditions (Villatoro 1994:13). Pay is often in kind rather than in money.

The midwife is usually respected within the community, but not always. She may have lower status in *ladino* communities than among indigenous communities (Acevedo and Hurtado 1997; Gonzales 1963). If she has a divine mandate she may also be feared because of her supernatural power and because of her intimate knowledge of people in the community. In Pustunich, Yucatan, respect is shown by using the term *"mah"* before the midwife's name (Güémez Pineda 1989). In some communities, the midwife is often chosen to be a godmother to the child, greeted by the term *comadre*, bowed to, and has her hand kissed when greeted (Cosminsky 1982a; Paul and Paul 1975).

Sargent and Bascope (1997:192) state that in Yaxuna, Yucatan, the "midwife's claim to authoritative knowledge derives from the respect resulting from her past successes and her position as a member of a family holding high status in the community rather than on technological expertise." They show that the extent of the midwife's authority during the birth process differs according to whether the parturient is a young inexperienced mother or a more experienced one who shares more of the knowledge of the midwife. The presence of other adults also affects the authority of the midwife.

Midwives are subject to pressures from community members if something goes wrong during a delivery. This is one reason the Ministry of Health urges midwives to get their certification. An unlicensed midwife has no recourse if something goes wrong. The family can bring formal charges against her. On the other hand, gossip, charges of witchcraft, and forms of ostracism are extralegal forms of social pressure that have been used against midwives (Day 1997; Faust 1988) and may be more powerful within the community than legal means.

Training programs have ambiguous effects on a midwife's status. Training can result in increased prestige by providing her with increased knowledge and a status symbol, thus strengthening her leadership in the community. Bilingual midwives can teach or communicate such things as the use of oral rehydration solution, distribution of family planning information and contraceptives, and sterilization of birth equipment. Other midwives, as in Ticul, criticize and may even report those that have not been trained, seeing themselves as being more legitimate. "Institutional recognition" constitutes an instrument of power for these midwives—and others fear being persecuted for not being accredited (Güémez Pineda 1997: 137).

On the other hand, the midwife's own authoritative knowledge is contested and often dismissed by biomedical staff and government officials, decreasing her autonomy and making her more dependent on the biomedical system and putting her in a subordinate status in relation to the biomedical personnel. Day (1996) argues that training programs actually created a "traditional" midwife whom they then put in a subordinate position, sometimes in areas where no or few midwives had existed before. On the basis of earlier ethnographic studies in Chiapas and interviews with elderly women, Day argues that midwives in Aguacatenango did not really exist until the 1950s, when they were created by midwifery training programs. In the past there were few or no midwives and family members managed the births themselves. A similar situation exists in the Maya community of San Antonio, Belize, where most Mayan women deliver on their own or with a family member assisting, without a midwife (Garber 1996). Some use a midwife for prenatal massage. Women also go to the prenatal clinic but rarely use a midwife for birth itself.

The Lacandón in Chiapas do not have a specialized position of a midwife, or at least there is no mention of any in the literature (Mellado Campos et al. 1994). Among the Northern Lacandón birth takes place in the home with female relatives (mother, mother-in-law, co-wife) and the husband assisting, the latter cutting the cord. Among the Southern Lacandón, only the first birth takes place in the home, with later births taking place in the forest with the woman's husband and mother accompanying her (Boremanse 1998).

The government has instituted midwifery training programs to train "traditional birth attendants" (TBAS), but the people are not using them. The term "traditional birth attendant," used by the World Health Organization and biomedical personnel to refer to local midwives who have little or no biomedical training, is ethnocentric and medicocentric in that it imposes a narrow biomedical definition on the midwife's role. These midwives do more than attend the birth. In most cases they also provide prenatal and postnatal care. That care is more than physical; it is also social, moral, and spiritual, and embedded within the larger sociocultural context.

Prenatal Care

The most important aspect of prenatal care performed by the midwives in every community throughout the area is the massage or *sobada*. It is still highly valued in urban areas such as Mérida (Maust 1995). Schulman (1975: 65) reports that in Yucatan, over 90 percent of women who have delivered in the hospital as well as the home agree that the massage is beneficial even if a woman plans to go to the hospital for delivery.

According to midwives, the exam and massage are used to determine the position of the fetus and due date, keep the mother warm, make both the fetus and woman more comfortable, and facilitate delivery. If the massages indicate a problematical position, the baby is turned externally. The midwife usually puts some cooking oil, balsam, or pomade on her hands so they will slide easily over the woman. She heats them over the fire so the mother and baby do not suffer from contact with cold, and then begins her exam and massage, moving her hands along the sides of the abdomen, across it, and palpating on the top. She feels the location of the head and measures the height to determine the size and age of the fetus. Some midwives also massage the legs, holding them up and rubbing downward toward the pelvis, thumping and rubbing the soles of the feet (Cosminsky 1982b). At least one midwife in Nahualá also massages the legs as well as the abdomen of high-risk mothers to avoid miscarriages and considers it a special skill which she paid to learn from another midwife. This midwife also prepares and administers various cups of *manzanilla* tea which are believed to soften the pelvis of the mother (Wilson forthcoming).

The time of the first visit and the number of visits during the pregnancy varies, but a primipara is visited earlier and more frequently than a multipara. A common pattern reported for several places, such as Nebaj, is monthly visits and then weekly in the last month. Multiparas may not seek a midwife until the fifth to seventh month (Villatoro 1994).

Both the mother and the mother-in-law of the parturient may play an important role in the birthing process, depending on whose house the woman is living in. Among the Ixil, the mother-in-law selects the midwife, makes the first visit to the midwife to solicit her services, accompanies her daughter-in-law to the first exam, and communicates the outcome to the husband (Villatoro 1994:14). In Aguacatenango, Chiapas, the midwife is also selected by the mother-in-law or mother, a decision based on personal relations, economic factors, past performance, and reputation. She requests her services bringing a gift, ideally around the sixth month. The midwife determines the due date. She calculates ten months from the end of a woman's last menstrual cycle if it is her first pregnancy and nine months for subsequent pregnancies. She visits twice a month to monitor progress, examines the fetus, tries to turn it if necessary, and advises the woman on proper diet and activities. She also tells the family what things are needed for the birth, such as alcohol, oil, Alka Seltzer, aspirin, candles, and strips of cloth (Day 1996).

In some Guatemalan villages, midwives give vitamins, pills, or injections. They also provide advice, such as not to carry heavy things, and dietary information. The latter often includes advice to eat "hot" foods. The midwife's visits are also a "social ritual" through which a relationship is set up to prepare for the delivery (Acevedo and Hurtado 1997).

Midwives are urged by government and biomedical personnel to advise their clients to go for prenatal exams at the local clinic or health center. Acevedo and Hurtado (1997) report that in indigenous villages, pregnant women who do seek prenatal care from a formal provider do so because the midwife suggested it. However, most visited the prenatal clinic only once during pregnancy. Mothers do not see any conflict between the midwife and prenatal clinic. In Nebaj, the midwife tells the pregnant woman to attend the prenatal clinic to get vitamins and accompanies her to the health center, whereas in one of the neighborhoods in that town the women do not go and indicated that their husbands do not approve of their going (Villatoro 1994).

During the 1970s in some parts of Guatemala, pregnant women received monthly rations of flour, oil, and powdered milk from the public health clinic if they went to the prenatal clinic and attended nutrition classes there. The food was donated through such programs as CARE and Catholic Relief Services. In one midwifery training session, midwives were told by public health nurses to *order* their clients to go to the prenatal clinic and to tell them that the midwives would not help them if they did not go to the prenatal clinic (Cosminsky 1982a). However, not treating someone who requests her services is a violation of the midwife's divine mandate, and she may be punished by God or by another supernatural being. Furthermore, nurses and doctors assume the midwife should have the same type of hier- archical relationship with the mother that they assume toward the midwife. This is contrary to the relationship that the midwife has not only with her client but with other members of the family, especially the mother and mother-in-law, who usually are the major decision makers in reproductive matters.

Prenatal exams and massages are carried out in the sweat bath in some indigenous villages (Marshall 1981:197; Villatoro 1994; Wilson forth- coming) whereas in others, as well as in *ladino* communities, they are not (Acevedo and Hurtado 1997; Cosminsky 1982a, 1982b). The frequency of prenatal use of the sweat bath, or *temazcal*, varies. Some mothers like to have every prenatal visit in the *temazcal*, but only certain midwives will do this. Wilson (forthcoming) says that of the fifteen examinations she attended in Nahualá, only two were in the *temazcal*. The sweat bath is believed to relax the mother, facilitate an uncomplicated birth, and give strength to the child (Marshall 1981:197). Heat is symbolically linked with life, and Ixil midwives indicate that "the heat of the sweatbath gives force, force is energy, and en- ergy is life" (Villatoro 1994:15).

Delivery

When a woman starts labor, the midwife is called to her home. She first determines when the woman will deliver, based upon how far apart the con- tractions are. One of the Nahualeño midwives mentioned various exercises to do which "prevent the woman from growing tired of the same position" and keep her mind off of the contraction pains so that she does not push too early (Wilson forthcoming).

Most of the Guatemalan studies mention that the husband should be present at the birth to assist, in addition to the midwife and female relatives. The relatives help prepare necessary materials, such as hot water or the sweat bath, and help support the woman. In Nahualá, various members of the family, including male relatives such as father and father-in-law and brothers and brothers-in-law, may be present during the birth. However, in "the more traditional families, no men are allowed in the room" (Wilson forthcoming). In Yucatan, the woman's husband, as well as her mother and other female relatives, are expected to be present during labor and birth

(Schulman 1975). Jordan (1993) says that this rule is explicit and the husband's absence may be blamed for a stillbirth. The husband may take the position of "head helper," with the woman bracing herself by putting her arms around his neck. If the labor is long and difficult, more female relatives, friends, and neighbors will come to provide emotional and physical support.

In Chiapas, however, some groups require men to leave. Thus, among the Tzeltal in Amatenango del Valle (Nash 1970) and in Aguacatenango (Day 1995), birth is attended by women of the immediate household, the mother of the woman giving birth, and the midwife. Children were kept out and men usually leave. Women are ashamed of husbands seeing the afterbirth because they joke about it with other men. Day (1996) mentions that she never saw a man present at a birth. On the other hand, Laughlin (1980) describes a birth in Zinacantan at which the husband assisted by holding his wife and pressing down on her waist when she had labor pains. The midwife also requested the husband to tie the cord. Similarly, among the Chuj and the Chol in Chiapas, the husband may be present and act as assistant to the midwife by supporting the woman during delivery (Mellado Campos et al. 1994).

Women usually deliver in a vertical position, either kneeling or squatting. The force of gravity and the position of the pelvic bones facilitates the birth. Kneeling is reported for the Tzeltal in Amatenango (Nash 1970) and the Tzotzil in Zinacantan (Laughlin 1980; Vogt 1969b), whereas squatting is the usual position in the Tzeltal community of Aguacatenango. The woman is supported by a female relative sitting in front of her and the midwife delivers the child from behind (Day 1996). Squatting is also the usual position in other parts of Chiapas, although according to Freyermuth (1988), one midwife, Doña Mati, who has had more contact with biomedicine than the other midwives, attends to women in a reclining position. The Chol also use the squatting position, supported by a rope attached to a beam in the roof or supported by her husband. This lets her exert more force than if lying down, although the mothers prefer reclining or leaning (Mellado Campos et al. 1994). Among the Chuj, Jacaltecos, Cakchiqueles, and Motozintlecos in Chiapas, and most Guatemalan groups, kneeling is the most frequent position; the woman is supported on the edge of the bed or a chair by the husband or another family member (Acevedo and Hurtado 1997; Cosminsky 1982a; Greenberg 1982; Mata 1978; Wilson forthcoming). The Chuj midwife presses the belly to help lower the infant. After the baby has come, she repeats the massage and gives her a cup of cooking oil to help lower the placenta. Among the Nahualeños, the woman can also lay down on a blanket on the dirt floor. She lies with her head close to the wall. During contractions she puts her hands over her head, pushing against the wall to gain leverage in pushing the baby out or placing her hands against her thighs, pushing against them. The midwife sits at her feet, waiting for the baby (Wilson forthcoming).

The Yucatecan woman may deliver in a hammock or by squatting or sitting on the legs of a wooden chair that has been laid on its side, with her arms around the neck of the helper and the helper's arms supporting her under her armpits. She can also pull herself up by holding onto a rope or *rebozo* slung from a roof beam. She is supported by the arms and body of the "head helper," who sits behind her on another chair (Güémez Pineda 1989; Jordan 1993). Sargent and Bascope (1997) also report that the woman delivers in the hammock supported by her husband, with the midwife and mother-in-law present. Jordan mentions one case in which the mother delivered sitting on her husband's lap. The midwife sat in front of the woman. Everyone present becomes part of the birth event, encouraging the mother with "birth talk," which changes in response to the contractions.

A number of midwives use the horizontal or supine position, which they have been taught to use in midwifery training classes (Hinojosa 1998; Withnall 1993). In one course, the midwives were told that the baby might hit his head on the ground and become brain damaged if the mother gave birth kneeling (Cosminsky 1982a). The statistical probability of this occurring is likely very low.

One midwife from Finca San Felipe in Guatemala said patients had to deliver lying down instead of kneeling or squatting. She said she would not let them disobey her. "I do not allow them to kneel because . . . they sometimes faint at the hour of giving birth . . . Thanks to God, I have not had any problems with my patients." In contrast, her mother, who was a midwife, would let the patient try out different positions with her and use whichever one the patient preferred, even though she would encourage them to lie down as she had been taught in the course. The daughter is taking a more authoritarian position toward her patients than her mother had, possibly as a result of the medicalization process (Cosminsky 1997).

Some midwives use hot drinks, oil, and external manipulation during labor to facilitate delivery. The midwife may also give various herbal teas to the woman to accelerate contractions and stimulate the birth, such as *piixoy* (*Guazuma ulmifolia*) in Yucatan (Güémez Pineda 1989; Mellado Campos et al. 1994:385). The Chol midwife gives the woman some water to drink or rubs alcohol on her neck, often giving her some to smell with the aim of fortifying the woman's body. The Mam midwife administers a *"vitamínico"* tea prepared with cinnamon, *manzanilla* (chamomile), or *yerba buena* (mint); *aguardiente* (liquor); and Esencia Maravillosa (a commercial mixture bought in stores) to increase the woman's strength during labor (Mellado Campos et al. 1994:358).

Other midwives do vaginal massage and stretching and internal manipulation during labor to facilitate delivery (Sibley 1993; Sargent and Bascope 1997). In Santa María Cauqúe, Guatemala, 76 percent of study mothers reported that the midwives did vaginal examinations (Bartlett and Paz de Bocaletti 1991). In Yucatan, when the midwife arrives, she prays to God, Mary, or a saint, such as Santa Rita de Casia, who is the protector of pregnant women. She entrusts herself to them and asks for success in her work. She may clean the patient, rub alcohol on her hands, apply a little oil, and massage the woman around the vaginal canal. At the moment when she sees "the red tear," the section with blood, she gives the woman an injection of Syntocinon Sandoz to hasten the birth (Güémez Pineda 1989).

Both the practice of vaginal examinations during labor and administering oxytocin injections have been adopted inappropriately from biomedical practice and have been associated in Guatemala with intrapartum mortality (Bartlett and Paz de Bocaletti 1991). The use of injections is becoming increasingly common. For example, in Santa María Cauqúe in 1971, no drugs were employed to precipitate or accelerate delivery (Mata 1978), whereas by 1986 intramuscular injections of oxytocin were extremely common and used in over 50 percent of births. These are given by midwives and requested by mothers to "give more force" to the mother's contractions (Bartlett and Paz de Bocaletti 1991) and sometimes to speed up labor. One midwife from San Antonio Aguas Calientes said many pregnant women ask for injections to help with delivery and will seek only those midwives who give them (Willats 1995:15). Freyermuth reports that in Chiapas, one midwife systematically administers oxytocin injections during the "expulsive period."

One of the midwives in Yaxuna, Yucatan, also uses oxytocin injections. She adopted this practice in 1990, having learned it from someone who had been a pharmaceutical salesman in a neighboring village. She started to use it after she broke her wrist and felt she no longer had the grip or strength needed to expedite labor (Sargent and Bascope 1997:191). Jordan (1993: 36) also mentions that the midwife Doña Juana gave vitamin B injections during the birth to increase contractions. Sargent and Bascope (1997:191) suggest that the use of oxytocin injections fits into the preexisting notions that labor may need to be accelerated and that a rapid delivery is desirable because it means less exposure of the mother and child to risk at a dangerous time; they also note that midwives do not perceive the injections as potentially dangerous.

Faust (1988:318) describes a case of a midwife in Campeche who was considered a witch in part because of her incorporating practices from biomedicine. She had participated in a training program and gave an oxytocin injection to a mother in labor. The baby was born healthy but died several hours later. The midwife was accused of being a witch who had deliberately killed the child. An important factor in this accusation was that she had not consulted with the woman's kin group before giving the injection. She now confines her practice to prenatal and postpartum care, and no longer does deliveries. Acevedo and Hurtado report that one doctor sued two midwives in court for inappropriately administering Syntocinon (oxytocin), causing the deaths of the mother and her infant twins. Villatoro (1994) reports that in the Ixil area, death of mother or baby is accepted as divine will, and the midwives are not blamed, but this was not so in the aforementioned cases. In these cases, the midwives were held accountable by the family, community, and biomedical system, with serious results for their future practice. The death of a patient may also have a drastic psychological impact on the midwife. Day (1996) presents a case in Aguacatenango, Chiapas, of a midwife who after twenty years of practice was traumatized after a patient died from a retained placenta and hemorrhaging. Now she encourages and at times demands that her patients be reviewed by the doctors at the Mexican Social Security Institute (IMSS) clinic prior to birth. This has resulted in a rise in the number of her patients giving birth in the hospital in San Cristobal, where three of four patients were given caesareans. The midwife in this case has also decreased autonomy, decreased self-confidence, and increased dependency on the biomedical system.

Cord and Placenta

The umbilical cord is usually not cut until after the placenta is delivered for fear that the placenta will rise up in the body and choke the woman if there is nothing to hold it down. The midwives know that in the hospital the cord is cut immediately after the birth and they are told to do this as well. The doctor does not have a problem because he uses clamps which prevent the placenta from rising, but most midwives do not have such clamps. Some Yucatecan midwives who have been given clamps and scissors said they had problems using them and thus did not do so (Güémez Pineda 1997: 134). The movement and displacement of organs is related to the image of the body as a tube. This body image is part of the more general ethnomedical model and is important in understanding certain concepts of illness causation and treatment. Recent scientific research has demonstrated that it is beneficial to wait at least until the cord stops pulsing before cutting, which maximizes the amount of oxygen going through the cord to the baby, although waiting too long may be detrimental to the baby (Grajeda, Perez-Escamilla, and Dewey 1997). Midwives have also been told to use gloves during the delivery, but said these made manipulation more difficult and they feared that the baby would slip from their hands (Güémez Pineda 1989).

Many midwives use massage, exerting downward pressure on the abdomen to facilitate expulsion of the placenta. They also use various techniques to cause gagging, which promotes muscular contractions to expel the placenta, such as the mother swallowing an egg, putting a braid in her mouth, drinking cooking oil, and drinking various herbal teas. In Aguacatenango, if the placenta has not descended after thirty minutes, members of the family will call a doctor or another healer.

The midwife may cut the umbilical cord with a knife, scissors, or razor blade. Although midwives are taught in the training courses to sterilize these instruments with boiling water, this practice is rarely reported. Jordan (1993:35) mentions that the midwife Doña Juana pours hot water over the scissors to "sterilize" them. Fifty percent of midwives who had been in a training course in Belize, compared to 45 percent who had not, boiled the scissors used to cut the cord (Sibley 1993:220). The biomedical training did not have much impact with respect to this particular practice. Neonatal deaths from *alferecía*, neonatal gangrene, were found in Chiapas children whose cord had been cut with household scissors which had also been used in agricultural work (Freyermuth 1993).

In many groups the midwife cauterizes the cord with a candle or hot knife (Cosminsky 1982b; Freyermuth 1993; Jordan 1993; Lang and Elkin 1997; Laughlin 1980; Mellado Campos et al. 1994). The baby has less chance of getting neonatal tetanus from this cauterization, which leaves the stump sterile and dry. However, in training courses, midwives are taught not to use a candle but instead to use alcohol or Merthiolate as a disinfectant. In some cases, the midwife combines these. For example, the Chuj midwife applies Merthiolate on the umbilical wound and burns the cord with a candle so that it dries rapidly and falls off in three days. Among the Tojobales, Jacaltecos, Cakchiqueles, and Motozintlecos, some still cauterize the cord. Today, however, many put Merthiolate, *aceite copai*, or Pomada 666 in addition to or instead of burning the end of the cord (Mellado Campos et al. 1994). On the Finca San Felipe the midwife first burns the cord with a candle and then applies alcohol and Merthiolate. The stump is then covered with a cloth bandage (Cosminsky 1982b). In Aguacatenango, the candle used to cauterize the cord is also lit to honor Saint Mary (Day 1996).

The midwife gives the baby its first bath and swaddles it. Among the Jacaltecos, Cakchiqueles, and Motozintlecos, the baby is bathed with *ruda* (rue) and *hinojo* (fennel) so that it will not get *pujo*, an illness of newborns characterized by inflammation of the intestines. This illness is believed to be caused by lack of cleanliness, or by a person who carries bad air (*mal aire*) from the bush and comes too close to the child. The Tzeltal believe that if the baby is not swaddled, the child will snatch at everything and eventually become a thief. The body remains bound for fifteen days. In the first twenty days, the child's contacts with the world are limited to the immediate family in order to guard against soul loss and illness from "hot" glances of outsiders (Nash 1970) or envy-related illness (Day 1996). The mother is also supposed to spend those twenty days in bed and abstain from housework.

The Aguacatenango midwife stays for about an hour to monitor the condition of mother and child. She expects to be served a meal and offered drinks (Day 1996:83). Most midwives give dietary advice, such as drinking lots of hot chocolate and coffee and eating chicken and foods classified as "hot," which are thought to give a woman strength after childbirth and facilitate the development of breast milk.

Postpartum

The length of postpartum care varies from five days to twenty or forty days; the number of times the midwife visits the mother and child during this period also varies (Cosminsky 1982b; Villatoro 1994). During these visits, the midwife massages and binds the woman, gives her a sweat bath or herbal bath, changes the dressing on the baby's umbilicus, and gives advice concerning diet and behavior to promote recovery.

The midwife puts an abdominal sash or binder (*faja*) on the mother shortly after the birth. According to the midwives, the binder "closes the bones" that opened up for the delivery, helps the uterus contract and keeps it in place, "disinflames" the uterus, slows bleeding, lessens pain after the birth, and enhances the physical strength needed for lifting heavy loads, carrying water, and carrying children. The binder is worn for twenty to forty days, depending on the community. In Yaxuna, Yucatan, the forehead as well as the abdomen is bound right after the birth (Sargent and Bascope 1997), whereas in Chan Kom (Fuller and Jordan 1981; Jordan 1993), the abdominal binder is put on twenty days after the birth when the midwife massages the mother. In Pustunich, Yucatan, the midwife massages and puts a binder on the mother on the twelfth day. The doctors try to prohibit this practice, which they say can cause circulatory problems. Güémez Pineda (1989) points out that one midwife who is seventy years old and who has been practicing for forty years has never had any complications with her patients from this practice. The twentieth day marks the end of the childbirth process, which is related to the Mayan ritual calendar, whereas the forty-day period is related to the Spanish and biblical *cuarentena*.

The postpartum use of the sweat bath varies but often starts on the third day, coinciding with the let-down reflex for the flow of breast milk. The sweat bath cleanses the woman, lowers the swelling of the womb, heats the body, which has become cold from the delivery, heats the breast milk, and stimulates its flow. The time spent in the sweat bath depends on the judgment of the midwife and the condition of the mother. The midwife rubs the mother with branches of orange leaves or other plants in the sweat bath and massages her. Bathing the breasts with orange leaves, but not using the sweat bath, was a custom in Mérida but is not done anymore (Maust 1995). One midwife in Santa Lucía Utatlán who uses the sweat bath says that "the sweat bath is my medicine." The same expression is used in the neighboring town of Nahualá (Wilson forthcoming). Another Luciano midwife who has converted to Protestantism will sometimes give the sweat bath but will not do the rituals or say the prayers associated with it. A third midwife, who is *ladina*, does not use the sweat bath because she is not used to it, and instead gives an herbal sitz bath or *bajo*. Greenberg (1982) says that in some Guatemalan communities a *bajo* is given which consists of a heated rock placed on the floor in between a woman's legs. Water with herbs is poured over it to create vapor to "cook" the milk, heat the uterus, and strengthen the woman.

A similar type of steam bath called a *pusel ton* (rock steam bath) has replaced the sweat bath in the Tzeltzal community of Aguacatenango since the introduction of piped water into household yards in the 1950s. The midwife administers several of these baths and massages the woman and infant during the postpartum period. The bath is a social affair, involving the midwife and nearly all the woman's older female relatives. Day (1996:45) believes that younger women are embarrassed and frequently refuse the baths, but according to the midwife, they may fail to develop breast milk if they do not have the baths.

A similar herbal bath is given on Finca San Felipe but without the rock and the steam, in which certain plants are heated up and the woman is bathed and massaged with the plants, especially her breasts. The first bath is given on the third day and is considered essential for the proper quality and quantity of breast milk. Plants are placed on parts of the body that are considered possible points of entry of *aire* (cold airs), such as the knees, soles of the feet, and the vagina. These plants are all classified as having a "hot" quality.

Some midwives wash the soiled clothes from the birth and the family's clothes, allowing the mother to rest (Cosminsky 1982a; Greenberg 1982; Lang and Elkin 1997). Villatoro (1994) says that in San Felipe Cotzal, this is done so that neighbors do not see the blood.

Complications

The midwife treats malpresentations such as a breech or transverse position by massaging the woman and performing an external version. Among the Chuj, a pomade like Vaporub, Balsamo Compadre, or Reuma is used to heat the womb. Others simply use alcohol or egg white. Having located the head of the baby, midwives push toward the bottom with one hand while with the other raise the feet. When finished, they prepare a tea from *chayote* and add Alka Seltzer to lessen the pain. They do this for three days. Sometimes, the child assumes an irregular position moments before birth, and they turn it to the correct position, but when it is difficult, the clinic doctors help them. If necessary, midwives insert their hand to adjust the child or to untangle the cord. Transverse or incorrect position of the baby is attributed by the midwives to various causes: mother worked too much; the husband drank too much and abused the woman, causing the incorrect position of the baby; the woman slept on one side, most often during the seventh month, which can change the position of the baby; or the woman did not get a massage each month. Midwives recommend that their patients abstain from working in the *milpa* and refrain from carrying heavy objects and avoid sleeping on one side. They also tell the husband to take care of the woman during this period (Mellado Campos et al. 1994:219–220).

In Yucatan, a midwife may solicit the help of another midwife for some problem births, such as foot presentation. If she anticipates a difficult delivery, she may resort to a clinic in Ticul, preferably one that she knows respects her activities. If possible, the midwife will go with the woman to the clinic and participate as an assistant or helper to the doctor (Güémez Pineda 1989).

Delayed birth is another problem midwives face. Among the Jacaltecos, Cakchiqueles, and Motozintlecos, midwives believe delayed birth happens when the clothes of the patient are "cold." To treat this, they apply egg white that has been rubbed together with the palms of the hands to the neck of the uterus. The white represents the sperm of the man's semen, providing heat in the vaginal neck, thus loosening it (Mellado Campos et al. 1994). Other methods midwives use to treat delayed birth or prolonged labor were mentioned above, and include massage, teas, injections, and techniques to make the woman gag. In some cases, a shaman may be called to perform rituals to facilitate the birth.

According to Lang and Elkin (1997:28) the Guatemalan midwives in San Miguel Pochuta whom they interviewed and observed had few skills to handle obstetric complications. They were not familiar with the technique of fundal massage to control postpartum hemorrhaging and believed nothing needed to be done or could be done to stop the bleeding.

Ritual Specialists

Many midwives are also ritual specialists and perform various rituals throughout the pregnancy (Cosminsky 1976a). These include praying and lighting candles for the protection of the mother. Hinojosa (1998:353) emphasizes that the Comalapa midwife interprets the spiritual dimensions of bodily signs. These begin prenatally with the ensoulment of the fetus, food cravings, and sensitivity to soul perils outside the womb and continue postnatally with interpreting the drops of blood in the cord and proper disposal of the placenta and cord. Midwives in many communities observe and interpret birth signs, such as being born with a caul or veil, which for a female baby may indicate that she should become a midwife. They also interpret signs in the umbilical cord, such as the number of nodes or drops of blood indicating the number, gender, and spacing of the mother's future children (Santa Lucía Utatlán, Santa María Cauqúe, San Juan Comalapa, Zinacantan). The midwife may place objects in the hands of the infant, which differ according to the infant's gender and symbolize his or her adult role (Cosminsky 1976a; Hinojosa 1998). According to Hinojosa (1998:387), these signs are all visible consequences of the "animating essence" or fetal soul, which the midwife is able to track, interpret, and treat because of her divine mandate and own spiritual embodiment as well as that of the fetus.

After birth, the midwife in the Ixil community of Cotzal places chili that is not spicy with some grains of salt in the mouth of the baby, so that as an adult the person will not be a gossiper. She also passes the child over *copal* smoke and lights candles saying various prayers to the child, for example, "Now you have come to this world, here you come to serve God" (Villatoro 1994). At the end of the postpartum restrictive period, a ritual may be held involving an herbal bath of the mother and child. In San Pedro la Laguna, such a bath is performed after eight days, whereas in Santa Lucía a ritual bath and celebration is held twenty days after the birth. The midwife cleans out the bed and the sweat bath; buries the accumulated material; lights candles, incense, and *copal;* and spreads flowers inside the sweat bath while praying to Saint Ann, God, Jesus, Mary, and El Mundo, giving thanks and asking protection for the child (Cosminsky 1976a, 1982b). These feasts and rituals serve to mark the integration of the baby and reintegration of the mother with the family and community, and end the midwife's duties.

Multiple Healing Roles

Midwives treat a variety of illnesses of women and children, and often occupy multiple healing roles, such as spiritists, diviners, herbalists, masseuses (*sobadoras*), or shamans, as well as midwives. Day (1996) shows how healers with multiple roles, especially midwives who are also spiritists, have important political and social meaning in the community. In addition, in certain communities in Yucatan, there are midwives who specialize in treating the *cirro* or *tipté*. The *tipté* is an organ in Yucatecan Maya ethnoanatomy that is located beneath the navel and regulates most of the internal functions of the body. The *tipté* can be displaced during birth or from bad winds that can accumulate on one's navel. The midwife treats it by massage and putting on a binder to hold it in place (Beyene 1989:4; Fuller and Jordan 1981; Mellado Campos et al. 1994).

Midwives also treat various gynecological conditions, including menstrual problems (delayed menstruation), miscarriage, abortion, hemorrhage, fallen or prolapsed uterus, lack of breast milk, as well as children's illnesses, including fright, evil eye, fallen fontanelle, *pujo* or *pujido*, and gastrointestinal and respiratory illnesses. One of the more common problems women have, especially after having several children, is a fallen uterus (*caída de matriz*). Among the Chuj (Mellado Campos et al. 1994:216), diagnosis is confirmed by palpating the abdomen. The treatment consists of raising the uterus manually to its proper place and maintaining it there with a band. The treatment is repeated at various times if necessary. The woman should not carry heavy things, make her womb cold, or have sexual relations during this time.

Midwifery Training Programs

Midwifery training programs are intended to lower maternal and infant mortality rates by teaching indigenous and local midwives the basics of biomedical obstetrics. They are one of the main mechanisms through which medicalization occurs. The government of Guatemala has been licensing midwives since 1935 and offering training programs since 1955 (Acevedo and Hurtado 1997). Training programs have been given in the Yucatan since 1888 (Morfit 1998). However, they were expanded in Mexico and Guatemala during the 1970s, supported by policies of international organizations (e.g., World Health Organization) that incorporate midwives into family planning and health promoter programs and into the official health system. Midwives are often the only type of indigenous or "traditional" healer with whom the formal health providers have contact.

In Mexico many of the programs were carried out by the Mexican Social Security Institute (IMSS) together with the National Indian Institute (INI) (Güémez Pineda 1997; Parra 1993). Several programs were attenuated or eliminated in Guatemala during the early 1980s at the height of the violence. Since then, various training programs have been and continue to be offered in different parts of the country (Hurtado 1998; O'Rourke 1995b; Willats 1995). These have proliferated and been supported by governmental policies, international organizations, nongovernmental organizations, and relief agencies.

The impact or effectiveness of these training programs is open to question. As Lang and Elkin (1997) point out, although the Guatemalan Ministry of Health has been offering training programs for over forty years, no systematic evaluations have been done to determine their impact on midwives' practices. Programs that have been offered by other agencies or organizations, usually as pilot programs, have used various criteria or measures of evaluation. Three that have been used are (1) change in midwives' knowledge, attitudes, or practices (of biomedicine), especially risk factors; (2) increase in referrals by midwives to a clinic or hospital; and (3) change in maternal and infant mortality rates.

Knowledge and Practices

One common method used to assess the impact of training programs is to administer questionnaires about midwives' knowledge, attitudes, and practices. Sometimes these are pre- and posttraining surveys testing midwives' biomedical and obstetrical knowledge. Training programs have tended to focus on hygiene and asepsis, especially with respect to hand washing and cutting and dressing the cord, as well as identification of risk factors and complications indicating referral to a clinic or hospital. The midwives' own ethnomedical knowledge and practices are usually not included, and if they are, they are evaluated negatively. Many of their standard practices, such as massage, external version of the fetus, administration of herbs, vertical delivery position, cauterization of the umbilical cord, the postpartum use of an abdominal binder, and the use of the sweat bath have been criticized and condemned by many biomedical personnel and programs.

Some of the changes associated with medicalization include the increased use of the horizontal delivery position instead of kneeling or squatting, decline in the use of sweat baths, increased use of patent medicines (especially oxytocin injections), increased use of alcohol and Merthiolate instead of cauterizing the cord, decreased use of the abdominal sash, decline in supernatural calling as necessary for recruitment to the role of the midwife, and increased use of washing hands and instruments.

An example of this type of program was the MotherCare Project, in which midwives were trained and then tested six months after the training concerning knowledge of various signs of danger. As is the case in almost all evaluation studies, no observations were made. Hurtado (1998) reports that according to the posttest, the training had a positive effect on the knowledge and practices concerning complications reported by the interviewed midwives. More than half knew some danger signs in pregnancy, and one-third or more knew danger signs of birth, postpartum, or of the neonate. Three-fourths of the trained midwives said they would refer women with these complications to health services. However, additional research would be needed to investigate actual referrals as opposed to the intention to refer.

Referrals

One of the underlying rationales of the training programs is that increased and earlier referrals to hospitals by midwives of women with "risk" factors and various types of complications would result in lower maternal and infant morbidity and mortality rates. Many midwives are reluctant to refer their clients to the hospital because of local perceptions that the hospital is a place where people die, as well as because of mistreatment and scolding of patients and midwives, lack of communication and language barriers, shame of exposure in front of male doctors, fear of sterilization, and fear of surgery. This last factor has become especially relevant because of the increase in caesareans performed in the hospital. Morfit (1998) found that in a private clinic in a town in the Yucatan, the doctor said that approximately 80 percent of the deliveries are caesareans. Maust (1994) reports that the caesarean rates in Mérida in large public hospitals are between 30 and 50 percent of all births. There has been a sharp increase in caesareans and a decline in deliveries attended by midwives not only in the city of Mérida but in many towns in Yucatan. On the other hand, for some women, asking a midwife to attend their births is regarded as a way of saving them from caesareans (Maust 1994, 1997). Hurtado (1998) found that most of the midwives were unfamiliar with the hospital and therefore did not refer women to it. One of the recommendations she made was to have organized, guided visits to the hospital in the area of the project.

Negative attitudes of hospital staff toward midwives, including condescension and scolding, are another factor affecting referrals. One program carried out in Quetzaltenango was unusual in attempting to deal with this problem because it not only trained midwives ("traditional birth attendants," or TBAS, as they are referred to in this program), but first had a training program for hospital staff. The staff were taught about local midwifery practices, how they contributed to patient well-being, and the importance of being supportive and understanding of the midwives and mothers referred by them (O'Rourke 1995a). "Results indicated a significant increase (200 percent) in the number of referrals following hospital staff training, approximately eight months following the hospital intervention, with no differences for women referred by trained or untrained TBAS" (O'Rourke 1995a:97). Hospital training resulted in a decrease in waiting time of patients and increased patient satisfaction as well as more positive and respectful interaction with the midwives and their patients. "The TBA training program had the greatest impact on timing of referrals—that is, after training, TBAS were more likely to initiate referrals when complications were first identified" (O'Rourke 1995a:96). Late referrals by midwives resulted in significantly increased perinatal mortality whether or not the TBA was trained. The study indicated that the hospital staff training program was an essential precursor to the midwifery (TBA) training program and that together they had a synergistic effect (Kwast 1996).

Parra (1993) reports evidence of success of midwifery training programs in Mexico based upon Mexican Social Security Institute (IMSS) referral data for 1985. Rural midwives referred 50,708 women with problems during pregnancy to the rural clinics or hospitals; they referred 2,744 women to rural hospitals and clinics to give birth because of complications they recognized they could not handle. They also referred children for vaccination as well as for malnutrition and gastrointestinal problems. In addition, midwives have been successful in incorporating mothers into family planning programs. Comparable data for Guatemala in this area is not available.

Day (1996: 39) presents a different view of a program in Chiapas. Despite IMSS attempts to make training courses as attractive as possible (paying for hotel, food, transportation, as well as a daily wage for their time attending the course [20 pesos/day for a week]), not a single midwife from Aguacatenango had attended the courses in either 1994 or 1995. Only two of the eight "official" midwives ever attended training courses in the past, and they kept this a secret from other members of the community. One course in 1992 was solely in Spanish and thus the midwife said she did not get much out of it or enjoy it. The other midwife had mixed feelings about these programs. She speaks Spanish and enjoyed meeting other midwives, but found the course content to be quite irrelevant to her practice. However, she is the only one who encourages her patients to go to the local clinic for prenatal exams.

Mortality

Maternal and infant mortality are very high in the rural and indigenous areas of both Guatemala and Mexico. As mentioned above, an assumption underlying midwifery training programs is that by training midwives, these rates will improve—that is, that the midwives are partially responsible for these rates. There seem to be few studies of the impact of training on maternal or infant mortality. Such studies need to be carried out to improve the effectiveness of these programs.

In Guatemala, maternal mortality for the country ranges from 280/ 100,000 (Hurtado 1998) to 132.5/100,000 (Kestler 1995). Neonatal mortality is 29/1,000 live births and infant mortality is about 73/1,000 live births (Hurtado 1998). These rates vary according to source and database, and differ widely among the different areas of the country, being highest among the rural indigenous populations. One of the few studies to have evaluated a training program by looking at changes in mortality rates found that training appeared to have had little effect in reducing perinatal mortality (deaths from the twenty-eighth week of pregnancy until the first week after birth).

There was some decrease due to earlier referrals, but it was not statistically significant and the rates of the trained midwives compared to the control group of "untrained" did not differ (O'Rourke 1995b).

Schieber, O'Rourke, Rodriguez, and Bartlett (1994) found that one-third of Guatemalan infant deaths occur in the first twenty-eight days of life. Prematurity, malpresentation, and prolonged labor accounted for a significant proportion of this mortality. Thus, if the midwife is taught to recognize these risks and refer them early enough to a hospital, the outcomes should improve. However, most infants in this region do not die from complications related to birth. Day (1996) found that in Chiapas the most common symptoms reported for newborn deaths were diarrhea and vomiting, associated by residents with the gastrointestinal disorders often caused by the local water and sanitary problems. Midwife training programs ignore these important causes of infant and maternal morbidity and mortality.

Control

Midwife training programs are not only aimed at improving birth outcomes and mortality rates but have a subtext of controlling the midwives and their patients. In Guatemala, a midwife is required to receive a license to practice, which usually involves taking an officially approved training course. In addition, the government requires a licensed midwife's signature and official seal on the birth registration form if the baby is not born in the hospital. The midwives are given the forms and official stamps at a health center or clinic, where they are supposed to report monthly the number of births attended and the outcomes. One midwife said the nurse "gave us the *order* not to give the form to the mother until she pays." The midwife is also supposed to take an annual blood test and receive a health certificate. These trips can be a hardship because of the transportation expenses and the loss of time and work. These policies are reinforced through the training programs and impose a subordinate position on the midwife. In many parts of the country, these policies are unrealistic, and unlicensed midwives ignore them or find a licensed midwife to sign the form. Otherwise, the birth may go unregistered. Some medical personnel regard the threat of taking away the license, the threat of not giving the midwives the birth registration forms, and the periodic meetings in the health centers as mechanisms for controlling the midwives (Acevedo and Hurtado 1997). Other medical personnel express their assumed control in different ways, such as scolding. For example, a nurse in a health post in a Guatemalan *ladino* village regarded the teas or infusions that midwives give to pregnant women as probable causes of urinary tract infections, but she noted that the midwives do not tell her if they have administered teas. She said, "They never say . . . because they are under my control, the midwives . . . They don't say because I have scolded them" (Acevedo and Hurtado 1997).

Midwives are also recognized as important links to controlling population size, and training programs have included expanding the midwife's role as a family planning promoter and distributor of contraceptives (Morfit 1998; Willats 1995). The term people use for both visiting the prenatal clinic and for using contraceptives is "control." They perceive both these biomedical practices as controlling.

Most of the midwives in Aguacatenango have little or no contact with doctors or nurses. Day mentions that one of the doctors tried to get midwives to call her to be present at births so they could get materials they needed from her—but they avoided her. She said she wanted to collaborate "so that together we can *control* the patient. This is so the midwives can serve in some capacity also" (1996:40). The biomedical personnel assume the midwife has more authority than she actually has. In the programs, the midwives are not only being taught biomedical knowledge and practices, but also a different type of social relationship with the patient—a more hierarchical and authoritarian one than usually is culturally appropriate and acceptable. This relationship ignores the family context and the role of other relatives in the birth process. An underlying assumption is that the midwife can "control" her patient, just as the government or nurse tries to "control" the midwife.

Conclusion

Over the past several years, anthropologists and other social scientists have described and analyzed training programs and made various recommendations to improve their effectiveness (Cosminsky 1982a; Freyermuth 1993; Greenberg 1982; Güémez Pineda 1997; Hurtado 1998; Jordan 1993; Parra 1991, 1993). Very few of these have been incorporated into actual programs. Instead, the content of these courses continues to be based on Western medical obstetrics. If the midwives' practices are mentioned in these pro-

grams, they are usually regarded negatively and condemned. Positive reinforcement of their knowledge and practices is virtually nonexistent. Biomedical knowledge is the only knowledge that is authorized and promoted
in the courses.

The methods used to teach this knowledge, moreover, are often inappropriate and ineffective. Instruction and educational practices are based
on Western-style didactic techniques, whereas midwives learn their skills
through apprenticeship, observation, their own experience of giving birth,
and divine intervention. Some of this knowledge is an embodied knowledge
which is based on possession of the divine gift and is thus spiritually based
(Hinojosa 1998). Jordan (1993) has analyzed these different learning techniques in reference to training programs in Yucatan. Most midwives in the
area are illiterate and many do not speak Spanish. Teaching methods need
to be adapted accordingly. Lang and Elkin (1997) discuss the ineffectiveness of the government training programs in Guatemala and contrast them
to a program developed by an indigenous organization, Centro Cultural y
Asistencia Maya (CCAM), which employs innovative, visual, interactive techniques. Another organization, the Association for Education and Training
for Health (ACSECSA), has developed programs training midwives as health
promoters; it has also incorporated into the program knowledge of herbal
remedies and a more holistic framework (Hopkinson 1988). A third program, in Totonicapán and Quetzaltenango, Guatemala, developed under
the auspices of Project Hope, uses trained midwives to train and supervise
other midwives. They visit them in their homes and use laminated posters
illustrating danger signs of pregnancy or childbirth. They also have the midwives provide family planning information and encourage women to go for
family planning. The latter so far has been unsuccessful (Nicolaidis 1993).
More detailed analyses and evaluations of these innovative programs would
be very useful.

Most evaluations of training programs use only biomedical criteria, such
as mortality rates, hospital referrals, and midwives' biomedical knowledge
(Jordan 1993). They look at the kinds of biomedical practices the midwives
have adopted or not adopted, with emphasis on the latter. Programs generally emphasize the introduction of new practices or changing old ones. No
consideration is given to existing positive practices of the midwives. Either
the characteristics of the midwives (illiterate, older, etc.) or their culture is
blamed for the ineffectiveness of the programs. The medical model tends to

see cultural factors as negatives—as "barriers" to overcome. However, the biomedical culture, as well as the indigenous culture, involves barriers as well as opportunities to improve birth outcomes. The continuing high rate of female illiteracy and lack of access to medical facilities also reflects the larger context of poverty, marginalization, national educational policies, and lack of investment and development in these regions.

Ironically, two of the new biomedical practices that midwives have adopted are ones they have not been taught in the programs: the use of oxytocin injections to speed up delivery, which make women push before they should, and internal vaginal exams. In fact, they have been told by biomedical providers not to use injections during labor and not to do vaginal exams. Studies have shown that these practices are dangerous and are associated with increased mortality rates (Bartlett and Paz de Bocaletti 1991). The adoption of these practices is an indication that some aspects of medicalization, ones that have had a considerable impact on midwives' knowledge and practices, are occurring outside of the training programs. One of these is pharmaceuticalization, which is facilitated by the ease of obtaining oxytocic medications and injections, for which prescriptions are not needed.

In the medicalization of reproductive practices, researchers and program developers are in danger of falling into the trap of "blaming the victim," focusing too narrowly on biomedical solutions, and ignoring the more holistic context of birth within which midwives function. This context includes a model of health based on concepts of equilibrium and balance: physical, emotional, and social. A balance must be maintained between degrees or states of hotness and coldness, which refer to qualities of substances and the body, as well as physical temperature. A pregnant woman is considered to be in a "hot" state, whereas after delivery she is in a "cold" state. The baby is also considered in a "cold" state and thus vulnerable to illness. To restore and maintain balance, the midwife heats her hands before massaging, administers herbal teas, gives herbal baths or sweat baths, covers the mother, swaddles the baby, and gives dietary and behavioral proscriptions and prescriptions. Balance also means tranquility and the avoidance of strong emotions. Sadness, fright, and especially anger can cause miscarriages, pain during pregnancy, premature labor, and cessation of breast milk. Emotional upsets are treated by the midwife with massages and herbal teas to restore the internal imbalance caused by the emotion (Cosminsky 1982a, 1982b). Disruption of emotional states is usually due to conflict in relations within the family, especially associated with a husband drinking too much alcohol.

The biomedical model upon which the training programs are based focuses on the individual midwife and the individual patient, and ignores the sociocultural, economic, and political contexts of poverty, inequality, and underdevelopment that underlie high maternal and infant mortality rates.

CHAPTER 9

Relations between Government Health Workers and Traditional Midwives in Guatemala

Elena Hurtado and Eugenia Sáenz de Tejada

Introduction

Nearly half of Guatemala's 10.8 million inhabitants have limited access to government health services. A history of social inequity, geographic isolation, and institutional inefficiency, plus decades of political conflict, have combined to produce a low level of preventive and curative services, especially to rural indigenous populations. Despite the network of hospitals, health posts, and centers, official public health services have too few personnel and experience chronic shortages of equipment, medicine, and supplies. Moreover, health services follow a Western, highly medicalized model of facility-based delivery without sufficient regard for the local cultural context and the needs of the impoverished indigenous populations, especially women.

Many Guatemalans utilize "alternative" health resources and treatments, including home remedies, traditional healers, bonesetters, herbalists, and midwives as well as Spiritualists, injectionists, pharmacists, traveling vendors, and private clinics and physicians (Cosminsky and Scrimshaw 1980; De Valverde 1989). These resources come from different health systems and cultural traditions. For example, among the indigenous Mayan population, the traditional midwife (*ilonel* or *iyom* in the K'iche' and Tzutujil languages, respectively) has provided obstetric care since pre-Hispanic times and continues to do so today.

The work of the traditional midwife is challenging. Guatemala has consistently reported very high maternal and neonatal mortality rates. The maternal mortality rate was estimated at 248 maternal deaths per 100,000 live births by the Ministerio de Salud Pública y Asistencia Social (MSPAS 1993b) and at 220 maternal deaths per 100,000 live births by the Demographic Health Survey (Instituto Nacional de Estadística [INE] et al. 1996). However, in most rural areas, especially among Mayan women, maternal mortality is notably higher than in urban areas, with rates estimated at 446/100,000 live births for Sololá and 289/100,000 live births for Totonicapán (U.S. Agency for International Development [USAID]/Guatemala–Central American Programs [G-CAP] 1995). Coverage of the tetanus vaccine is also very low.

The major obstetric causes of maternal mortality—hemorrhage, infection, obstructed labor, eclampsia—require hospital-level emergency care. At present the Ministry of Health in Guatemala attends only 20 percent of all births, and its capacity cannot be extended beyond that level. Therefore, the approach to have obstetric or perinatal complications attended at the hospital and normal births attended at home makes sense. However, this approach requires effective linkages between local, traditional health care providers such as midwives and hospital personnel. Specifically, it requires that women who experience complications be referred to the hospital by their midwives.

This chapter discusses the relations between traditional indigenous midwives and practitioners from the official health system in Guatemala. The introductory section provides a general description of both types of health practitioners and attempts of the official system to regulate the practice of traditional midwives. The central part of the chapter uses data collected during the implementation of the USAID-funded MotherCare Project in four departments in Guatemala. Relations between government health workers and traditional midwives are more closely examined in light of materials collected during ethnographic and survey interviews, and two special meetings of midwives and government health personnel. The chapter concludes with a discussion of recommendations for improved cooperation between these two types of health care providers.

The Government Health System

The Ministry of Public Health and Social Assistance (MSPAS) in Guatemala was founded in 1944 when the Revolutionary government reorganized public administration. The MSPAS had three general directories: public assistance, mother and child assistance, and public sanitation. In 1969, they collectively became the General Directory of Health Services (DGSS). The DGSS had responsibilities in two basic fields: public health and social assistance (Rivera Álvarez 1996). Since its founding, the DGSS has been the operative arm of the MSPAS. In the field of public health it organized national campaigns of education, prevention, and treatment.

Administratively, the DGSS divides the country into health areas which correspond to departments, except for the department of Guatemala, which is divided into three health areas: north, south, and Amatitlán. A network of health centers and health posts have been established in health areas throughout the country. The impact of institutionalized political violence of the late 1970s and the 1980s on the utilization of health services and on the health of the population has not been extensively studied. However, it is informally known that extension activities of community health workers and other forms of community participation in health were diminished or repressed, and that several health promoters were killed for their supposed links with the guerrillas (e.g., providing them with medicines and health care). In addition, the indigenous population became apprehensive and suspicious of any services provided by the government during this time.

In 1993, the MSPAS operated 787 health posts—188 type B health centers (with no beds), 32 type A health centers (with some beds, primarily for maternity care and laboratory facilities), and 35 hospitals. There were 53 state pharmacies, 104 municipal medicine stores, and 609 posts for malaria control (MSPAS 1993a). Current reports indicate that there are 857 health posts and 254 health centers (MSPAS 1999). In the department of Guatemala there are three times more hospital beds than in the rest of the country, and approximately 70 percent of human and financial resources is allocated to hospitals.

Physicians and professional nurses are found in hospitals. The health centers are typically staffed by a physician, a professional nurse, an auxiliary nurse, a rural health technician, administrative personnel, and at times a laboratory technician. The health posts are generally staffed by an auxiliary nurse and at times by a rural health technician. In addition, since 1970 the MSPAS has recruited and trained volunteers as health promoters, most of whom are male. MSPAS services have been provided at practically no charge to the users, although hospitals have started to apply some cost-recuperation schemes.

The Association of Physicians was founded in 1947, when the number of physicians was 192. In 1990 there were 7,970 registered physicians, of whom 7,420 were active. Professional nurses were the first paramedical human resource to be trained in the country. The National School of Nursing was opened in 1940 and was moved to its present site at the Roosevelt Medical Complex in 1949. The School of Nursing in Quetzaltenango was established in 1946 and a nursing school in Cobán was established in 1976. In 1990, registered professional nurses numbered 2,945. Auxiliary nurses started to train in 1952 under the auspices of the Guatemala Institute of Social Security (IGSS). The 1954 and 1955 courses were taught in private hospitals. The first official course took place at the San Juan de Dios Hospital, where an auxiliary nurses training center was established. After this center was closed in 1961, a national office for auxiliary nurse training was developed by the School of Nursing. Similar schools operate in Quetzaltenango, Jutiapa, and Mazatenango (Rivera Álvarez 1996). The Health Personnel Training Institute (INDAPS), located in Quiriguá, Izabal, has been the training center of rural health technicians (TSRS) since 1975, when it was established. This program is unique to Guatemala.

Most health practitioners of the MSPAS are *ladino*[1] and most physicians are men. In a 1988 representative survey of all "modern" health care providers, Enge and Harrison found that 89 percent were male and that only 15 percent could speak a Mayan language. Moreover, the investigators concluded that since only 17 percent of physicians had served at two or more posts inside a health area, they were less likely than other health personnel to get to know in-depth and extensively the population that they served.

According to a more recent survey of all providers (Macro International Inc. and Instituto de Nutrición de Centro América y Panamá [INCAP] 1997), of a total of 5,110 health care providers of maternal and child health care in four departments in western Guatemala, 3,467, or 68 percent, are traditional midwives, 12 percent are "others" (presumably other kinds of traditional practitioners, and pharmacists), 12 percent are paramedics, 6 percent are physicians, and 1 percent are professional nurses. This means that in these four departments there are 0.17 physicians per 1,000 inhabitants compared to 2.1 midwives per 1,000 inhabitants.[2] The total number of midwives in the country was estimated to be 20,000 in 1989 (Putney and Smith 1989) and 15,000 in 1995 (USAID/G-CAP 1995).

In 1996, the MSPAS reported that 46 percent of the population did not have access to basic government health services, 40 percent had access to services from the MSPAS or the IGSS, and 14 percent resorted to private practitioners. With respect to its services, the major problems identified by the MSPAS (1999) were lack of human resources and inadequate distribution and management of financial resources. Also, the distribution of resources between preventive and curative services was found to be inadequate, with the health budget primarily dedicated to hospitals (Centro de Investigaciones Económicas Nacionales [CIEN] 1992).

These assessments spurred the official health system to extend the coverage of basic government health services by means of subcontracts with nongovernment organizations, or NGOS (MSPAS 1999). The Integrated Health Care System, or SIAS, as the model is known, has added two new members to the basic health team, the ambulatory physician and the institutional facilitator. This model has started to be implemented in the departments of Alta Verapaz, Chiquimula, and Escuintla. Alta Verapaz is the only one of these three departments to have a predominantly indigenous population. The progress to date has been slow, although the MSPAS claims that the percentage of the population without access to government health services decreased from 46 percent in 1996 to 24 percent in 1998 (MSPAS 1999).

Traditional Midwives

Since pre-Hispanic times, Mayan midwives have had a prominent place in their communities, providing care to women during pregnancy, delivery, and the postpartum period. Traditional midwives have been regarded as both ritual and obstetrical specialists, mediating between their patients and the supernatural by performing rituals to safeguard their patients (Paul 1974; Paul and Paul 1975). However, their role as sacred and ritual specialists has been attenuated in the process of changes in medical practice and official training (Cosminsky 1982a).

Results of the last demographic health survey (INE et al. 1996) show that traditional midwives continue to be the most important source of prenatal, delivery, postpartum, and newborn care in rural indigenous communities. In fact, it is very likely that most pregnant women seen by a physician are also seen by a midwife. The existence of a plurality of systems of health care during pregnancy has been well documented in Guatemala (Acevedo and Hurtado 1997; Cosminsky 1977a, 1982a; Hurtado 1984, 1995, 1997b).

According to the same survey, 88 percent of births to indigenous women occurred at home, and 72 percent of births to indigenous women were attended by a midwife.[3] These percentages are higher in rural Mayan communities, where it is believed that more than 90 percent of deliveries are attended at home by a traditional midwife.

Since 1945, the government of Guatemala has attempted to regulate traditional midwives by requiring them to be trained through a licensing program. Midwives refer to their licenses as their identification "papers" or *carnet*. Articles 98 and 99 of the Government Decree of April 16, 1945 delegate the responsibility for granting permits to midwives to the General Directory of Public Sanitation, stipulating that permits were to be granted after an examination. This decree also says that any midwife who fails to attend a training course after being summoned is prohibited from attending deliveries (Putney and Smith 1989). There seems to be no information on the kind of training courses that midwives underwent at that time.

In 1953, additional regulations for granting licenses to traditional midwives were introduced. Section F, Article 15, Decree No. 74, dated May 9, 1955, authorizes the MSPAS to extend authorization certificates to traditional midwives after an aptitude examination. Annual medical exams were required for the renovation of the licenses. Training courses consisted of two classes a month over one year, the costs of which were absorbed by the midwife.

With the creation of the Division of Maternal and Child Health in 1969, the training of midwives increased dramatically. By 1975, 6,000 midwives had been trained. However, only 905 kept a relationship with the MSPAS after being trained (Harrison 1977), which reflected the lack of continuity and supervision that has afflicted these programs. MSPAS officials estimated that there were another 10,000 untrained midwives providing services in the country during the 1970s (Putney and Smith 1989).

In the 1980s, the Guatemalan Ministry of Health, like other health ministries in Central America, adopted the model recommended by the World Health Organization (WHO), which recognizes the importance of traditional health care providers and of incorporating them into government health services. This model required that the MSPAS formally recognize midwives, establish a system of registration for them, grant them licenses, administer a midwife training program, and train midwives to promote the use of family planning methods (Leedam 1985).

The United Nations Children's Fund (UNICEF) and USAID have been the major financial supporters of the training of midwives in Guatemala. Besides the MSPAS, several international and local NGOs have participated in their training. In the 1980s the training of midwives was fifteen days long and professional nurses were officially responsible for it (Putney and Smith 1989). However, most training of midwives has been the actual responsibility of auxiliary nurses, who have limited or no experience in delivery. From the midwives' perspective, training courses have been about washing their hands, disinfecting the scissors, using the supine position for delivery, using alcohol and Merthiolate on the umbilical cord, giving dietary advice, promoting the consumption of colostrum, and cleaning out the baby's nose and throat (Cosminsky 1977a).

In the 1990s the focus of the training of midwives shifted to their referring pregnant women and women with obstetric complications to the hospital. Specifically, the USAID-funded MotherCare Project has trained midwives in the recognition of "danger signs" during pregnancy, delivery, and the postpartum and neonatal periods that could lead to the death of the mother or the baby unless they are referred to the hospital. The SIAS—the new model of basic health service delivery being implemented in Guatemala—regards midwives as part of the basic health team and plans to train them in the recognition and referral of dangerous events during pregnancy, delivery, and the postpartum period.

Data and Methodology

The first author collected data between 1995 and 1997 when she was working in the USAID-sponsored MotherCare Project in Guatemala. The project took place in the departments of Sololá, Totonicapán, Quetzaltenango, and San Marcos in western Guatemala with a predominantly indigenous population. She collected information from four independent sources:

1. ethnographic interviews of twenty midwives from eight rural Mayan communities in three of these departments,

2. a survey of 106 midwives who had recently been trained by the MotherCare Project in Guatemala for the recognition and management of obstetric and perinatal complications,
3. interviews with fifteen public health care practitioners in the same areas, and
4. meetings that the MotherCare Project in Guatemala facilitated between hospital and other government health care providers and traditional midwives in two of the departments.

In the data analysis, we paid particular attention to topics such as the midwives' referrals to health services for prenatal care, referrals of complicated cases of delivery to hospitals, compliance with referral, relations with government health service personnel, and recommendations for improving prenatal care. In the formal health care providers' interviews, topics included relations with midwives, role of the midwives, and recommendations for improving relations with midwives. Manual tabulations were made of interviews to obtain an idea about proportions or trends in the data. The survey was analyzed with a statistical program.

Findings

THE MIDWIVES

The information from the ethnographic interviews of midwives and from the survey can provide a picture of the "typical" midwife as well as variations among midwives. The ethnographic study focused on traditional midwives living and working in eight small rural communities[4] (see Table 9.1).

Note that all of the midwives are women. The group of twenty midwives studied in 1995 had a mean age of 57 years with a range of 38 to 85 years old. With the exception of one, all identified themselves as *naturales*, that is, Mayan. The literacy rate among rural Mayan women is one of the lowest in the entire continent, at less than 20 percent. Not surprisingly, only two of the midwives interviewed had attended school and none of them knew how to read or write. Except for the one who said she was *ladina*, all said they could only speak the Mayan language of their community (either K'iche' or Mam).

All of the midwives had started practicing before receiving any training course by the Ministry of Health and six of them had never received a training course. Midwives were asked about the main manner in which they were

TABLE 9.1: DEMOGRAPHIC CHARACTERISTICS OF THE MIDWIVES

Characteristics	Ethnographic Study		Survey	
Mean Age	57		52	
Age Range	38–85		24–85	
Mean number of years practicing	21		17	
Manner of recruitment				
By herself	1	(5%)	18	(17%)
With mother	3	(15)	12	(11)
With another midwife	6	(30)	10	(9)
Requests for help	6	(30)	21	(20)
Supernatural calling	4	(20)	18	(17)
By health services	—		21	(20)
Other	—		6	(6)
Attended school	2	(10)	32	(30)
Knows how to read	0		34	(32)
Trained by the MSPAS	14	(70)	106	(100)
Language usually spoken				
K'iche'	15	(75)	56	(53)
Mam	4	(20)	20	(19)
Mayan language & Spanish	0		8	(8)
Spanish	1	(5)	22	(20)
Ethnic group				
Mayan	19	(95)	95	(90)
Ladino	1	(5)	11	(10)
	N = 20		N = 106	

recruited: one midwife said she had learned all by herself, two had a midwife mother from whom they had learned, four had served an apprenticeship with another experienced older midwife, six had responded to requests for help during delivery from relatives or neighbors, and for six it was their "destiny" or "fate" to be midwives, or they had received a "divine call," which means they were born on a day which, according to the Mayan divinatory calendar, was favorable for them to become midwives. The process of being born a midwife has been described for the Lake Atitlán area (Hurtado 1984; Paul and Paul 1975). These forms of starting a practice are not mutually exclusive; a woman may be born on a propitious day, but only start her practice after successfully attending an unexpected urgent call. Also, midwives often have relatives, usually grandmothers or mothers, who were midwives.

Much more so than midwives in the Mam linguistic area, K'iche' midwives expressed a strong sense of responsibility, commitment, "law," or "mandate" that forces them to provide care "from the moment that a pregnant woman or her relatives go talk to them to ask them the 'favor' to see a pregnant woman to the time when she is 'normal' again [after delivery]." One midwife said, "We don't have a salary, some people pay us, others do not." Midwives may be offered food during prenatal visits, but they receive their payment, if any, at the end of the postpartum period.

In the survey, the mean age of midwives was 52 years old. Ages ranged from 24 to 85. The majority (68 percent) was illiterate and only 30 percent had attended school. Also, most of them (62 percent) said they only spoke the Mayan language, although 20 percent, mostly those living in Quetzaltenango, said they communicate with their patients in Spanish. Only eight midwives in Quetzaltenango and three in Comitancillo, San Marcos, said they were *ladina*, while the rest (95 midwives) identified themselves as indigenous or *naturales*. The survey results probably present a more realistic picture of the diversity of midwives in the western Mayan areas of Guatemala.

The midwives surveyed had attended deliveries for a mean of 17 years. About 20 percent of them said that they had learned midwifery from a government health program, another 20 percent started with an urgent call to attend a case, 17 percent felt they had learned all by themselves through dreams and visions, 17 percent said they either had a divine calling or knew they had been born on a particular day, 11 percent had learned from their midwife mother, and 9 percent had learned from another traditional midwife. The practices of these midwives during pregnancy, delivery, and the postpartum have been described elsewhere (Hurtado 1995, 1997a).

Public Heath Care Providers

As previously mentioned, the government health system divides the country into health areas that are generally equivalent to departments. Health areas are subdivided into health districts, which correspond to one or more municipalities. Health centers are established in districts and are responsible for one or more health posts. Posts are found in villages (*aldeas*). Figure 9.1

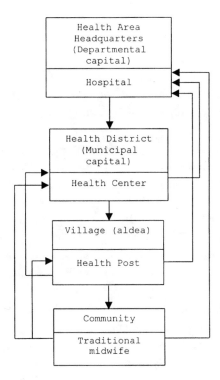

FIGURE 9.1: Health system structure and ideal referral patterns in Guatemala.

shows the hierarchical organization of public health services and the ideal referral patterns from the community and health post upward. The midwife is asked to refer pregnant women to a health post, if they are living in a small village, or to a health center, if living in a municipal seat. The midwife is also trained to refer obstetric complications to the health center or directly to the hospital.

The public health care providers who were interviewed work at hospitals, centers, and posts, to which the midwives ideally refer their patients. Three physicians from the hospitals, four professional nurses and one rural health technician from the health centers, and four auxiliary nurses and two paramedics from the health posts were interviewed. All of them were in charge of providing prenatal care or had relationships with the traditional midwives of their health facilities.

Prenatal care was provided in these facilities once a week (in one health center and one hospital), twice a week (in one hospital, one health center, and two health posts), three times a week (in one health center and two health posts), and five times a week (in one hospital and five health centers).

According to the MSPAS, all health facilities should provide prenatal care on a daily basis, or in any case, the larger facilities should offer prenatal consultations every day. However, this was not the case in two hospitals. This inconvenienced pregnant women who traveled a long distance only to find out that the facility did not offer prenatal exams on that day. The hospital doctors interviewed said that obstetric emergencies were attended around the clock and seven days per week, but health centers and posts closed after 4 P.M. or earlier, and on weekends.

The interviews tried to establish the degree of bilingualism of government health personnel. Out of the fifteen respondents only three (20 percent) could speak the Mayan language of the community in which they worked. Two-thirds of them answered that there was someone else in their facility who could speak it, and this was usually the concierge. The bilingual personnel said they had never received any incentive (material or otherwise) for being able to speak Spanish and a Mayan language, or any training as translators or as cultural interpreters.

There are varying degrees of bilingualism in public health facilities. For example, in the hospital in San Marcos, less than 1 percent (two people) of a staff of 226 speak Mam, about 25 percent speak K'iche' in the hospital in Totonicapán, and about 50 percent speak K'iche', K'aqchikel, or Tzutujil in the hospital in Sololá.

Table 9.2 compares and contrasts selected demographic characteristics

TABLE 9.2: COMPARISON BETWEEN SELECTED DEMOGRAPHIC CHARACTERISTICS OF TRADITIONAL MIDWIVES AND GOVERNMENT HEALTH CARE PROVIDERS

Traditional Midwives	Physicians and Nurses
Women	Most physicians are men and most nurses are women
Mayan	Most are *ladino*
Illiterate	University, high school equivalent
Speak a Mayan language	Most speak Spanish
Are from and live in the same community as their patients	Live outside their patients' communities

of health care providers and midwives. For example, physicians and professional nurses have university degrees, and auxiliary nurses have a high school equivalent. Since the time of the Conquest, asymmetric relations between Mayans and *ladinos* have existed in Guatemala. Therefore, it is not hard to imagine the potential for double discrimination toward traditional midwives, for being Mayan and for being women, to be aggravated by their impoverished socioeconomic status.

Relations between Midwives and Government Health Care Providers

As mentioned above, one of the most critical elements in reducing maternal and neonatal mortality in Guatemala is the establishment of an effective referral and counterreferral system between traditional midwives and hospital personnel. In this section, particular attention is paid to referrals during the interviews and during the two meetings held between midwives and hospital personnel in Totonicapán and Sololá. Both the midwives' and the public health care providers' perspectives are presented.

Referral and Utilization of Health Services

MIDWIVES

In the smaller ethnographic study, most midwives (fourteen out of twenty) said they had worked with personnel at the health service facility closest to their community. However, six midwives said they never go to a health service facility because they "do not have their papers" and "they get scolded." Midwives who have not been trained by MSPAS also avoid referring their patients to hospitals for fear that the patients will be rejected and that they will get scolded. One midwife said she had been forbidden to attend deliveries because she had not been formally trained. She tells public health care providers that she "doesn't attend deliveries, she has no strength, and she is cold," although she does attend births for relatives and close neighbors. Out of fear, untrained midwives either restrict their practice or do not report it to the MSPAS. This fear could be partly responsible for anecdotal reports that at present fewer women are inclined to start a practice as midwives.

Other reasons for midwives not going to health service facilities is that they "don't like to go" because they do not feel welcome, or the long distance to the facility makes it hard to travel as well as costly. They also say they lack the time or have too much work since they work at home and in the fields. In addition, if midwives live far from a facility, they are sometimes not told about meetings.

Midwives said that health personnel never visit them in their communities. Some midwives resent this because they feel their relationship with government health care providers only serves the purposes of the health care providers and not theirs. The midwives may refer patients, bring their patients to a health post, and provide health care workers with information. Yet, they feel that they get nothing in return. One midwife in particular said: "They only come when there is a vaccination campaign and to look for servants for their homes."

Usually, midwives receive telegrams requesting their presence at a health facility for meetings, brief orientations, training courses, vitamin distribution, and reporting of information on pregnant women and deliveries. In general, midwives report that when they go to a health care facility they are "treated well" or that "they don't treat us too bad." Their criteria for being well treated includes the following: they know us, they greet us, they ask us questions, they explain, they explain well or slowly so that we understand, they give us ideas, they train us, and they repeat what they say so that we remember well. However, one said that "they get angry when we ask them when there will be training."

Most midwives in the ethnographic study (sixteen out of twenty) said that they refer pregnant women to a health service facility for prenatal exams. However, the relationship they have with government health personnel is a factor affecting referral; all four midwives who said they did not refer pregnant woman for prenatal exams did not visit the health services themselves. Midwives said that even if they recommend to pregnant women that they should go to health services, about half of them do not comply. Among the reasons for this, they mentioned that women are afraid of vaccines because they think they can cause an abortion or make the woman swell, and they are ashamed because they cannot speak Spanish and because of exams performed. Some women are also afraid because of rumors about sexual abuse during gynecological exams and because of beliefs that the "pills" provided can produce an abortion, function as a contraceptive, or sterilize them. Some midwives also express fear that the vitamins provided "can make the baby grow too big and make a delivery difficult."

Reasons for noncompliance with referral for prenatal care also included fear of health service or *ladino* personnel (48 percent), the husband not allowing the woman to go (46 percent), shame because of exams (40 percent), long distance to the health service (20 percent), perceived bad quality of care (20 percent), language (10 percent), and other reasons (34 percent) such as lack of economic resources to pay for transportation, lack of confidence in health service personnel, and having more confidence in their midwives. Also, in both studies more than half of the midwives reported that they do not accompany pregnant women to health facilities either because of lack of time or because the pregnant women did not ask them to go.

Even if midwives tend to say that there is nothing that health centers and posts should change, the recommendations that they gave during the interviews highlight the obstacles they face in their relationship with government health personnel. For example, with respect to prenatal care, they said that a woman should examine pregnant women, that the nurse or physician should speak K'iche' or Mam, that a midwife should be present in the facility and during exams, that medicines provided should be appropriate for pregnant women (i.e., medicines that cause an abortion or illness should not be administered), and that pregnant women should receive explanations of procedures performed and treatments prescribed. Other changes they suggested regarding treatment for themselves included welcoming them with a friendly face or smile and good manners, extending the hours of health care service to the pregnant woman and midwives, giving them medicine and informational materials for pregnant women, attending to them and giving them medicine when they fall sick, and speaking to them in their Mayan language because they do not understand Spanish well.

Midwives in the survey also provided recommendations for training courses, such as receiving a personal invitation to attend them (rather than hearing through other people). They also recommended that training courses be carried out in the Mayan language spoken by them, that they be compensated per diem for transportation and food when they have to attend an all-day workshop, that they be provided equipment and materials, that they receive medical treatment in health services while attending courses, and that they get their identification cards promptly after training.

Turning to hospital referrals for obstetric complications, one-half of the midwives in the ethnographic study had been to the hospital with a patient. They reported that they were treated "well" at the hospital. Criteria of good treatment mentioned are that they were allowed in the hospital, that the gate-keeper had not demanded "papers" but only asked "who is the midwife," that they were let in despite not having "papers," that their patient was attended quickly, and that their patient had received treatment and was well. Midwives who complained about bad treatment said that they were not allowed in the hospital, they were not received in a friendly manner, they were not allowed to stay with their patient, or relatives were scolded. Also, suggestions given by midwives to improve their relationship with the hospital are telling: being let in the hospital and being permitted to accompany their patient into the delivery room to provide information and emotional support.

An important finding from these studies was that only half (in the ethnographic study) or fewer than half (in the survey) of the midwives had actually been to the hospital where they were supposed to refer emergencies. Midwives said that "we cannot recommend what we don't know"; for midwives it is too risky to take the responsibility of referring patients to an unknown place.

Public Health Providers

The Ministry of Health in Guatemala makes a distinction between an "empirical midwife," who carries out her practice on the basis of experience, and a "trained midwife," who has received training via the public health system. As mentioned, it is the latter who the MSPAS formally recognizes. This demonstrates the dominant position of the biomedical system since the MSPAS legitimizes knowledge and practice. Moreover, government health care providers also distinguish between active and inactive trained midwives. The active ones are those that are enrolled in the government health service and attend monthly meetings.

Health care providers recognize that they see fewer pregnant women than do traditional midwives, and in fact, say that the reason most pregnant women do not go to health service facilities is because they prefer and trust their midwives. They also mentioned other reasons for the low coverage of prenatal services, such as long distances, bad roads, women not knowing the benefits of prenatal care, women's lack of formal education, their monolin-

gualism, their low status, their husbands' and families' opposition, their feelings of fear and shame, and the health care providers' language barrier to
communication with patients.

Health care providers view midwives as responsible for the high morbidity and mortality among pregnant women and newborns. Their goal is to
have them "change their ways." At the same time they recognize that "their
customs and culture" are a considerable obstacle to change. Specifically,
providers mentioned that they are against dangerous practices that they believe midwives carry out extensively, such as abusing liquor while attending
births, using injections to speed up delivery, making the woman push too
early during labor, and using the traditional sweat bath (*tuj* in K'iche', *temazcal* in Spanish) during pregnancy and the postpartum period. Also, massages that frequently take place in the sweat bath are believed by some health
personnel to be too strong.

The interviews and survey showed that most midwives do not take liquor, although they may be offered a drink after the delivery in celebration.
Only 11 percent of midwives surveyed said they use an oxytocin injection
(although they do not apply injections themselves) and 4 percent more said
that, even if they do not recommend injections, women ask for them and
someone in the community administers them. Midwives who use injections
say that they "give strength" or "feed" the woman during delivery and thus
they "hasten delivery" (*apurar el parto*). It should be noted that midwives
have learned about injections from hospital personnel (Bartlett, Bocaletti,
and Paz de Bocaletti 1993).

The traditional sweat bath is still widely practiced by traditional midwives in these departments. In the small ethnographic study all of the midwives said they gave prenatal and postnatal baths and massages in the sweat
house, and in the survey almost all midwives said that they use the sweat
bath during prenatal care, if their patients want, and 63 percent said they
use it for delivery, probably meaning in the immediate postpartum period,
because it has been observed that at present few deliveries occur in the sweat
house. In the K'iche' area the midwife is also known as *aj tuj* if she gives baths
in the *tuj*, or "*temazcalera*," as one of the field workers translated the term.

It may be that health care providers' opposition to the sweat bath is so
strong because the use of the *temazcal* is a reminder of the persistence of
traditional Mayan practices in the population. However, the reasons they
give for opposing its use are that it debilitates the pregnant woman and can

even be fatal for the anemic, already weak woman. They also mentioned that women and newborns are "burnt in the *temazcal*," which hints of Spanish descriptions of the sweat baths as stoves and furnaces (Orellana 1987). No cases of burnt women or newborns were reported as causes of maternal or neonatal death in ethnographic and other studies conducted by project members, however. The closest midwives came to recognizing a condition produced by the *temazcal* was the instance of midwives from Nahualá, who said that sometimes newborns get "*ru tuj*," or an illness from the *tuj* characterized by "red spots," "hot skin eruption," "difficult breathing," "grains in tonsils," or difficulty in swallowing or excessive crying. Curiously, women attribute *ru tuj* to a midwife's rushing the postpartum bath, not using all the wood required, or throwing a piece of half-burnt wood out of the bath house. The comparison of health care providers' and traditional midwives' practices presented in Table 9.3 highlights the numerous areas that make for tense relations between these groups.

Although most providers interviewed did not speak the Mayan language of the community, only one emphasized language as a major barrier in her relationship with midwives. Also, the health care providers tend to believe that most people in their areas can speak Spanish, which probably means that most people who go to health facilities can.

For health care providers, the ideal role for midwives is mostly "preventive" and includes the promotion of prenatal care in health services, use of the tetanus vaccine, use of prenatal vitamins, and the promotion of "hygiene during pregnancy." Also, midwives should practice "clean delivery" in the homes and refer women with complications to the hospital. Finally, midwives should also help them recruit other midwives who are practicing but have not been trained.

Government health care providers said that they speak with active midwives about once a month, when midwives are summoned to provide information on deliveries and pregnant mothers under their care. Sometimes midwives are given talks or training. Providers see a number of limitations regarding their relationship with midwives. Providers "can only offer training." Midwives "ask for things [equipment and supplies], but we have no resources." Providers almost never visit midwives in their communities and tend to believe that midwives do not want to be visited or supervised because "they dislike reprimands." Health providers regard traditional beliefs of midwives as "superstitions."

TABLE 9.3: COMPARISON BETWEEN TRADITIONAL MIDWIVES' AND HEALTH SERVICES' PRACTICES DURING PREGNANCY, DELIVERY, AND THE POSTPARTUM

Midwife Practices	Biomedical Health Practices
Pregnancy	**Pregnancy**
In the home of the woman	At a health facility
Midwives see and feel with their hands	Exams with instruments, sometimes a pelvic exam or no physical contact at all
Massage and bath in the sweat house (*tuj* or *chuj*)	Injections
	Vitamins/iron pills given or prescribed
Customary advice	Advice and reprimand
Delivery	**Delivery**
In the home of the woman	At the delivery room
Midwife and relatives present	
Dressed	Naked, hospital gown
Dark	Light
Own house, warm environment	Cold environment
Position preferred by the woman (kneeling or squatting)	Supine position
Postpartum	**Postpartum**
Placenta receives ritual treatment	Placenta thrown away
Massage and bath in sweat house	Cold shower
Warm environment	Cold environment
Hot food with appropriate, immediate care at home for 8–20 days	Cold food/no special food, on schedule Postpartum care for 10–24 hours

The First Meeting between Midwives and Health Care Providers

The first meeting was carried out in one of four participating hospitals with the objective of "bringing together the midwives and hospital" as a strategy to reduce maternal mortality. There were about thirty people at this meeting. More than half of them were health service personnel (mostly from the hospital, but also from some health centers and posts and one NGO) and eight were midwives, most of whom could speak Spanish. The meeting underscored the conflicts that were apparent in the interviews, which are summarized below.

MIDWIVES

Treatment

Midwives described the treatment that they and their patients receive from health personnel as "pedantic," nasty, and sometimes openly insensitive. For example, one midwife related that she was bringing a patient to the hospital but the patient delivered on the way. Since the patient was not feeling well (she had a "ball in her stomach"), the midwife took her to the hospital. To her surprise, hospital staff said, "Take back your patient; she is your responsibility, not ours."

Another point that midwives make is the mistreatment of their patients' clothing. Often the clothes are just "thrown away" by hospital staff. At other times "the clothes were not there," and they had to ask and look for them. Clothes are an important marker of ethnic identity among the Maya, especially among women, and woven motifs reflect to varying degrees their vision of the cosmos. One midwife said that they are discriminated against because of their "race, color, and the clothes we wear." Another one said that because they are indigenous, "We are not valued and our work is not recognized."

Some midwives resent that "there is no respect in addressing midwives" who are generally well-respected members of their communities. In the Sololá area, when people meet a midwife they kiss her hand. One midwife said that her patient received prompt attention in the hospital because of someone she knew there, but asked what would happen when midwives have no contacts in the hospital. Midwives also said that if they want to stay with their patients they are sent away: "Out! Out! They tell us." Not only midwives are treated badly but also their patients' families. One midwife recounted an incident where a patient's mother-in-law, who was thought to be the midwife, was scolded.

When midwives speak Spanish they use the verb "to supplicate" (*suplicar*) instead of "to explain" (*explicar*). For example, "I 'supplicated' the doctor what was the condition of the patient." The confusion in the use of these verbs is very telling of the submissive position that midwives have to assume with regard to health personnel, especially doctors.

Procedures and Quality of Care

Midwives say that many women have died in the hospital, and that this is a reason why women and their families do not want to go there. Also, the medical treatment patients receive at the hospital is harsh in their opinion. Often, they can hear patients delivering who scream and cry, and who are told by health personnel: "Now, bear it. You didn't cry when you were making this baby, did you? Why do you cry now?" Women are afraid of "operations" performed in the hospital, such as C-sections and involuntary sterilizations, which are rumored to have occurred. Another midwife said she accompanied her patient to have the C-section sutures removed but they did it in a "bad manner," harshly.

Midwives also mentioned that their patients are made to wear hospital gowns or to shower, and they feel cold. Pregnancy is considered a "hot" condition that must be maintained as hot through the use of massage and hot baths in the *temazcal*. The process of delivery is a transition to the cold of the postpartum period through the loss of blood and fluids, and because "the stomach becomes empty." Midwives believe that women in labor, delivery, and the postpartum period should be kept warm and avoid cold (cold air, cold water, cold food, and cold activities like washing).

Language

Midwives attributed bad or delayed treatment to the fact that they do not speak Spanish or do not speak it well. "I don't speak Spanish well, maybe that is why they do not pay attention to me quickly." In addition, they do not receive any or enough information about their patients.

Appearance and Hygiene

The fact that health personnel regard midwives and their patients as unhygienic and dirty does not escape midwives. "We are told that we are dirty (*chorreadas*), bad smelling (*apestosas, hediondas*)." However, the midwives explain that "we are dirty because we work in the fields" and "we smell of burnt wood from our fire."

Coverage

Midwives seemed to be very aware of the way their services differ from those of physicians. "We do not compete with doctors, we are not going to take away their patients. However, we go everywhere, to all parts, we get to the little houses with dirt floors, where they never go."

There were a few positive comments from midwives regarding specific members of the staff or specific cases in which the woman was treated well and came out healthy.

PROVIDERS

Manipulation

An expression that sums up many of the health care providers' complaints is "manipulated patients" (*pacientes manipuladas*). Health providers said midwives refer patients who are "very manipulated," meaning that the midwife has tried several maneuvers before deciding to seek care at the hospital. They describe severe conditions such as "abandoned transverse position, fetal death, severe edema of the vulva, rupture of the uterus." These conditions make it evident that the midwife has been exerting force. Also, health personnel tend to think that midwives make their patients "push" earlier than they should.

Referral

Another complaint of health personnel was that midwives "wait to the last minute to refer patients." They attribute untimely referral to "lack of awareness of the midwives" or "lack of knowledge" of complications. Also, there were complaints that midwives do not refer patients to prenatal care where some conditions could be identified early on. However, some health care providers at community health posts disagreed, saying: "We don't treat [midwives and patients] the way we should; we do not take into consideration distance and poverty." Community personnel also mentioned that midwives never receive written counterreferral information from the hospital. In fact, these personnel encouraged self-examination regarding the treatment of midwives, and urged the hospital to change.

Mortality in the Hospital

Hospital personnel said that the kinds of "last minute" cases midwives refer to the hospital are desperate and it would be very hard for these women to survive. They recognize that hospital deaths reinforce "negative feelings" toward the hospital.

Training

One physician asked: "With due respect, what kind of training do they [midwives] have [to attend women]?" They all agreed that midwives should be trained to recognize their limitations in the management of complicated cases. Midwives should understand that timely referrals prevent deaths in the hospital.

Treatment

According to hospital personnel, midwives should distinguish between the hospital and the emergency room; they tend to generalize to the hospital as a whole the things that happen in the emergency room. Midwives come to the emergency room demanding that things be done their way, and that is why midwives and families are sent out. Another reason not to have midwives in the hospital or the delivery room is fear of their contaminating patients.

Characteristics of Midwives

Providers also noted that characteristics of midwives such as their advanced age, illiteracy, and monolingualism are obstacles to effective training. Older midwives "go to sleep during training courses," cannot understand instructors, or forget what they are taught.

Limitations

Providers noted limitations in the number of health service personnel, with only one physician sometimes covering all emergencies. One participant further noted that the hospital maternity ward has the same number of personnel it did fourteen years ago even though the population has increased. They say their salaries are low and they are tired because they have to stay up all night.

The NGO member who participated in the first meeting made a series of petitions to the hospital that were later submitted in writing and responded to by the hospital's director. Some of the requests are presented to emphasize problems mentioned above. For example, to the request that "K'iche' be spoken to pregnant women," the hospital director responded that "not all personnel speak K'iche' and nobody here is forbidden to speak a dialect."

The request that "for warmth patients be allowed to use a sweater underneath the hospital gown" was answered by saying that "it depends on the degree of hygiene of each patient." The request that patients "be allowed to change clothes in the room (which is warmer) and not in the bathroom (which is colder)" was "not understood" by the hospital director. The request that the midwife be allowed to enter the maternity ward to check her patient was responded to by saying that "we don't think the midwife is qualified to check her patient; in any case, she can observe."

The Second Meeting between Midwives and Hospital Personnel

The second meeting between midwives and hospital personnel took place outside of the hospital in a village in Sololá. The first author designed a series of group discussions for hospital personnel and midwives separately to analyze their views on what makes it difficult for women with obstetric and perinatal complications to reach the hospital. Also, they were to discuss positive and negative experiences and develop a report to present at the meeting.

MIDWIVES

Midwives reported on the problems that they face in taking their patients to the hospital. These were as follows:

Transportation

Patients from some of these communities have to be brought "down" from distant hamlets (*caseríos*) to the towns on the lakeshore and be transported across the lake to the hospital. Although there are daily boats, transportation is scarce or nonexistent at night or dawn, when emergencies can occur.

Economic Resources

In addition, transportation is expensive and families do not have the economic resources to pay for it. Sometimes families want to take their relatives to the hospital, but they do not have the money to do so.

Knowledge of the Hospital

Although most midwives had seen the hospital when they went to the market in Sololá, more than half of them said they had never been inside the hospital. Again, they said they "cannot recommend what they don't know."

Influence of Husband and the Extended Family

Midwives explained that decisions to take a woman to the hospital are made by the family (e.g., husband, parents-in-law) and not by the woman herself. Although the midwife can influence the decision, it is the husband who usually has the last word. Reasons husbands and family members give for refusing referral to the hospital can be expenses, fear that the woman will die, and the suffering and expenses associated with her death, should this occur.

Knowledge of Midwives

Midwives said that not all of them recognize "dangers" during pregnancy, delivery, and the postpartum.

Knowledge of Women

Midwives also pointed out that women and their families do not recognize "dangers" during pregnancy, delivery, and the postpartum.

Hospital

Some midwives recounted positive experiences at the hospital, such as when they are received by amicable and attentive personnel and when their patients "come out healthy and alive" from the hospital. However, they noted specific conditions at the hospital which make it difficult for them to refer and accompany their patients to the hospital:

"We are not allowed in the hospital."

"There is no place for us to spend the night. At 10 at night we cannot be wandering around Sololá looking for a place to stay. We don't know anybody there and we are poor; we don't have money to pay for a hotel."

"Health personnel reprimand us."

"They don't give us information about our patients."

"The stay after delivery is too short."

"If the patient dies, there are many steps to get her out of the hospital and transportation is more expensive."

"Registering children born in the hospital is more difficult."

GOVERNMENT HEALTH CARE PROVIDERS

Problems identified by government health care providers were the following:

Identification

Midwives often do not have their identification cards with them, so it is difficult to let them in the hospital at odd hours. Midwives should always have their cards when they come to the hospital. Midwives fear reprimands for bringing patients to the hospital at a late hour.

Language

Nurses said that only a few of them speak the Mayan language, which makes it difficult to communicate with midwives and their patients. Most health personnel recognized that "the fact that midwives do not speak Spanish is a problem."

Manipulation

Again, the midwives were said to manipulate their patients for a long time before referring them to the hospital. Midwives are expected to perform a "clean" (hygienic) delivery without manipulation, without conducting vaginal exams.

Referral

Untimely referrals by the midwives were again mentioned.

Culture

Health personnel recognized that they do not know the "customs of the communities." Therefore, hospital procedures clash with community expectations and practices. Also, they think it is due to cultural reasons that relatives of indigenous patients do not want to donate blood as the hospital requires. Table 9.4 provides a summary of the different types of factors mentioned by both midwives and official health care providers that affect their relationship with each other.

Out of the discussion of problems came a series of suggestions given by both midwives and public health care providers to improve the relationship between them and contribute to the reduction of maternal mortality. Midwives asked to visit the hospital and to have a room in the hospital where

TABLE 9.4: FACTORS AFFECTING RELATIONS BETWEEN
TRADITIONAL MIDWIVES AND GOVERNMENT HEALTH CARE PROVIDERS

Traditional Midwives	Government Health Care Providers
PHYSICAL FACTORS	
Distance	"We do not take into consideration distance and poverty" (biomedical, facility-oriented approach)
Cannot go to health services	
Neither called nor visited	
Lack of transportation	
ECONOMIC AND OTHER RESOURCES	
Poverty	Lack of resources
No money for traveling	to give *per diem* to midwives
Transportation is expensive	to give supplies to midwives
Too much work	Too much work; Few personnel
ETHNIC DISCRIMINATION	
Clothes we wear	Language as an obstacle to communication
"Race"	
Skin "color"	
Language	Mayan language as a "problem"
(Hygiene) "dirtiness"	
SOCIOCULTURAL FACTORS	
The midwife is *aj tuj* (performs baths in *tuj*)	Customs and culture as an obstacle to change
	Beliefs are "superstitions"
Midwives do not regularly use liquor, only for celebration	Midwives' practices opposed
	Use liquor; get drunk
	Use of injections
Some midwives use injections; families request them	Make woman push too early in labor; Use of *tuj* or *temazcal*
QUALITY OF CARE FACTORS	
Midwife is not allowed to accompany or check patient; no place to stay	High maternal and neonatal mortality is midwives' fault
Hospital is a place you go to die	High hospital maternal and neonatal mortality due to late referral by midwives
Hospital procedures are harsh, "operations"	Manipulation of patients by midwives
"Don't know the hospital"	Midwives' characteristics (lack of knowledge, advanced age, illiterate, monolingual) not conducive to learning and good quality care
They do not give information about patients	
Stay after delivery is too short	

they can spend the night. Midwives said they would refer patients with complications promptly, but everybody involved should seek solutions to transportation problems across the lake. Midwives also said they would accompany their patients to the hospital.

Health care providers promised the midwives a room in the hospital to stay overnight as well as food during those stays. Also, an interpreter would be available to facilitate communication. During the meeting, the midwives discovered that although only a few of the health staff could speak the Mayan language, there were people in the hospital—in charge of the laundry and the kitchen—from their own villages who could act as translators. Hospital personnel suggested visiting communities to learn their ways.

Upgrading services, such as health centers, that women can reach was proposed. A radio communication system and an inventory of available boats from several NGOs working in the region were suggested. Community participation was deemed essential for the establishment of an emergency transportation system. A communication campaign informing the population about the joint work of the midwives and the hospital was proposed, as well as information on improvements in the quality of care at the hospital. The functions of the hospital should be made known to both health care providers at the community level and the population. Also, men should be involved in social communication efforts so that they know about major "danger signs" and the need for referral to the hospital.

Discussion

Conflict between the medical profession and midwives has occurred in many societies. For example, in the United States at the beginning of the twentieth century (1910–1930), there was a heated debate in medical circles and even in the popular press about the role midwives should have in a modern society (Litoff 1978, 1986). Two factors contributed to the attack on midwives. First, there was general concern about an oversupply of recent graduates from medical school and a perception that this problem could be reduced if midwives were prohibited from providing care for pregnant women. Furthermore, maternal and infant mortality rates in the United States were higher than those in European countries, and, as in Guatemala, midwives were blamed for these problems.[5] Nevertheless, midwives became more acceptable as health care providers when waves of immigrants from southern and eastern Europe arrived in the United States. The arrival of immigrants from countries in which midwives were socially respected figures gave a new boost to this type of provider (Litoff 1978, 1986). To date, the tension between traditional and biomedical belief systems of care during pregnancy and delivery has not been reduced much, even in "developed" countries (Jordan 1983).

In Guatemala, the tensions between traditional and biomedical systems of health care are complicated by the coexistence of indigenous and *ladino* ethnic groups, and by ethnic discrimination based upon language, appearance, and other characteristics. Tensions in the area of health care have to do with these elements of ethnic discrimination, with specific conflicts resulting from practices derived from different systems of health beliefs in these groups, and from geographic barriers.

It must be noted that as a result of the strategies promoted by the MotherCare Project and implemented by the MSPAS, the relationship between biomedical health care providers, especially hospital personnel, and midwives has improved in recent years. The very fact that the meetings between them have taken place would have been unthinkable a few years ago. As a result of these meetings, midwives in western Guatemala have participated in guided visits of all hospital departments, where they have been greeted by the director and the staff, and have been offered lunch in the hospital. Also, prenatal care is now offered daily in many health care establishments. However, this process is by no means complete, as ethnic discrimination is very rooted in Guatemalan society.

Recommendations that midwives be trained in the detection of complications and when to refer patients to health facilities are currently being implemented by the MSPAS in Guatemala and supported by USAID through the MotherCare Project. In addition, we have other recommendations that can promote understanding and improve relations between traditional midwives and biomedical health care providers.

Training courses for government health care providers should include not only an interpersonal relation component but also an interethnic and intercultural relations component. Health providers should understand the history of ethnic discrimination in Guatemala and that beliefs and practices of midwives and their patients are not necessarily superstitions or problems. Rather, they represent another way that people have faced pregnancy and childbirth, and they should be respected. The peace accords signed by the government and the former guerrillas in 1995, especially the one on the identity and rights of the indigenous peoples, provide a starting point.

Together with epidemiological data, the knowledge and practices of traditional midwives and their concerns and interests should define the content of future training courses. Many well-intentioned courses tacitly assume that midwives do not know anything prior to training. Health care personnel do not regard as valid the knowledge that midwives have acquired from their extensive experience with childbirth. Instead, they unilaterally teach the biomedical approach (for example, the recognition of "danger signs" during pregnancy, delivery, and the postpartum, and the referral of women to health services if these occur). They do not strengthen the midwives' traditional knowledge or address their concerns. For example, midwives have many questions regarding the use of traditional herbal medicines.

Monthly meetings with midwives should likewise respond to the midwives' needs and concerns, rather than only serving to provide the data that health services need for their information systems. The use of the midwives' language in these meetings is very important.

Although, as mentioned, some midwives have been taken to visit the hospital, it is important to provide more practical courses. Courses have tended to be too theoretical, and on occasion, the instructors had no experience themselves in providing prenatal or delivery care. Midwives would like hands-on experience in pregnancy examination and deliveries at these health facilities. Furthermore, midwives have learned their profession by observing, imitating, and doing. This is a mode of learning that works well with them.

We are promoting the concept of a traditional midwife or "traditional birth attendant (TBA)-friendly hospital," modeled on the WHO-UNICEF (n.d.) baby-friendly initiative and the Coalition for Improving Maternity Services (CIMS) (1996) mother-friendly childbirth initiative. A TBA-friendly hospital

1. Offers the midwife access to the hospital and to her patient during labor and delivery, except when the situation does not permit. Also, the midwife should have access to a place where she can stay overnight when for reasons of distance, transportation, or lack of resources she cannot return to her home.

2. Provides the midwife with descriptive information regarding its delivery practices and procedures, especially regarding the midwife's patients.

3. Values and takes into account any information provided by the midwife, either verbal or written.

4. Provides the midwife with the opportunity of guided visits of the hospital, and especially of the maternity ward in the hospital.

5. Provides the midwife with culturally competent treatment that is sensitive and responsive to the beliefs, values, and customs of the midwife.

6. Allows the midwife to counsel her patient in relation to walking and moving about during labor and to adopt her preferred position during labor and delivery, except where there are restrictions related to resolving a complication.

7. Has clearly defined policies to collaborate and consult with the midwife when the patient has to be moved or when another intervention has to be performed. Also, it should link the mother with the child and the midwife for follow-up of pregnancy, the postpartum, and support of breast feeding.

8. Provides counterreferral information.

9. Does not routinely combat practices and procedures of the midwife, including but not limited to giving massages, administering baths in the sweat house, keeping the mother warm, and tying a scarf around the mother's head during and after delivery. It has been reiterated in the anthropological literature that traditional practices such as the use of the sweat bath, prenatal and postnatal massage, beverages of medicinal plants, the kneeling or squatting birthing position, and cutting the umbilical cord with a heated instrument when the placenta has been born are usually beneficial or innocuous and should not be combated without scientific evidence.

10. Collaborates in training the midwife in the recognition, management, and referral of obstetric and perinatal complications.

11. Encourages the midwives to touch, hold, and participate in the decisions affecting the newborns, to the point compatible with their condition.

Notes

The first author wishes to express her gratitude to the MotherCare Project in Washington, D.C., and Guatemala for the opportunity to work in the project in Guatemala both as a consultant and a permanent staff member from July 1995 to September 1998. However, the content of this chapter does not necessarily reflect the policies or points of view of USAID, the MotherCare Project/John Snow Inc., or the MotherCare Project in Guatemala; it is the sole responsibility of the authors. This work would have not been possible without the dedication and profes-

sionalism of our fellow field-workers. We would like to also gratefully acknowledge the interviewees and the participants in the meetings—hospital staff and
traditional midwives—who shared their experiences and opinions with us.

1. The Guatemalan population is divided into two ethnic groups of roughly equal
   size: the indigenous population, who are descendants of the Maya and other pre-
   Conquest groups, and *ladinos*, who regardless of ethnic origin or phenotype, speak
   Spanish, wear European-style clothes, and view themselves as descendants of the
   Spanish and other European groups or of mixed indigenous and European descent;
   the *ladinos* constitute the nonindigenous population of Guatemala. The distinction
   is not rigid. However, ethnicity has been closely tied to socioeconomic status: the
   indigenous population is, with few exceptions, poor, while *ladinos* are members of all
   social classes.
2. Based on population information obtained from the 1996 census carried out by the
   National Institute of Statistics (INE) in Guatemala.
3. These are slightly higher than the national averages of 65 and 55 percent, respectively.
4. The survey interview was administered to midwives who were trained in obstetric
   and perinatal complications, including a few midwives from urban Quetzaltenango.
5. Paradoxically, a series of studies during that period demonstrated that the maternal
   mortality rate was lower in areas where the proportion of deliveries attended by midwives was greater (Litoff 1978, 1986).

CHAPTER 10

Mesoamerican Bonesetters

Benjamin D. Paul and Clancy McMahon

Introduction

Broken bones and dislocations are part of the hazards of life in native Meso-american communities, where the terrain is often rough and paths are steep, and where pickers can fall from fruit trees or builders from roofs of houses under construction. Among the debilitating physical problems that may beset an individual, these injuries are perhaps the most easily recognized and understood, with the occurrence of damaging physical force and the resulting pain and impediment often clearly connected. However, appropriate methods for treating bone injuries are not common knowledge, and for this reason medical specialists concerned with this type of healing have come to occupy an important niche in traditional medical systems. Bonesetters can be found in most communities across Mesoamerica, ministering to the victims of accidents and even to sufferers of chronic musculoskeletal problems. Bonesetting is an art that to some of its practitioners is strictly a natural endeavor, while to others it is a calling or mandate from the realm of the supernatural. There are naturalistic bonesetters in all but a few of the indigenous groups and mestizo communities that form a complex ethnic patchwork over most of the provincial land of Mexico. Spiritually driven bonesetters mostly belong to Maya communities of the Yucatan peninsula and the highlands of Chiapas and of Lake Atitlán. These two contrasting approaches to bonesetting are related to status. A diverse set of materials and therapeutic techniques employed in naturalistic methodology does little to enhance the status of practitioners; the use of sacred objects and ritual, together with naturalistic therapy, by contrast, secures a measure of status for bonesetters who are mindful of supernatural influences. The latter group also tends to utilize fewer materials in their work. To illustrate the major characteristics of these two approaches to bonesetting in Mesoamerica, we will primarily draw from our personal encounters with bonesetters in San Pedro, Guatemala, and from the three volumes of *La medicina tradicional de los pueblos indígenas de México* (Mellado Campos et al. 1994), which documents the treatment of bone disorders in indigenous communities throughout Mexico.

Bonesetting has escaped much notice in ethnographic work until recently, but it has maintained its presence within the larger and everchanging health care landscape. The health systems in hamlets, villages, and cities throughout the Mesoamerican region have developed into amalgams of health professionals, traditional specialists, and lay curers informed by medico-scientific or culturally specific etiologies and theories for the understanding and treatment of illness and injuries. Herbalists, midwives, bonesetters, shamans, and specialists that treat specific folk illnesses such as *susto* and *aire* operate in the midst of a growing number of nationally sponsored health posts, hospitals, and privately owned pharmacies. The region has, since European contact five hundred years ago, experienced an increasing stream of medical knowledge and technology that has been met with acceptance or ambivalence by its inhabitants (see Woods and Graves 1973: 23–26). As a result, it is often difficult to determine where the medico-scientific paradigm ends and the traditional Indian, or even *ladino* folk, medical beliefs begin when looking for origins of practices. Traits of Old World medicine show up in some of the choices of materials used in bonesetting, and at times the use of North American ointments and painkillers is a recommended part of treatment, but for the most part, bonesetting fits within the framework of the health care systems in which it is reported as a traditional (folk) specialty, informed by traditional Indian ways of life.

Bonesetters recognize and treat an extensive list of musculoskeletal disorders, maintaining a domain that has little overlap with those of other traditional specialists (Álvarez Heydenreich 1987:196; Douglas 1969:141), although there are individuals who practice another specialty, such as midwifery, in addition to bonesetting (Huber 1990a: 173; Huber and Anderson 1996:25; McMahon 1994:81), and there are also curers and midwives known to treat some musculoskeletal problems (Mellado Campos et al. 1994). At times bonesetting gets competition from the medical services extending from urban centers into the rural areas and municipalities. Most villages have health posts occupied by auxiliary medical personnel and a resident physician that administer vaccinations, provide public health information, give primary care, and refer patients with ailments or injuries beyond their capacity to treat—such as orthopedic cases—to the nearest hospital. In the health care systems of which bonesetting is a part, it may not be a patient's only choice for orthopedic care; but a patient may decide, for reasons of accessibility, affordability, and perceived efficacy, that it is his or her best choice. We have found that people in highland Guatemalan villages of the department of Sololá often view state-operated hospitals with dread, and private clinics and doctor's visits are considered to be far more costly than even the most expensive treatment obtainable from traditional bonesetters.

Recruitment and Training

Effective bonesetters have a combination of assets that make their work possible. They know the healing properties of the medicinal plants and commercially available materials specific to the cures they provide. They understand the structure of the human musculoskeletal system and how to diagnose a range of problems it may suffer. They exercise a sensitive touch that enables and enhances their diagnostic and healing abilities. They must have strong resolve in order to perform their treatments, often subjecting patients to enough pain to make bodily restraint necessary.

Some bonesetters voluntarily choose to serve their communities by providing their critical services. Others claim that they were chosen—in essence given a mandate from a higher power—to heal and thus help those around them. Difficult circumstances usually lead to one's initial involvement in bonesetting. Stories abound of individuals who, when suffering a fracture or dislocation, must help themselves. Discovering their latent healing abilities, they begin learning the specialty in an empirical fashion through trial and error. Many bonesetters claim to be self-taught: acquiring their knowledge by being willing to work on people in need of help. Precise

TABLE 10.1: MODES OF RECRUITMENT AND TRAINING OF BONESETTERS BY LINGUISTIC GROUP

	From Family	Self-Taught	Apprentice-ship	Dreams or Signs
Amuzgos	XX	XX	XX	
Cakchiqueles*				
Chatinos		XX		
Chichimeco–Jonaz	XX	XX		
Chochos	XX	XX		
Choles*				
Chontales	XX			
Chujes	XX	XX		
Coras			XX	
Cuicatecos	XX			
Huastecos		XX	XX	
Huaves*				
Ixcatecos			XX	
Jacaltecos*				
Lacandones*				
Mames		XX	XX	
Mayos		XX	XX	
Mazahuas			XX	
Mazatecos		XX	XX	XX
Mexicaneros		XX		
Mixes		XX	XX	
Motozintlecos*				
Nahuas	XX	XX		XX
Otomíes	XX	XX	XX	
Pames	XX	XX		
Popolocas		XX	XX	XX
Purépechas	XX	XX		XX
Tepehuanes del Sur	XX			
Tlapanecos		XX	XX	
Tlahuicas			XX	
Tojolabal		XX		XX
Totonacos		XX	XX	

TABLE 10.1 (cont.)

	From Family	Self-Taught	Apprentice-ship	Dreams or Signs
Triquis			XX	
Tzeltales			XX	XX
Tzotziles			XX	XX
Tzutujiles	XX	XX		XX
Zapotecos*				
Zoques de Chiapas	XX			XX
Zoque-Popolucas	XX			

*No available information.

numbers are not available for all groups, but in twenty-one of the thirty-four ethnic groups of Mexico that have practicing bonesetters, one or more of the bonesetters used this method of learning (Table 10.1) (Mellado Campos et al. 1994). In the Nahua village of Hueyapan, all bonesetters reported that they were self-taught, all but one having had no occasion to observe and learn from another bonesetter at work (Huber and Anderson 1996:27). However, in half of the Mesoamerican indigenous groups, a novice's exposure to an experienced bonesetter is a vital part of learning the specialty. Some bonesetters are influenced by a role model to take on the practice, and learn by apprenticeship. Often the mentors who teach them the secrets of the trade are family members—parents, grandparents, uncles, or aunts—but in some cases, the mentors may be nonrelatives of the same village (Mellado Campos et al. 1994).

Some bonesetters have birth signs that predispose them to their future calling. However, this is very uncommon in Mesoamerica. There are Nahua villages where some bonesetters profess this type of calling to their work, albeit infrequently, since 50 percent of those interviewed have learned by apprenticeship to elders in their family, and 37 percent are self-taught (Mellado Campos et al. 1994:532). The absence of birth signs and other mystical influences, such as dream sequences that indicate a future in bonesetting, for Nahua bonesetters of Hueyapan (Huber and Anderson 1996) speaks of the heterogeneous nature of recruitment experiences from individual to individual, and from village to village.

Supernatural signs—though not necessarily birth signs—play a role in the recruitment of bonesetters among the Purépechas, the Zoques of Chiapas, and the Mazatecos (for whom the mandate is obtained through the consumption of hallucinogenic mushrooms). The healing techniques, however, are learned from family members, for some Zoque and Purépecha bonesetters; by apprenticeship to someone in the village, for some Mazateco bonesetters; or are learned through self-teaching, for some bonesetters among the Purépechas and the Mazatecos.

Dream experiences that reveal a special calling to heal are common among Mesoamerican curers (Huber 1990b:55–56; Huber and Anderson 1996:26). Dreams reportedly figure in the recruitment process of bonesetters mainly in the Mayan areas of Chiapas and highland Guatemala, namely, among the Tojolabal, Tzotzil (Mellado Campos 1994) and Tzutujil-Maya (McMahon 1994; Paul 1976)—but also among the Nahuas, Popolocas, and Huaves of Puebla, Guerrero, and Oaxaca. In a way similar to the experiences of Tzutujil midwives (Paul and Paul 1975:711), the dreams strongly influence a healer's acceptance of his or her role and they also provide instruction in the methods to be used for curing patients. This type of recruitment has a universal pattern in which dreams are a part of a sequence of events including acute pain and illness for the reluctant initiates, who, as a way to end their suffering, ultimately decide to assume their mandated roles.

The narrative below provides a glimpse of the series of occurrences that not only were responsible for the recruitment of three generations of bonesetters in San Pedro la Laguna, Guatemala, but that also have contributed to the town's recognition as a regional bonesetting center.

In 1941 Benjamin Paul and his wife, Lois Paul, were routinely making a community study of San Pedro la Laguna. An accident yielded an unplanned episode of participation—emergency recourse to a native curer to treat Lois' painfully dislocated ankle—and abruptly brought attention to Ventura Quiacaín, the town's only bonesetter, previously unknown to the researchers.

Ventura was a wizened old man with a quiet air of almost saintly humility. He slowly passed a kerchief around the injured ankle and applied pressure. Hidden in the kerchief, it developed, was a special object, a little bone that guided the movements of Ventura's hand and thus the responsible agent for repairing the dislocation. Then Ventura massaged the sprained area with beef-bone marrow, wrapped a heated tobacco leaf around the ankle, causing a smarting sensation, and applied a tight bandage before leaving. He returned a few times to re-dress the ankle, which healed quite satisfactorily. He charged no fee but accepted a gratuity. He was seventy-seven years old at the time of this incident, and had been healing bones for over fifty years. The story of how he began his career as bonesetter (*wekol bak*) has come down through the generations.

Not long after getting married at around age twenty, Ventura was troubled by a dream in which he saw a bone hopping about. The next morning, as he was in his field, he perceived a strange object in the path. On closer approach it turned out to be a shiny bone. It leaped toward him. He recoiled in fright, but the object kept jumping toward him. Full of fear and finding his way blocked, Ventura returned home, covering the disturbing cause of his retreat by feigning illness and going to bed.

The next night he had another strange dream. A little old man, a dwarf, came to demand, "Why didn't you pick me up? If you keep refusing you will die." In the morning he set out to work with new determination. Once again he encountered the jumping bone. Now unafraid, he picked it up, wrapped it in his kerchief, and tucked it into his sash. At home he placed the object in his shoulder bag and hung it up. He was unaware of the strange bone's purpose, but instructions followed in dreams. It was Ventura's destiny, the dwarf told him, to aid humanity by caring for the afflicted "because they are our children." The dream visitor taught him a secret song and at night Ventura would sing it.

One night in a dream the dwarf appeared with a skeleton. He handed Ventura a whip and ordered him to strike the skeleton down. He did so. The skeleton collapsed in a heap of bones. The dwarf demanded that Ventura put the skeleton back together, threatening to whip him if he failed. Ventura protested, "Señor, I cannot." "Where is the bone I gave you?" asked the dwarf. Ventura fetched it. With its help he began to recognize the various parts, starting with the toes and proceeding to the larger bones. After Ventura had reassembled the entire skeleton, the dwarf said, "With this little bone you will cure our children." Ventura still did not know just what he was to do, but he continued to receive instructions in his dreams.

The bone told Ventura to guard it carefully. He put it in a little chest. Getting on his knees, he could hear the object making sounds as of people talking inside. He wrapped it in a silken cloth, blew on it repeatedly, and replaced it gingerly. No other person must see or touch it, he was warned, or else he or his children would perish.

The bone announced that Ventura's young wife would give birth to a boy who would die. Their first child, a boy, was born and lived only a short while. Ventura fell to quarreling with his wife, who expressed fear that because of his *fortuna*, his magic object, all their future babies were destined to die. He replied that his call came only from God, that its true purpose was to give life, and that he and his wife were due to live better and longer on earth. But he made no use of his mystic bone for a year. Meantime, Ventura fell ill; his head and his heart ached and he was on the point of death. Only by exercising his God-given gift as a healer could he regain his health.

A boy he knew suffered a broken leg. In a dream the dwarf commanded Ventura to heal the boy by making use of the bone. He complied; the boy's break was mended and in three days the patient was able to walk again. Ventura told no one what he had accomplished, but word slowly spread. His practice grew and he regained his good health. He never charged for his services. Grateful patients gave what they could; if very poor they gave only a few pennies. Ventura became increasingly in demand, healing the bone injuries not only of fellow Pedranos but also of accident victims who came from out of town.

It is likely, given the need, that there were bone menders in San Pedro la Laguna before 1900, when Ventura began to practice, although tradition holds that he was San Pedro's first, as well as finest, practitioner. During his lifetime Ventura was the town's only bonesetter, but since the time of his death, when the town had about two thousand inhabitants, eleven or twelve part-time practitioners, male and female, have appeared on the scene, their increase outpacing the fourfold growth of the population, which stood at over nine thousand inhabitants as the century ended.

The number of practitioners may be a response, in part, to San Pedro's current fame as the nation's center for effectively curing bone injuries. Practitioners are sometimes summoned to travel out of town by launch and bus to do their work, charging only the cost of transportation and keep. Indian and *ladino* patients, Catholics and Protestants alike, from communities all around the lake from Guatemala City and from as far away as the border areas of El Salvador and Mexico come to San Pedro, sometimes on improvised stretchers or litters, to remain in town enough days to complete a course of treatment.

There is a story, possibly apocryphal, that President Jorge Ubico (1933–1944) once slipped, sustaining an injury, while traveling in the country. Informed that a young man in San Pedro named Ventura Quiacaín could fix his foot, the president repaired to Sololá near the lake and summoned Ventura, who paddled across the lake in a dugout canoe and skillfully repaired the injury. Impressed, the president—so the story goes—issued a general advisory that one Ventura in San Pedro la Laguna is a skilled curer of bone injuries.

Many of the people injured in the catastrophic earthquake that shook Guatemala before dawn on February 4, 1976—a quake that touched San Pedro only lightly—were rushed to San Pedro to be treated by bonesetters, some of whom hastily set up cane shacks to house the patients.

With the exception of one contested case, all of the current bonesetters, like the venerable Ventura, owe their calling to divine election. In this they resemble San Pedro's midwives, a parallel category of sacred professionals (Paul and Paul 1975). In both cases the recruitment process is protracted and proceeds by stages. It begins by discovery of a significant object. The future midwife, for instance, may find in her path a conch but is afraid to touch it. In a dream the spirits of departed midwives, like the dwarf in Ventura's dream, rebuke her for failing to pick up the magic object, commanding her to go back and take possession of her "power," an object akin to the bonesetter's magic bone. (It is believed that scrapings from the midwife's sacred conch can later be dissolved in water to cure a woman of sterility).

Both types of sacred professionals, bonesetters and midwives, learn their destinies in dreams. But they are afraid to practice and their delay results in a series of misfortunes such as life-threatening illnesses or the death of children in the family. Finally induced to practice, they learn how to proceed by dream instruction. Once they start, they must exercise their profession without fear or hesitation, for timidity would endanger the practitioner or the patient.

Practicing one's sacred profession restores one's health; it also helps avert misfortune. One Pedrano bonesetter, the owner of a marimba band that traveled to many towns, remarked significantly that he had been in four road accidents without ever being injured. A bonesetter who was also a midwife and who occasionally had to hurry over difficult paths, often at night, to attend women in labor, was prone to slipping and spraining her ankles, but became nimble and sure-footed after she began her long-delayed practice as a divinely accredited bonesetter (Paul 1976:79).

In native conception it is not the bonesetter but his or her magic bone that works. Hidden in a kerchief, the bone searches for the exact site of the injury as its owner keeps moving the kerchief around until the magic bone, like a magnet, clamps tightly onto a certain spot. After thus locating the critical site, the bone directs the practitioner how to perform the necessary manipulations and massages.

When Ventura died a curious thing occurred. His magic bone did not disappear with him. It went to work for Rosario, one of his children. In time she became a well-regarded bonesetter, addressed respectfully as "Doña Rosario." Before she died she recounted how this came about to Butler and Rocché Bixcul (1973), and this story has been retold by McMahon (1994).

When she was growing up, Rosario occasionally could hear movement within the little chest containing her father's mystic object. When she asked her mother about it she replied that she did not know. Rosario recounted that she had a dream in which she cured broken bones for many people. In this prophetic dream the divine object told her where the patients would come from and whether they were *ladinos* or Indians.

On his deathbed Ventura turned the sacred object over to his daughter Rosario, saying that she could not evade the responsibility of curing people after he died; that she must never charge for her services; that she must keep the object locked up in its little chest and never let anyone see it.

After Ventura died, people came to ask about his famed object. Two men tried to rifle through the dead man's pockets. On the way to the cemetery, one of them demanded to know where the thing was, offering to buy it. Rosario said it had no price, that the sacred bone itself had forbidden her to sell it.

Two years later, after having endured illness and having rejected the pleas of people who came begging to be cured, Rosario was reassured by the sacred object: "Do not be afraid; I am with you."

Moved by the plight of a badly injured boy and by the beseeching of his distraught father, Rosario took on her first case. She asked the boy whether he could endure the pain that would be involved and he said he could. Others held him while she applied pressure. When the object was just over the tip of the boy's spinal column it made a noise, indicating that his injured bone had been set in its proper place.

Rosario agreed to return the next day to continue the cure on condition that her work would not be made public lest others would rush to her for help. But they came anyway. Gradually she gained confidence in herself.

The object told Rosario, "It is I who enter the body, not you." In her dreams it assured her that when she died it would go nowhere else but would let itself return to earth.

Rosario practiced her curing craft for about forty years. After her death the sacred object, contrary to assurances, moved on to work with another person: José, a grandson of Rosario's brother and thus a great-grandson of Ventura. José refers to Rosario, his great-aunt in point of fact, as his grandmother, "*mi abuelita*," perhaps to promote the belief that he and the sacred object are in the direct line of descent from Ventura, reputedly the original bonesetter.

José does work with the sacred object to remedy bone injuries, but whether his calling is truly legitimate is subject to some doubt in San Pedro. It is not clear just how he came into possession of the bone. Did it come to him willingly? José has been accused of stealing it when Rosario was dying, but he claims that she gave it to him, and that he must use it to cure the injured even should people accuse him of theft. If it was really his destiny to become a curer, people asked, how come he did not, like his predecessors Ventura and Rosario, experience fear and suffering and allow considerable time to elapse before starting to practice? Some Pedranos think that he is motivated less by the urge to fulfill a spiritual mandate to assist his fellow man than by the possibility of substantial economic gain. San Pedro does, after all, attract patients from a wide area because of its favorable reputation as a bonesetting town. Some Pedrano bonesetters have been known to see at least one patient a day nearly every day during a three-week period.

Despite the demand for the bonesetters of San Pedro la Laguna it appears—for them as well as for all other indigenous groups of Mesoamerica—to be uncommon for either male or female bonesetters to make healing patients their primary occupation. Throughout the region women most commonly are involved in household activities. Men mostly pursue agricultural production or a trade, spending part of the day working away from the home in their fields or as wage laborers. Bonesetting is a medical specialty that they can readily do, since compared to other traditional medical specialties, it tends to have a light patient load; days often pass between patient visits. Based on the sample sets of healers that were interviewed (Mellado Campos et al. 1994), fourteen of the Mesoamerican groups are reported to have only male bonesetters; in one they are all female (see Table 10.2). Female bonesetters outnumber males in nine of the different ethnic groups;

TABLE 10.2: GENDER DISTRIBUTION AMONG BONESETTERS
BY LINGUISTIC GROUP

Amuzgos	M	F = All female;
Cakchiqueles	NA	M = All male.
Chatinos	M	F > M = More females
Chichimeco–Jonaz	F > M	than males.
Chochos	NA	M > F = More males
Choles	NA	than females.
Chontales	F > M	M = F = Males and
Chujes	M	females in equal numbers.
Coras	F	NA = No available
Cuicatecos	M	information.
Huastecos	M	
Huaves	NA	
Ixcatecos	M	
Jacaltecos	NA	
Lacandones	NA	
Mames	F > M	
Mayos	F > M	
Mazahuas	M	
Mazatecos	F > M	
Mexicaneros	M	
Mixes	F > M	
Motozintlecos	NA	
Nahuas	M > F	
Otomíes	M	
Pames	M > F	
Popolocas	M	
Purépechas	F > M	
Tepehuanes del Sur	M	
Tlapanecos	M > F	
Tlahuicas	F > M	
Tojolabal	M	
Totonacos	M > F	
Triquis	M	
Tzeltales	NA	

TABLE 10.2 (cont.)

Tzotziles	M
Tzutujil Maya	M = F
Zapotecos	M = F
Zoques de Chiapas	F > M
Zoque-Popoluca	NA

males outnumber females in six; in two their numbers are equal. No information on gender ratios was available for nine of the groups.

Bonesetters are usually not wealthy people, but their occupation does create additional income. Most bonesetters that were recruited by a supernatural mandate assert the philosophy that, since their ability to heal is a gift from God, they must never charge for their cures, although it is acceptable to take money that is freely offered by the patient out of gratitude.

Therapeutic Techniques

There appear to be two major types of bonesetting practiced in native Mesoamerica: spiritual and naturalistic. Spiritual bonesetters—principally from the mountainous Maya area of southern Mesoamerica—are normally initiated to their position through a life-changing supernatural experience. Their ability to cure is attributed to God. Although they carry out their duties with humility, they gain elevated status from recognition of being a divinely elected healer. Spiritual bonesetters typically charge nothing for their work, but willingly accept donations from grateful patients. Naturalistic bonesetters—throughout Mesoamerica but primarily in the western and northern areas—commonly are self-taught (although some are recruited via supernatural experiences) and work with an array of medicinal materials. But with no connection to the spiritual realm, they rank low in status compared with other types of traditional healers that do have the spiritual connection. With no divine sanctions to consider, naturalistic bonesetters are not reluctant to charge for their services. Despite differences, a strong common denominator of the two approaches to bonesetting is the importance of the healer's hands in the diagnosis and treatment of bone problems. Rubbing and massage are part of every cure.

Spiritual Practice

Depending on the community, the status of people who repair bone injuries can range from persons of little recognition and social standing to professionals with divine attributes and elevated social status. Although exceptions exist, in Mexican indigenous communities bonesetters are normally fewer in number and lower in social standing than other types of traditional healers. Status is related to the degree to which healers act as intermediaries between the supernatural and natural worlds. Tzotzil (Laughlin 1969:166), Tzeltal (Mellado Campos et al. 1994:830), and Yucatan Maya bonesetters have been observed to be magico–religious practitioners (Villa Rojas 1969: 262). The more recent information on Yucatan Maya bonesetting is that it is known to be a specialty of people who undertake the traditional healing roles of herbalist (*hierbero*) and shaman (*h'men*) and is thus highly regarded (Mellado Campos et al. 1994:387, 424).

The relationship of status and mystic knowledge is notable in Tzotzil communities, where the naturally curative approaches of bonesetting are diverse but make up only a part of the total treatment. The participation of supernatural forces in curing is believed to be essential to bonesetters. In the material aspect of their treatments, they have various remedies for fractures, all of which entail heating the injured area, setting, and then immobilizing the bone. Heat is applied with leaves from plants such as *sisil*, *higuerilla* (*Ricinus communis*), and *mano de león* (*Chiranthodendron pentadactylon*[1]) that are warmed on coals. Massage directed at reduction of the fracture is given over the herbs and these remain in place for their analgesic and anti-inflammatory properties even beneath the bandages and splints used for immobilization. During the therapy, the bonesetter recites orations to "*los dueños del cerro*" (lords of the hill) requesting their benevolent intervention in the cure on behalf of the patient. They also invoke the help of certain plant species with great root systems, asking that their essence pass over the break, inducing it to knit together.[2] Some prayers are directed at *pukuj*, a malevolent spirit that is considered to be the cause of all misfortune (Holland 1963; Mellado Campos et al. 1994:852). In the Tzotzil town of Zinacantan, the most highly regarded bonesetters rely mostly or exclusively on spiritual curing methods, while those whose knowledge of healing bones includes only techniques of physical manipulation are considered inferior (Fabrega and Silver 1973:41–42). Yet even bonesetters that employ spiritual techniques have been found to occupy the lowest rank in an informal hier-archy of healers—the upper two ranks are held by shamans and diviners—since compared with the others they have a lesser degree of contact with the spirit world (Holland 1963; Laughlin 1969:173).

Although in the distant past Nahua bonesetters performed a variety of invocations to the spirit world petitioning its help in curing (López Austin 1988:165–166), today they have a secular approach to healing. Nahua bone-setters in Hueyapan, Mexico—mostly men—have a lower status than cur-ers, who are mostly women (Huber and Anderson 1996:25). In Hueyapan, bonesetters give normative diagnoses and treatments, with little variation from healer to healer, whereas curers have more leeway in their diagnosis—observation combined with divination—and treatment (often with strong ritualistic content) of illnesses. It is not simple for patients to empirically verify a curer's efficacy, the healing rituals being characteristically subjective (Huber 1990b:59–60).

Central Mexican bonesetters, along with *curanderas*, practice as secular healers that make no claim to supernatural powers. As a result their popu-larity has lessened concomitant with the growth in numbers of practic-ing Spiritualist curers, who derive their legitimacy through the control and sanction of supernatural figures from the Christian religion (Finkler 1985:43).

The magico-religious elements of the bonesetting done in the Tzutujil community of San Pedro la Laguna on the southwestern shore of Lake Ati-tlán in Guatemala have factored greatly in the status and recognition ac-crued to the practice today. The Tzutujil bonesetters have moved away from the naturalistic approach of the majority of their contemporaries with their use of a *"hueso"* (bone)—an object considered to be of considerable healing power given to them by God—to move broken bones back into place. The medicinal products that they use are quite sparse in comparison to those used by bonesetters elsewhere. They have, however, developed a rich oral history that provides strength to their image in the eyes of patients. In the highland region where they work, the cures that they provide are generally acknowledged as effective for the types of problems that they face.

We now return to the consideration of a special case involving the al-leged improper use of sacred material. When José in San Pedro la Laguna began curing people several months after acquiring the revered bone, some people accused him of violating tradition by making money on his practice.

They noticed that he would return from out-of-town curing visits laden with goods he had purchased for his family. He was accused of extracting a sizable sum of money, for instance, from an out-of-town petitioner who had sought out José and accompanied him back to the petitioner's home to cure an injured man who was waiting there. It was José's claim in self-defense that his client was so pleased with the treatment that he happily and voluntarily handed him the money. But some people called José a thief, asserting that he was robbing the poor.

Tired of enduring constant disparagement, José resolved, after seven years of practice, to abandon bonesetting and stick to agriculture, but he was dissuaded of his resolve by a timely dream. The dream told him that he must not quit, that he and his bone must continue to help suffering people. José then decided to continue but to charge openly for his services. For adults he set a fee of 10 *quetzales* (about $2 US) for each visit, and for children he charged 5 *quetzales*.

Some people in San Pedro, even though they may question his credentials or criticize the commercialization of his practice, nevertheless admit that they would go to José if they suffered a fracture because of the fame of the sacred curing instrument in José's possession—the best bone in town. One informant said that he would go to José because he had been successfully healed earlier by the same bone when it was still in the hands of José's "grandmother" Rosario (McMahon 1994:63).

José enjoys a lively patronage and this may be because he attracts not only clients who respect the power of the sacred bone but also clients of a different kind, mainly out-of-towners, who believe that money talks, and that one gets only what one pays for. They prefer José precisely because he charges, unlike his colleagues in San Pedro la Laguna, who are obliged by destiny to provide their curing services freely as a sacred duty.

It may turn out that José is inaugurating a secularization trend that will eventually lead to the decline or elimination of sacred professionals in San Pedro, a relatively prosperous and rapidly modernizing town, in favor of secular practitioners.

In the meantime, however, every bonesetter in San Pedro la Laguna works with a supernaturally provided object variously known as one's *suerte*, *cuento*, *aparato*, *material*, or, most often, as one's *hueso*. The injunction that the object, always hidden in the folds of a cloth during healing sessions, must never be exposed to view is supported by cautionary stories. One bonesetter said that a young child of hers once played with the forbidden object, and that shortly thereafter the child died.

The narratives told by and about Pedrano bonesetters and their *huesos* are often constructed to have an awe-inspiring effect on the listener. They add to the mystery and power that is attributed to these small objects that purportedly recruit their users and give them a sacred mandate to become healers. Perhaps the commonplace reality that keeps patients coming to see Pedrano bonesetters is, however, that most of them consistently satisfy their patients' needs by providing a good cure. The *hueso* narratives are simply meant to explain how they are able to do it. This was the experience of one of the authors (Clancy McMahon) when undergoing treatment by a Pedrana bonesetter.

In 1992 Clancy McMahon fractured the distal end of his fibula (part of the ankle) and was treated successively by orthopedists and by a bonesetter in San Pedro. The story of his treatment has been documented in detail (McMahon 1994).

The fracture occurred in Antigua. The injured ankle was encased in a half-cast in an Antigua hospital. Soon Clancy's toes became so swollen and discolored that he removed the half-cast. He next visited a private clinic in Antigua and was advised to allow four days for the swelling to go down before having his leg encased in a full-sized cast. He was to remain in bed with his leg propped up.

Supported by crutches, Clancy then traveled to Santa Cruz la Laguna on Lake Atitlán, having earlier arranged to participate in an anthropological training project there. While propped up for four days in the local hotel, he had ample time to be urged, first by a gardener and then by a health education promoter, that he should go to San Pedro la Laguna to be cured by one of the expert bonesetters in that town. He had not previously heard about them. He received contrary advice from a young woman doctor who was completing her obligatory year of public health service in Santa Cruz. She believed that native bonesetting was effective for minor fractures and bruises, but not for breaks like Clancy's.

One week after his accident, Clancy traveled to the Herrera Llerandi hospital in Guatemala City, where his ankle was X-rayed and then examined by a doctor trained at the Duke University Medical School. He determined that the ankle should be immobilized for a month, and had a cast applied that extended from below the knee to behind the toes.

Clancy returned to Santa Cruz la Laguna, where he was befriended by Andrés, the town's last practicing shaman, who noticed the cast and commented that casts do not cure broken bones. One week after getting the cast, Clancy, annoyed by a painful ankle, accepted the shaman's offer to take him to San Pedro to get cured, naively assuming that the treatment would not involve removing the cast, but that if it did he would refuse.

In San Pedro the two visitors were led to the house of an aged bonesetter named Juana Ixmatá. Surrounded by grown daughters and their children, she was set to begin work immediately. First she wanted to remove the cast so that she could locate the break and determine its severity. To remove a cast—not a new experience for her—Juana softens it by immersion in a tub of hot water and cuts it off with a razor. The cast would be discarded, she explained, and replaced with a tight bandage to keep the bone from moving.

Learning from Andrés that Clancy had gone to a hospital where they took an X ray and put on a cast, Juana remarked, "I do not use X rays. None of that. I use a bone and the bone tells me if it is a bruise or a fracture, and where the fracture is. The bone is a magnet. It grabs where it is fractured. If it is just a bruise it does not indicate anything."

Clancy protested that he still needed to keep the cast on his leg as the doctor had ordered. With the cast and his crutches he could walk, he explained. He asked Juana whether he would have to be in bed for a number of days. She replied that from the second day on he could put force on the leg, but only a little at first, and that he would be well in two weeks. One of the daughters said, "Today, tomorrow, and the day after, you will need to come." She and Andrés kept urging Clancy to start right away with Juana's treatment.

Clancy was inclined to accept treatment but asserted that he needed time to think things over. Juana said, "Let him go and think on it, so that later he can come back. I do not want him to regret it." Juana's daughter offered last-minute advice: he should stand on his leg instead of carrying it in the air "so that the veins do not shrink." Andrés, clearly disappointed at the delay, accompanied Clancy back to Santa Cruz la Laguna and advised him to have the cast removed in the Sololá hospital, not far away, and to return to San Pedro for treatment when he was ready.

A week later, having slowly removed the cast with his pocketknife and wrapped the ankle in an Ace bandage, Clancy was ready. He went back to San Pedro, taking three people with him. One, Rolando, was an interpreter, whose description of how his left scapula, broken in a fall from a roof, had been successfully remedied by a San Pedro bonesetter, reinforced Clancy's decision to be treated by Juana. The others were two colleagues, a man and a woman, who were to videotape and photograph the curing process.

The trio entered the bonesetter's house and positioned themselves. Clancy sat on a chair to remove the bandage. Juana sat down on the floor, her legs folded beneath her, and placed his foot on her knees. From a pocket in her apron, she extracted her small curing bone, wrapped in cloth, and began probing the ankle with it.

When Clancy pointed to the part that was broken, she slid the covered bone above it and forcefully applied pressure. Pain jumped through Clancy's body. Juana continued searching, pressing, pushing, and massaging with the bone in her left hand, her right hand holding the ankle steady. As the pain intensified, Clancy pleaded, "Take it easy!" Rolando, who had been holding the patient's arm, loosened his grip as everyone, including Juana, chuckled at Clancy's reaction.

After a brief pause, Juana resumed her work with solid purpose. Neither Clancy's jerking back against the chair, nor stiffening his leg against the pain, nor his groaning broke the steady rhythm of the pressure she applied to his ankle with her bone. George, the videotape operator, joined Rolando in restraining Clancy in the chair.

After one and a half more minutes of using her bone, Juana stopped and put it back in her apron pocket. She produced a container of GMS, a mentholated salve, and rubbed some of it on the ankle. This was followed by thirty seconds of massage around the area of the break. Then she wrapped the ankle with Clancy's Ace bandage. The pain subsided. Rolando, interpreting, said that Juana wanted Clancy to gently begin using his foot. He stood up and took a few careful steps. The visit was over in fifteen minutes.

The next day Clancy returned for his second treatment. George came along to videotape the session. Clancy removed the Ace bandage. Juana knelt on the floor as she held his ankle with her left hand and worked on it with the miraculous object held in her right hand. The cure consisted of massaging the inside of the ankle, opposite the broken bone. Juana worked on this part of the ankle without any conscious cue from Clancy. It was, in fact, the stiffest area of the ankle, causing the most resistance to free pivotal movement. The work lasted only a minute and was painful; but it relieved the ache that had been bothering this part of the ankle. After putting the curing bone back in the pocket of her apron, Juana rubbed mentholated salve onto the ankle.

Through a daughter, acting as interpreter, Juana told Clancy that he no longer needed to return for a third treatment unless the ankle was bothering him. He was told to stop relying on the crutches and to walk on the injured foot.

Back in Santa Cruz, he did so gently, using the foot as though walking, but carrying the greater part of this weight on the crutches. Five days later he quit using his crutches completely, and returned once again to San Pedro, with Rolando as interpreter, to interview Juana about her work and history as bonesetter. Juana expressed interest in the state of Clancy's ankle. He removed the Ace bandage so she could examine it. Clancy informed Juana that he felt much better. She was pleased with the results and took occasion to say that he should have trusted her to cure him earlier and that there is no need for operations and examinations.

Clancy's evaluation of the outcome of his treatment matched Juana's: it was effective. On the basis of any number of curing instances that came to Clancy's attention following his treatment by Juana, he judges that most evaluations on the part of both the bonesetters in San Pedro and their patients are equally favorable. An X ray taken later in the United States indicated that the bone was properly healed. As for possession of a miraculous object—a sine qua non of healing bone injuries in San Pedro—it can be viewed as providing the curer with necessary self-confidence, and the believing client with confidence in the curer.

In progressive and relatively prosperous San Pedro la Laguna, two features dominate the bonesetting system: recruitment of practitioners by *divine election* and a *sacred bone* that communicates with its possessor in dreams and actively aids in the hands-on cure of injuries. The use of a sacred bone has not been recorded elsewhere in the Mesoamerican region, although there are other societies whose bonesetters call upon benevolent assistance from the supernatural world in order to effect their cures. It is apparent that healers who employ supernatural means experience a higher measure of respect in their communities than those who do not. Most bonesetters with naturalistic approaches to their work thus enjoy little prestige associated with their work. They do, however, command a great knowledge of medical materials and methods that are effective against a wide range of musculoskeletal problems experienced by their patients.

Naturalistic Therapy

For almost all of Mesoamerica, bonesetters conceptualize the causes of broken or fractured bones, dislocations, sprains, bruises, and chronic joint pain in naturalistic terms. Etic symptomatology is identical to the bonesetters' emic terms for skeletal health problems (see Huber and Anderson 1996:29). An exception is the case of the Chatinos of southwest Oaxaca, for whom bone lesions are caused by a wind (*aire*) that enters the patient and must be removed by massage (Mellado Campos et al. 1994:108).

Following is a grouping of the most common types of disorders suffered by bonesetters' patients. Each disorder is treated in various ways by bonesetters among the different indigenous groups in Mesoamerica. For each disorder, we give examples of treatments from one or more of the indigenous groups. Unless otherwise noted, the descriptions are representative of the methodology of healers that have a naturalistic philosophy of bonesetting. The notes list the indigenous groups from which bonesetters responded with information about each disorder.

BROKEN BONES AND FRACTURES

Musculoskeletal injuries[3] are recognized for the intense pain that is suffered by the patient. If the injury consists of a bone broken (*hueso quebrado, quebradura, fractura*) in one of the extremities, it will be apparent because of the noise of the break, the misshapen bone, and the restriction of movement (Mellado Campos et al. 1994:90). Bonesetters also note symptoms of intense pain, swelling, burning sensation, and loss of feeling in some cases. The Chujes of Chiapas recognize headache and abdominal pain as associated symptoms (p. 221). Chinanteco bonesetters of northeast Oaxaca believe that broken bones also result in *susto* (fright), a condition that must be cured before continuing with bone treatment (p. 146). Diagnosis is carried out via conversation with the patient to learn how the accident occurred and examination of the area with the pads of the fingers to feel the nature of the bone lesion.

The next objective in the treatment process is to relieve pain and swelling in the area of the lesion. Tlapanecos of southeast Guerrero use oil of *arrayán* (*Gaultheria acuminata*) mixed with ground flowers and tubers of *florifundillo* (*Datura candida*) to serve as an anti-inflammatory (p. 775). Hot salt water is used to reduce swelling by Chatinos (p. 117) and Mazahuas (p. 462). In Guanajuato, Chichimeca bonesetters use a preparation of arnica (*Arnica* sp.) or *cuachalalate* for this purpose (p. 135). The Tojolabal in southeast Chiapas relieve pain and heat the area of the lesion with a boiled preparation of red salt, five mango (*Mangifera indica*) leaves, and five heads of *malva* (*Malva* sp.) applied with a cloth (p. 787). Cuicateco therapists wrap injured areas that are too swollen for reducing the fracture in (*Annona* sp.) leaves greased with beef fat under a bandage overnight (p. 91).

The processes of reducing broken bones, of setting them back into place, are specific to the location and type of lesion. Chontal healers in southeast Oaxaca claimed to dislodge the blood that aggregates around a broken bone before setting it, but did not explain how (p. 202). Otomí bone-setters use a cloth pulled back and forth across the injured area to remove any flesh from inside a severed bone before it is reduced. This is done by massaging the bone into place with a salve of *sebo de borrego, camote de gato,* and tobacco (*Nicotiana* sp.) from cigarettes (p. 582). Other salves used to add heat to the lesion during massage are of a mentholated variety bought from local pharmacists. Most bonesetters use their hands to massage and reduce fractures. The Cuicatecos massage with a hot tile or brick wrapped in *pega-josa* leaves. This kind of leaf is also used in a poultice that is kept applied to the injured area until the bone fuses, at which time it is replaced with a bandage soaked in turpentine of burned *ocote* (*Pinus sp.*) or with a mixture of turpentine and lamb's wool which must be worn until the cure is complete (pp. 90–91).

To set broken ribs Chinanteco bonesetters begin with a gentle massage first with their hands and then with their fingertips. They gently work their fingers in between the ribs to manipulate them into proper position. In some cases they will cover a patient's mouth with their hand and then blow forcibly into his nose to fill the lungs and push out the broken rib (p. 147). Chatino healers locate rib lesions by having their patients lie on their uninjured side while they push against the thorax, using a wide cloth with gradual movement as the patient informs them of increasing pain intensity. They use the cloth to move broken ribs back into place with a pressing and loosening motion. If they suspect internal problems, they will administer penicillin to thwart infection. Teas are another aid against infection, such as one made with leaves of *ítamo real, tepeguaje* (*Lysiloma watsoni*), or avocado (*Persea americana*) (pp. 117–118). Otomí bonesetters use a salve to massage the rib cage while the patient blows into a bottle to reset broken ribs. Then they put a cataplasm of *sacasil* tuber ground with cumin (*Cuminum cyminum*), cayenne pepper (*Capsicum* sp.), and cloves (*Eugenia caryophyllus*) over the lesion, cover it with a cloth, and wrap it with cardboard and a bandage. They advise their patients to avoid pork, spicy foods, and wine for forty days, the time it takes to heal (p. 572).

Once set, bone lesions are immobilized in various ways and to different degrees. In cases involving the extremities, Chichimeca bonesetters apply a poultice of ground *sacasil* tuber and a splint for two to three weeks. If there is a cut associated with the bone injury, then it must be washed with a preparation of arnica two more times during the course of healing (p. 135). For broken leg bones, some Mazahua therapists use a cloth with plaster to create a cast, while others apply a poultice followed by a bandage soaked in tar. If they treat a compound fracture, they will typically use commercial antibiotics on the wound for three days before immobilizing the leg (p. 462). Mazatecos use splints of *ocote* (pitch pine) the size of the bone that is broken to immobilize it, first heating the area with a hot brick over leaves of *mantecoso*, then applying a mixture of turpentine, honey, and white *copal* (*Bursera* sp.) that is covered with *chirimoya* leaves. The splint is secured with a bandage. Some healers add spider web to the poultice (p. 480).

An alternative to bone immobilization is practiced by bonesetters who only apply a movable bandage to breaks that are in the extremities. The Tzutujil and Chatino bonesetters that practice this approach believe that the ability to use the muscles of an injured limb while it is healing will allow the bone to gain strength gradually, avoid stiffness, and keep the limb from atrophying. Compound fractures can be treated against infection with the easier removal of a bandage compared with a splint (p. 118).

DISLOCATED BONES

The symptoms of a dislocated bone (*zafadura, desviadura*)[4] are swelling, heat, bruising, and occasionally a headache. The bone usually makes a popping noise when it is forced out of joint. Bonesetters diagnose this type of problem by palpating to feel if a bone is out of place in the affected articulation. Therapy for dislocations is generally easier the sooner the patient seeks treatment. If much time has elapsed, Tzotzil bonesetters will require a patient to warm up the injury by applying herbs to it while in a *temazcal*, or sweat bath (Mellado Campos et al. 1994:848).

To correct dislocations of the heel, wrist, and collarbone, Chuj bonesetters of Chiapas use a gentle pulling motion until the patient feels the pain lessen. Once the bone is almost in place a more vigorous pull is given to pop the bones of the joint together. Then two heated leaves of white *higuerilla*

(*Ricinus communis*) with salt or vinegar are wrapped around the injury. This poultice must be changed once a day for four days (p. 220).

Throughout native Mesoamerica dislocated—as well as fractured— bones are thought to be "cold" in the Hippocratic sense, and therefore call for "hot" treatments and materials in order to restore the balance. Before putting a bone back into joint, it must be heated. This is done by massage with an ointment, like Vicks or Iodex, or with friction from rubbing with the hands (p. 201).

Zoque-Popoluca healers begin the treatment of a dislocated hip with a hot compress made by dampening a cloth with a preparation of the leaves of *corazón, malva de cochino,* and arnica. They then wrap the patient around the hips with a porous plaster and a wide bandage that will maintain pressure on the joints. The patient must wear the wrap for three months (p. 909).

To correct a dislocated vertebra in the spinal column, Zapotec boneset- ters of Oaxaca begin with careful diagnosis of the problem. First they have the patient walk and observe the body's movement. Then, using their fin- gertips, they begin with the cervical vertebrae in an examination of the spi- nal column. They locate the dislodged vertebrae by touch and determine the direction of slippage. The healers then move the vertebrae back into place with great care to ensure that it is done correctly. This maneuver is done slowly, according to how well the patient handles the pain. If it be- comes unbearable the work is interrupted and the spine is massaged toward the lesion to calm the uneasiness until work can resume. If much time has lapsed since the injury, the Zapotec bonesetters observe that some fusion of the bones will have occurred and must be loosened with massage. They ap- ply a poultice after setting the spinal column. This is made of 40 grams of *chapopote,* 30 grams of *ocote* resin, 10 grams of wood glue, 10 grams of *cola,* and 5 grams of *copal* cooked and soaked into a bandage that is applied to the injured part of the spine. It conforms to the shape of the back to provide support, keep it warm, and speed healing (p. 886).

SPRAINS

In cases involving a sprain (*torcedura*),[5] the patient displays insupportable pain, contracted muscles and ligaments, and swelling. Mestizo healers in Acamixtla make a careful diagnosis of the sprained area, looking for *botones* (lumps) and *nudos* (knots) associated with the disarrangement of tendons, muscles, or nerves resulting from the injury. These are massaged with beef or pork lard (Perez 1978:76). Tlapaneco bonesetters rub sprains with *arrayán* oil combined with the flower and tuber of *florifundillo*. They wrap the sprain with a bandage to retain heat on the affected area. This is left in place for three days (Mellado Campos et al. 1994:775).

A related musculoskeletal problem involving the injury of muscles and tendons is called *falseado*, and is caused by accidental falls or by blows to the body, or by straining to lift or carry heavy loads. Purépecha healers treat *falseado* of the hand by massaging from the shoulder to the elbow, and then from the elbow to the wrist. Then they apply a compress of *hierba del golpe* twice a day to relieve swelling. For *falseado* of the foot, a compress of boiled turpentine and *ocote* soaked into a rag is applied and covered with a bandage for eight days (p. 672).

RHEUMATISM

Rheumatism (*reumas*)[6] is thought of as a coldness that affects the muscles and joints that is primarily brought on by exposure. The Cora find that its pain and stiffness result from a patient's getting cold and wet when convalescing from a fracture; or from a person crossing a river while still hot from a long walk. They treat this disorder using a tea made with three splinters of *cuamecate* boiled in water, and taken at room temperature. They also give massage with hot ointments of arnica, *fresno* (*Fraxinus* sp.) leaves, *ocote*, *chuchupato* (*Ligusticum porteri*), *colcolmeca* (*Salix mexicana*), *san marcos*, and *palomulato* (*Bursera grandifolia*) (p. 78).

Yucatan Maya bonesetters prescribe a treatment of 75 ml of lemon juice to be drunk on an empty stomach two hours before breakfast for twelve days. They also give palliative local applications of wildcat, duckling, or rattlesnake grease or oil. The patient should eat the fried meat as well as the toasted and ground skin of the same animal for relief of pain. To rub the patient, they use preparations of ground *guaco* fruit or *kakaaltuun* in rum; camphor and marijuana (*Cannabis sativa*) in alcohol; and the leaves and roots of *paay chí*, *teresita* leaves, *ortiga* (*Urera caracasana*) roots, a head of garlic (*Allium sativum*), and a small handful of marijuana ground up in rum (pp. 424–425).

Conclusions

Bonesetters have an important part to play in the diverse medical care system that has evolved in Mesoamerica. Quite often they provide the only source of a remedy for broken bones, dislocations, sprains, and so on, within their communities—a job which is physically demanding and requires skillful hands. Bonesetters come into this knowledge through a variety of ways, with the most common approaches involving the secular acquisition of knowledge through self-teaching or apprenticeship to another bonesetter. This is normally the path of the naturalistic bonesetter, the type that is especially common among the majority of ethnic groups in the western and northern areas of Mesoamerica.

In the Maya areas to the south a typical form of recruitment involves dreams or supernatural signs that direct the usually reluctant initiate to assume the role of bonesetter. With their knowledge and ability being attributed to a divine source, these spiritual bonesetters traditionally perform their work as an act of charity, and thus may not charge, although they will accept payment voluntarily offered by the patient. As a class of healer, bonesetters do not rank as high as shamans, diviners, and specialists, who heal almost strictly through mediation between the patient and the spirit world. But because of the divine influence in spiritual bonesetting, it has higher status than its naturalistic counterpart. However, spiritual bonesetters have a sparse medical kit in use during treatments. This is especially so in the Tzutujil town of San Pedro la Laguna, Guatemala, where the bonesetters rely on a small supernaturally powered object—presumably a bone— wrapped in cloth, which they use to diagnose and cure bone injuries. In contrast, naturalistic bonesetters utilize a great number of plants and some animal products in combinations they deem appropriate for the various injuries or ailments they must treat. It is difficult to predict if one or the other will ultimately prevail in Mesoamerica. They both provide the hands-on manipulation that is so effective in treatment of bone injuries. But each also provides something in addition to that: naturalistic methods use the empirically proven healing properties of their *materia médica* to enhance a cure; spiritual methods tap into the beneficial effects of faith in a higher power to get patients' involvement in their own healing.

Notes

1. Scientific nomenclature for plants, when provided, is taken from Martínez (1959) or Ford (1975).
2. The use (whether invoked or actually applied) of materials with physical properties akin to the problem at hand, e.g., plants with a mass of roots, or even in some instances, spider web, for knitting bone is a trait that is similar in concept to the Doctrine of Signatures. This medical concept originated in China and was widespread in Europe during the Middle Ages (Lewis and Elvin-Lewis 1977).

3. Amuzgos, Coras, Cuicatecos, Chatinos, Chichimeco-Jonaz, Chinantecos, Chochos, Chontales, Chujes, Huastecos, Huaves, Ixcatecos, Mames, Mayos, Mazahuas, Mazatecos, Mixtecos, Nahuas, Otomíes, Popolocas, Purépechas, Tepehuanes del Sur, Mexicaneros, Tlapanecos, Totonacos, Tzeltal, Tzotzil, Zoque-Popoluca (Mellado Campos et al. 1994), Chortí (Wisdom 1940:356), Cakchiquel (Marshall 1986:337–366), Tzutujil (Douglas 1969:143–144; McMahon 1994:133–169; Paul 1976).
4. Cuicatecos, Chatinos, Chichimeco-Jonaz, Chinantecos, Chochos, Chontales, Chujes, Huastecos, Ixcatecos, Mames, Mazahuas, Mazatecos, Mixes, Mixtecos, Otomies, Pames, Popolocas, Purépechas, Tepehuanes del Sur, Mexicaneros, Tzotzil, Zoque-Popoluca, Zoques de Chiapas (Mellado Campos et al. 1994), Tzutujil (McMahon 1994:85–86; Douglas 1969:143).
5. Coras, Cuicatecos, Chatinos, Chichimeco-Jonaz, Huastecos, Ixcatecos, Mayos, Mazahuas, Mazatecos, Mixes, Mixtecos, Nahuas, Otomíes, Pames, Popolocas, Purépechas, Tlapanecos, Totonacos, Tzotzil, Zoques de Chiapas (Mellado Campos et al. 1994), Tzutujil (Paul 1976).
6. Coras, Cuicatecos, Chinantecos, Huastecos, Mames, Mayos, Mixes, Mixtecos, Nahuas, Pames, Popolocas, Purépechas, Tepehuanes del Sur, Mexicaneros, Zapotecos (Mellado Campos et al. 1994).

CHAPTER 11

Mexican Physicians, Nurses, and Social Workers

Margaret E. Harrison

Introduction

"The health sector is an important part of [any] economy: employing huge numbers of workers, absorbing relatively large amounts of national resources" (Walt 1994:5), and contributing to the development of a healthy population. This chapter focuses on the biomedical health system of Mexico, with specific reference to the deployment and utilization of human resources. The three medical professions that form the basis of this study are physicians, nurses, and social workers. Together these professions are essential to the effective and efficient delivery of health care services. While each profession is important, I present a more detailed analysis of physicians because of the greater abundance of information on this group. Indeed, this imbalance in available information reflects the perceived greater value of physicians over other health sector workers.

In particular, I examine the spatial and structural aspects of employment in the Mexican health sector. Health care is provided by several public and private institutions, and I will review some of the factors that influence employment in these institutions. I investigate organizational requirements, financial constraints, and the personal needs and circumstances of employees in order to help explain the spatial and structural inequalities in Mexican health service. In addition, I provide a brief case study of Mexico City to highlight the concentration of physical and human health sector resources in this diverse urban area. I also explore the various tensions and problems within the health services at the end of the 1990s. Tensions include rising unemployment among physicians, the feminization of the workforce, the possible privatization of some institutions, and constant change and reform, as well as the ongoing financial difficulties of the health sector. While the focus of analysis in this chapter is the development of human resources in the modern health sector, I will place the study in the context of the changing nature of Mexican society and the evolution of Mexico's health sector. The primary period covered by the analysis is 1970 to the present. However, I will provide a brief explanation of the evolution of the health system since the 1940s, the start of the modern era of scientific medicine in Mexico.

I obtained the material used in this chapter from various sources. I gained access to published employment statistics for the main public health institutions as well as private institutions. Information from the Asociación Nacional de Universidades e Instituciones de Educación (ANUIES) and the Secretaría de Educación Pública (SEP) provides details on training courses available, numbers of university students studying medicine, and numbers of graduate professionals. I consulted the *Atlas de los profesionistas en México*, produced by the Instituto Nacional de Estadística, Geográfica e Información (INEGI); the Sistema Nacional de Salud yearbooks; and documents recently published by the Instituto Nacional de Salud Pública (INSP), a public research institute, and the Fundación Mexicana para la Salud (FUNSALUD), a private research institute. In particular, Julio Frenk and his associates at the INSP and later at FUNSALUD have investigated several major issues affecting the medical profession and the development of the health sector over the last thirty years or more. It should be noted that the quantity and quality of medical statistics have improved over the years, making the analysis of spatial and structural changes more precise. Finally, I present the preliminary findings of an ongoing investigation of the career and life course experiences of female physicians in Mexico.[1]

Mexico: A Developing Country

Dramatic events and changes occurred in Mexico during the twentieth century: a revolution, a shift from a rural, agriculturally based economy to an urban, industrial, and service-based economy, rapid demographic growth, rapid urbanization, the rise of a small middle class, and membership in the

North American Free Trade Agreement (NAFTA), the regional trade bloc. The Mexican Revolution ripped the country apart (Krauze 1997) and only by the mid- to late 1930s did Mexico obtain economic and political stability. The year 1940 represents a turning point in Mexican history because that is the start of the modern industrial era of Mexican development (Philips 1988). A brief overview of the changing character of Mexico's society and economy since 1940 forms a contextual backdrop to the study of health sector developments.

The demographic history of Mexico is quite phenomenal. The estimated population in 1900 was 13.6 million; by 1990 this figure had reached 81.2 million (see Table 11.1). A demographic transition has occurred in the country; death rates have declined dramatically since 1900, and birth rates started to decline in the 1980s. Because the decline of birth rates came after the decline in death rates, and because there is a high fertility rate, the Mexican population grew rapidly between 1950 and 1980. Rapid population growth in Mexico has been the subject of numerous studies (CONAPO 1982; Fox 1972; MacGregor 1984; Méndez Morales 1994). Such rapid population growth can be

TABLE 11.1: TWENTIETH-CENTURY DEMOGRAPHIC RECORD FOR MEXICO

Date	Population (in Millions)	Life Expectancy (in Years)	Birth Rate per 1,000 Pop.	Death rate per 1,000 Pop.
1900	13.6	29.5	34.0	31.0
1910	15.1	NA	NA	NA
1920	14.3	NA	NA	NA
1930	16.5	36.9	49.5	26.7
1940	19.6	41.5	44.3	22.8
1950	25.7	49.7	45.6	22.8
1960	34.9	58.9	46.1	11.5
1970	48.2	61.9	44.2	10.1
1980	66.8	64.9	35.0	6.3
1990	81.2	69.8	33.7	5.2
1997	95.7[1]	72.6[2]	27.0	5.0

Source: INEGI (1986, Vol. 1, Tables 1.5 and 1.13); Frenk et al. (1994); Population Reference Bureau (1985, 1995).

NA = not available.

[1] Estimate.

[2] Last recorded figure is for 1994, taken from Poder Ejecutivo Federal (1995).

explained by improvements in the social and economic life of the country as well as the application of scientific knowledge to the field of medicine. Immunization programs, advances in child and maternal care, vastly improved sanitation and environmental health care, and a better diet have led to an increase in the life expectancy in Mexico. By the mid-1990s, average life expectancy was reported to be 72.6 years (Poder Ejecutivo Federal 1995).

Mexico's drive to industrialize after 1940 did not benefit all Mexicans. The agricultural sector suffered in particular, and this fact partly explains the massive wave of rural out-migration which began in the 1950s. Population movements and a high natural birth rate led to the growth of large urban areas, for example, Mexico City, Guadalajara, and Monterrey. It is estimated that one-third of all Mexicans lived in these three cities by 1980. Yet, the absolute size of the rural population has remained significant. In 1990, 23.2 million, or 28.7 percent, of the population were classed as rural. This figure compares with 14 million people in 1950, which was then 57 percent of the population.

Rapid urbanization, internal and external migration, education, and the secularization of society have all had an impact on Mexican society. Hondagneu-Sotelo (1994:9) claims, "The daily lives of contemporary rural peasants and of working-class and middle-class urban dwellers in Mexico do not rigidly conform to traditional patriarchal cultural ideals." The conventional roles for men and women have been realigned and challenged, and the concepts of *machismo* and *marianismo* have been eroded. And as Chant (1991), González de la Rocha (1994), and García and Oliveira (1996) have demonstrated, the role of women, especially in female-headed households, is vitally important to an understanding of modern Mexican society.

Mexican Health Care System

On the basis of the work of Frenk et al. (1994) and Robledo Vera (1996), it is possible to identify six phases in the development of the Mexican health sector:

1. 1917–1943: establishment of the various health institutions
2. 1943–1958: growth of the institutions and specialization in biomedicine
3. 1958–1967: rapid growth of the institutions and consolidation of specializations
4. 1967–1979: crisis period

5. 1979–1988: health sector reform

6. 1988 to present: privatization in the health sector

Before the Mexican Revolution, most health care was provided by private, charitable, often religious, organizations and traditional healers. After the Revolution, the state became a central force in shaping the health sector. During the depression of the late 1920s and 1930s, efforts were made to create a national public health system. In 1943 both the Instituto Mexicano de Seguro Social (IMSS) and the Secretaría de Salubridad y Asistencia (SSA) were established. Later the SSA became known simply as the Secretaría de Salud. The SSA and IMSS attend to the needs of two distinct groups within the population. IMSS provides health care and social security for the predominantly urban industrial workers and their families, whereas the SSA covers those outside IMSS jurisdiction, essentially those known as the "open population." The IMSS is funded by worker and employer contributions, whereas SSA funds come from the federal purse. The SSA is seen as a "free" service to all Mexicans.

In 1960 the Instituto de Seguridad y Servicios Sociales de los Trabajadores del Estado (ISSSTE) was established; the ISSSTE covers all public sector workers. During the 1960s several national organizations were created, most of which were located in Mexico, D.F. (Federal District). Other organizations providing health care include charitable concerns: the Cruz Verde (Green Cross) and the Cruz Roja (Red Cross), as well as the many union- and industry-specific institutions such as Pemex (oil industry workers), FFCC (railway workers), and the services for the armed forces. In 1982 the FFCC health service was incorporated into IMSS. The other major provider of biomedical health care in Mexico is the private sector.

The 1970s were turbulent years for the health sector. Inscription to the IMSS doubled, but financial resources did not match this growth. By the 1970s it was quite apparent that there was a regional and spatial distributional problem in health care: a rural–urban divide. Health facilities and personnel were concentrated in the larger urban areas (Ward 1986), and the still sizable rural population was neglected. As a result, IMSS-COPLAMAR (Coordinación General del Plan Nacional de Zonas Deprimadas y Grupos Marginados) was created in 1979 to attend to the marginal rural population. In 1981, a program for the marginal population in the large urban areas was also introduced. These ambitious programs were affected by the debt crisis of the early 1980s. By 1989, IMSS-COPLAMAR was replaced by the IMSS-Solidaridad program. Federal funds, increased through the "sell off," or privatization, of various state-owned enterprises, were used to support the IMSS-Solidaridad program.

A key feature of the 1980s was health sector reform. As Ward (1986:129) pointed out, "The multiplicity of parallel and sometime overlapping organizations with responsibilities for health care is both wasteful of resources and inefficient"; reform was essential. The 1984 General Health Law "assigned major reform responsibilities to the new Ministry of Health" (Lassey, Lassey, and Jinks 1997:308). Reform was to include modernization, integration of units, community participation in planning, and decentralization. The policy of decentralization was implemented in the SSA. Initially, twelve states were decentralized, and two more were decentralized in the late 1980s. All developments could be seen as the first attempt by the government to restructure the health service.

Since 1988, the Mexican government has continued to pursue a policy of health sector reform, including privatization and the development of new forms of private health care. This policy mirrors the changes occurring in other parts of the world as countries adopt neoliberal policies and attempt to meet the health needs of all while dealing with debt. Reform of Mexico's existing complex system, with its many provider institutions, is proving slow and difficult. Nigenda (personal communication) suggested that by the late 1990s, each institution was pursuing its own form of privatization, with little coordination between the institutions despite the government's stated aims for health sector reform. Mexican health care is still highly fragmented. In addition, only a small amount of the gross national product (GNP) is spent on health. In 1992 an estimated 2.76 percent of the GNP was spent on public health and 2.06 to 2.97 percent of the GNP was spent on private health resources (Frenk et al. 1994).

The *Progama de reforma del sector salud* (Poder Ejecutivo Federal 1995) presents the various aims and objectives of Mexican health sector development for 1995–2000. The main objectives have been to improve the quality and efficiency of the service; to increase coverage to include the nonwaged and informal-sector, to continue the process of decentralization of the SSA, and to increase access to health care for marginal urban and rural populations. Mexico is seeking to ultimately provide all citizens with health care and thus reach the World Health Organization (WHO) target of "health for all by the year 2000." Soberón-Acevedo, Langer, and Frenk (1988) believe the provision of primary health care (PHC) via the national health system is the way to achieve this goal. Health sector reform should aim to have 50 percent of the population in some form of social security system and the other 50 percent covered by a decentralized "free" national health system. Frenk et al. (1994) assert that a reformed health sector should aim to provide some form of national health insurance, place the work of the SSA central to any reform, encourage a link between public and private provision, recognize the needs of both rural and urban populations, and overcome problems of inequality and standards (Soberón-Acevedo, Langer, and Frenk 1988).

In Mexico, the establishment and delivery of curative care facilities appears to have taken precedence over preventive care in the early stages of the development of the system. Medical education systems have been criticized for perpetuating this emphasis. Curative care responds to an actual illness or health complaint, while preventive care emphasizes promotional services designed to educate and reduce the incidence of illness. In the 1970s Mexico had a health system that was dominated by curative care: the focus of attention was on the hospitals and specialist treatment centers in Mexico City and the larger urban areas. The principle of PHC was incorporated into the Mexican health sector via the IMSS-COPLAMAR and the marginal populations in large urban areas' programs. Mexican PHC aims to improve the health and welfare of society though the incorporation of preventive and promotional health care activities linked to curative systems.

The introduction of PHC in the late 1970s made it necessary to integrate PHC with existing health care structures; this was not always easy for medical personnel or patients. The medical division of labor acts as an obstacle to the delivery of PHC (Frankel 1984). PHC medical personnel are usually trained to a specific level of competence and may not have "formal" qualifications. In Mexico, however, PHC staff receive training beyond that needed to deliver preventive and promotional health care. They have an education equivalent to that of workers in other areas of health care (e.g., curative care). In spite of public health care workers being trained to a high level of competence, PHC work is perceived by many health care professionals as inferior to secondary and tertiary care (Harrison 1991).

Mexican health care operates a hierarchical structure of primary, secondary, and tertiary care units. Primary care units or centers attend to minor and basic medical issues, including routine practices such as family planning, pre- and postnatal care, and injections, while more serious conditions are referred to a secondary or tertiary care hospital. Curative care is provided principally in secondary and tertiary care units; these units also provide some preventive care. Secondary care units are general hospitals while tertiary care units represent specialist hospitals. Specialist hospitals are only found in Mexico City or one of the other major urban areas in Mexico. By 1995 it was clear that Mexico still invested far more in curative than preventive care. In 1995 62.5 percent of the health budget went to curative care, 5.7 percent to preventive care, 4.6 percent to social benefit, and 24 percent to other programs, including administration, policy, and planning.

A complex form of inequality exists within and between the various health institutions. Medical employment with Pemex, the armed forces, and the private sector is recognized as very good and prestigious. Staff development and remuneration are often better than in public institutions. Of the three principal public institutions—ssa, imss, and issste—the imss is perceived as "better" and of higher status. Work in an imss tertiary hospital is considered far superior to work in an imss-Solidaridad unit. As a result of these internal and external differences, the medical labor market is highly competitive. There is a clear hierarchical scale of institutional preferences among the workforce. Jobs with the imss are eagerly sought, yet at a time of unemployment, gaining work with any institution is better than nothing.

Despite the growth and development of the Mexican health service since 1940, López Acuña (1980) estimated that in 1976 between 20 and 25 million Mexicans had limited access to biomedical health care coverage: nearly one-third of the population. By the early 1990s, it was estimated that the imss, ssa, and issste provided health care for 85 percent of the total population, while an estimated 10 million Mexicans, the poorest, were without biomedical health care. This represents about 12 percent of the Mexican population (Frenk et al. 1994; Poder Ejecutivo Federal 1995).

Illnesses and Treatment

As Mexico experiences the epidemiological transition, medical personnel must be equipped to deal with communicable and noncommunicable diseases and ailments in a whole range of situations and environments. Mesa-Lago (1992) noted that as a result of the imss-coplamar program in the 1980s, the incidence of influenza, enteritis, and acute tonsillitis decreased, while the incidence of scabies, human rabies, and typhoid fever stayed the same. Also, there was an increase in chronic diseases such as malnutrition and rheumatic fever. Morbidity records for the health sector in the early 1990s indicate that respiratory diseases as well as gastroenteritis are still the major medical problems in the country (Módena 1992; Secretaría de Salud 1994a) (see Table 11.2).

The Second National Health Survey provides a detailed examination of national and regional health service use, ailments by region, and patient requirements. For example, 75 percent of patients visiting a health unit within the two-week period prior to the survey went for reasons of finding a cure for a particular ailment or symptom. Thus, only 25 percent of visits were related to preventive care. When visiting the health unit, 86 percent of patients (both for preventative and curative care) saw a doctor, and those not seeing a doctor were attended to by a range of medical personnel such as nurses, health workers, and auxiliary nurses. Over 88 percent of patients used PHC units and attendance was for either a specific clinic or to see a doctor in his or her consultancy room. Few patients visited second- and third-level care units (12 percent), presumably because of physical distance from such a unit, the knowledge that "minor" ailments should be dealt with at the primary level, and the feeling that primary units would be adequate for their needs. Also, patients recognized that a referral system was operating and that patients would be transferred to higher level units if their condition necessitated such a move.

TABLE 11.2: THE FIVE PRINCIPAL AILMENTS BY REGION REPORTED IN THE SECOND NATIONAL HEALTH SURVEY

Ailment/Condition	North	Central	ZMCM	PASSPA	South-east
Respiratory problems	28.8%	29.2%	27.2%	18.4%	18.5%
Muscular and joints	16.5%	12.0%	9.7%	13.9%	12.1%
Gastrointestinal	10.4%	9.7%	9.6%	15.0%	11.2%
Headache	4.3%	3.7%	1.8%	5.8%	4.9%
Hypertension	4.9%	3.7%	2.8%	3.7%	3.2%

Source: Secretaría de Salud (1994a, Table 5, p. 18).

Note: These are percentages of the five principal health problems reported in the two-week period prior to the Second National Health Survey interview.

ZMCM: Metropolitan Zone of Mexico City.

PASSPA: The states of Hidalgo, Oaxaca, Guerrero, and Chiapas.

The survey identified the principal users of health posts to be women, people with little formal schooling, and people who come from larger households (i.e., more people in the household suggests a greater demand and need for health care attention). People living near a health post, such as those in urban areas, were more likely to use or access the service than people from rural communities. Certain groups of users reported specific health requirements, for example, students sought birth control and advice on sexually transmitted diseases; housewives and mothers had pregnancy and maternity needs, and the elderly came with illnesses related to old age. These three groups are part of the noninsured population who should use the services of the ssa. In addition, certain groups of users are encouraged to make use of specific health programs. Women between fifteen and sixty-four years of age should avail themselves of the cancer screening program. The healthy child program recommends biannual checkups, and a dental program for all school children suggests two visits per year. Most preventative health care programs are delivered at the primary unit (Secretaría de Salud 1994a).

Attendance at phc units, and thus health service usage, is dominated by visits for curative care for minor ailments. The medical team prescribes the appropriate medicines or treatment. Patients may purchase their prescription medicines from either the health institution pharmacy, which will supply medicines from a basic list if they hold them in stock, or from a private pharmacy where patients are probably guaranteed availability and choice. However, in an analysis of the Second National Health Survey by Bronfman et al. (1997), it was discovered that some patients doubt the advice of doctors. Doctors may prescribe the same medicine for two different ailments; patients perceive the ailments as different; or some medicines may be on sale and patients query their pharmacological properties. As a result of these factors, auto-medication occurs. Bronfman et al. emphasize the problems of auto-medication and the need for education, as well as the necessity of preventive care rather than curative care of "minor" ailments. Bronfman et al. also observe that some patients complain of doctors appearing to be in a rush to finish their consultations, thus not giving their full attention and time to patients. This may explain why a considerable number of patients access private care.

Private health care ranges from consulting traditional healers, bonesetters, and *curanderos*, to consulting doctors and nurses. Lower income households make considerable use of private health care (Secretaría de Salud 1994a). Tensions exist between private and public health care (Módena 1992); public health care doctors may view the traditions and beliefs of traditional healers as inappropriate or potentially harmful. Some private practitioners, especially those in rural areas, provide a variety of services to the community and are thus known by the community. For example, a private doctor may operate a clinic, pharmacy, shop, and bar from one building (Harrison, unpublished data).

Health Sector Workforce: Physicians, Nurses, and Social Workers

In the human resource pyramid of the health sector there are three horizontal bands. At the vertex or upper band are the university-trained personnel, in the middle band are the technically trained personnel, and at the lower band are workers with limited educational qualifications (Norgueira and Brito 1986). Physicians, nurses, and social workers represent two of the horizontal bands: upper and middle. In theory, these professions form the team that operates as a functional unit in PHC. Much of what is achieved in health care is the result of team work among physicians, nurses, clinical support staff, and administrative staff workers. Each part of the human resource pyramid is essential to the functioning of the health system. Improvements in the Mexican education system during this century, coupled with growth and development of the health sector, have resulted in the professionalization of health sector jobs and an expansion in the number of qualified personnel.

Socioeconomic Status of Medical Personnel

The medical profession does not come from a single class (Nigenda and Solorzano 1997). Students studying to be physicians tend to come from the "middle class," with parents holding professional, managerial, and commercial jobs; some parents may be physicians themselves (Garduño-Espinosa et al. 1995; Robledo Vera 1996). Robledo Vera (1996) found that 48 percent of parents of all physicians have secondary or higher education attainment levels, and that female physicians have the most educated parents on average. Nurses and social workers tend to come from a socioeconomic background similar to that of their patients' (Harrison, personal observation; Módena 1992).

The civil and family status of workers in the medical profession also differs slightly across groups. Robledo Vera (1996) observed, using the 1993 INSP study, that 62 percent of female physicians were married (official or in *unión libre*); the figure for male physicians was 87 percent. Also, there were more single female physicians in the younger age bracket than male physicians. One explanation is that a woman physician puts her career before marriage and a family. Douglas et al. (1996) reported that 68 percent of nurses were married, with a mean of 2.17 children (a range of 0–5). In their study of working mothers (nurses) in Mexico, D.F., Asunción Lara et al. (1993) recorded that 80 percent were married.

Training

Physician training normally consists of five years of medical school attendance, during which the length of time spent in clinical practice varies. A person may study to become a general practitioner, a general practitioner and homeopath, a general practitioner and gynecologist, or a homeopath practitioner and gynecologist. The most popular programs of study (i.e., those most widely available) are general practitioner and general practitioner and gynecologist (ANUIES 1995). On completion of formal clinical studies, students must undertake one year of social service (in accordance with the Ley Federal de Profesiones). This applies to all university students and during this social service year a trainee physician is called a *pasante*. Since the late 1970s, many trainee physicians have spent their social service year working in an urban or rural PHC center of the IMSS-COPLAMAR (later IMSS-Solidaridad), or with the SSA as part of the marginal urban area program. Critics of physician training claim students are given insufficient clinical experience for PHC work. Training prior to the year of social service does little to prepare a physician for work in PHC centers, which are often remote and poorly equipped. On completion of their social service, physicians may opt to secure work or attempt the national examination to gain admission to a speciality training course. Career development plans and personal family circumstances, as well as academic ability, may well determine what a physician chooses to do once qualified as a general practitioner.

Entrance to speciality training programs is very competitive, and some physicians may take the entrance exam several times. Certain specialities are only offered in certain places, for example, neurology in Mexico, D.F., Guadalajara, and Monterrey.

Nurses in Mexico can be classified according to level of qualification: degree, technical, and in training. Degree studies normally last four years. A technical program is undertaken if students have completed secondary education; the program lasts three years. Student nurses may study for a degree or technical qualification at either a university or a technical institution. As part of their study students will undertake hospital-based work. On completion of both degree and technical study programs, students are expected to carry out one year of social service. They too are subject to the Ley Federal de Profesiones and during their social service year they are also called *pasantes*. Fully qualified nurses have the opportunity to train in a particular speciality such as obstetrics, teaching, or administration.

A study by Soberón-Acevedo and Najera (1988) suggested that most technical and degree training programs for nurses fail to give students sufficient experience for primary-level care activities. Also, they pointed out that over recent years there has been a tendency to increase the academic requirements of most professions, but that nursing has been slow to accept these changes. This criticism applies to the whole of medical work. Valdez de Reyes and García Jiménez (1991) believe there is an urgent need to control what is taught in nursing schools and that the curriculum needs to change. In addition to degree and technically qualified nurses, there are many auxiliary nurses; they receive on-the-job training. An auxiliary should have completed nine years of general education before acquiring a position in a medical unit. By far the largest groups of nurses in Mexico are the auxiliary and *pasante* groups. An unusual feature of nursing is that students may secure employment in a health institution and be paid before receiving a degree (Martínez Benítez et al. 1993). Pay levels reflect the level of qualification, although years of practice without a degree may also secure a certain pay level (Harrison 1994).

A social worker may undertake degree-level or technical training. The degree in social work at the Universidad Nacional Autónoma de México (UNAM) was established in 1940 (Schmid-Dolan 1995). Degree-level students take nine semesters (4.5 years) and, as with all degrees, students are required to undertake one year of social service. A degree is obtained via a social science program of study and not in a faculty of medicine. Studies at a technical institution are shorter (three years), and the entrance qualifications are different. A qualified social worker has a whole range of possible job opportunities in both the private and public sectors: health, education, housing, social security and social assistance programs, industry, ecology, prison work, tourism, rural and urban development programs, and many other areas. This wide range of employment options may account for the limited number of social workers in health care. In particular, the potential to earn more and have a well-defined career structure are more obvious in other employment areas. As in nursing, social workers may practice their profession before completing their studies.

Statistical data on human resources in the health sector have become more detailed over the years. For example, in 1996 most of the major public health institutions recorded physicians by activity and qualifications, that is, in contact with patients or in administrative positions, as general practitioners, or as specialists. Furthermore, physicians are also recorded as fully qualified or as *pasantes*. The same type of professional classifications are given for nurses: in contact with patients or in administrative positions, general and specialist nurses, and auxiliaries and *pasantes*. Unfortunately, data on social workers are extremely limited, which may be indicative of the status of the profession in health care, and this lack limits the amount of detail that can be presented in this analysis. Also, very few statistics are available by gender.

Growth and Development in the Numbers of Physicians, Nurses, and Social Workers

Throughout this century there has been an expansion in the number of physicians, nurses, and social workers. Employment in the health sector is directly related to economic supply and demand factors, national expenditure and investment in health care, the popularity of health studies programs, and the needs of society. Although the numbers of physicians and nurses have increased over time, it was not until the 1970s that any dramatic increase occurred. Between 1970 and 1990 there was a threefold increase in the number of physicians and a fourfold increase in paramedical staff (see Table 11.3). Frenk et al. (1995) claim that between 1970 and 1990 there was a shift from physician scarcity to excess.

TABLE 11.3: INCREASE IN PHYSICIANS AND PARAMEDICAL STAFF IN MEXICO, 1970 TO 1995

Year	Physicians	Paramedical Staff
1970	24,989	43,319
1975	38,746	63,921
1980	61,084	102,058
1985	70,683	147,502
1990	89,842	186,866
1995	97,454	197,942

Source: INEGI (1986, Table 4.2); Secretaría de Salud (1994b:12, 1997:64).

In the 1970s the Mexican government supported a rapid increase in the number of universities, including the opening up of numerous medical schools. In 1970 there were twenty-seven medical schools in Mexico (Frenk et al. 1994), and by 1979 there were fifty-six schools. Between 1979 and 1987 a further three schools were created. There are both private and public medical schools: by far the largest public medical school is at UNAM in Mexico City. The largest private medical school is at the Autonomous University of Guadalajara. In the mid-1990s there were fifty medical schools, of which fifteen were private. Some universities have multisite medical schools, for example, the State University of Veracruz.

The government policy to channel students into higher education since 1970 may be seen as an attempt to delay an impending employment crisis: too many workers and too few jobs. However, the government's "open door" policy led some universities to rigorously sift out weaker students to maintain the standard of their medical degree (personal comments made by two directors of provincial medical schools). Growth in the number of medical schools was too rapid and the quality of medical education deteriorated. In addition, a hierarchical division between the schools, with some recognized as providers of good quality medical training and others seen as being of an inferior quality, was observed (Nigenda et al. 1990a). Rapid growth in the number of physicians graduating from medical schools started in the 1970s, a direct result of the government's "open door" policy. The late 1970s was a growth period in health service provision, with the introduction of various PHC programs. Thus, there was an increased demand for medical workers.

Student enrollment into the health sciences as a whole declined dramatically after 1980, and especially in the case of private universities (ANUIES 1995). Yet, the number of students entering medical schools to train as physicians increased between 1986 and 1992. Since then, numbers have declined. Also, exit statistics have declined (see Table 11.4). By the mid- to late 1980s, medical schools were responding to calls to curtail the oversupply of physicians. Other possible explanations for the decline in exit statistics are that students are choosing to switch careers, having become disillusioned with medicine, or that students are finding courses too hard. The gender split in intake and exit statistics is interesting. More women enter medical schools than in the past. As a result, equal numbers of men and women exited medical schools by 1994. The number of graduating male physicians has dropped considerably over time. These data provide some evidence of the feminization of the health service; this has been analyzed elsewhere (Harrison 1995). It should also be noted that students exiting a medical school do not automatically translate into practicing physicians.

The number of nursing schools in Mexico is quite phenomenal. In 1982, Martínez Benítez et al. (1993) reported that there were 141 nursing schools. However, Soberón-Acevedo and Najera (1988) recorded 214 nursing schools in Mexico in 1988. These schools are unevenly distributed. There is

**TABLE 11.4: INTAKE AND EXIT FIGURES FOR
MALE AND FEMALE MEDICAL STUDENTS, 1986 TO 1994**

Year	First-Year Intake			Exit Year		
	Male	Female	Total	Male	Female	Total
1986	5,631	3,460	9,091	5,876	3,619	9,495
1987	5,757	3,898	9,655	5,146	3,499	8,645
1988	6,128	4,662	10,790	5,522	4,084	9,606
1989	5,800	4,480	10,280	5,129	3,903	9,032
1990	6,293	4,933	11,226	4,693	3,751	8,444
1991	6,597	5,493	12,090	3,841	3,149	6,990
1992	6,615	5,865	12,480	3,613	3,313	6,926
1993	6,089	5,360	11,449	3,752	3,374	7,136
1994	5,762	5,297	11,059	3,634	3,607	7,241

Source: ANUIES (1995).

TABLE 11.5: INCREASE OF NURSING PROFESSION IN SSA, IMSS, AND ISSSTE, 1965 TO 1995

Year	No. Nurses[1]	Nurses: Population
1965	24,716	1:1,335
1970	26,642	1:1,839
1980	75,443	1:954
1985	102,758	1:768
1990	124,798	1:649
1995	175,624	1:529

Source: INEGI (1992); Martínez Benítez et al. (1993:119); Population Reference Bureau (1985, 1995); Secretaría de Salud (1994b:39, 1997:64).

[1] All categories of nurses.

a lack of schools in the north and south of Mexico, areas of considerable demand (Valdez de Reyes and García Jiménez 1991). On the northern border zone there are other options for female workers—*maquiladora* work and emigration to the United States. These factors, as well as low wage levels in the nursing profession, are used to explain the poor recruitment levels of nursing schools in the area.

There are numerous programs of study in the Mexican nursing schools. Soberón-Acevedo and Najera (1988) stated that in the 214 nursing schools there were 230 programs of study. Nearly 90 percent of programs were at the technical level, with the remaining 10.4 percent offering degree-level studies. By 1995 there were 260 nursing schools throughout Mexico, with 32 in Mexico, D.F. alone (UNAM 1995). The balance between technical and degree training remained the same. Most statistics on nursing do not differentiate between technical and degree-qualified nurses. Statistics do indicate the existence of specialist nurses (nurses who have undertaken an intensive program of study after completing their initial studies). Although not identified as such within the statistical tables, specialist nurses are most probably degree-qualified nurses.

As already indicated, the growth in paramedical staff has been phenomenal. Nurses represent a large proportion of paramedical staff. Details of the increase in the nursing profession in the three main public health institutions are given in Table 11.5. There was a sevenfold increase in nursing staff in the major public institutions between 1965 and 1995, and as a result, a dramatic decline in the ratio of inhabitants per nurse.

In 1994, twenty-eight institutions offered a degree program in social work. In addition, there are master's and specialization programs in social work (ANUIES 1995). UNAM offers a specialization in social work in the area of health. The number of students enrolling in and graduating from this particular higher degree program are low. The number of degree and higher degree programs in social work suggests that social work, and in particular medical social work, is not considered to be as important as other branches of medical studies.

Distribution of Physicians, Nurses, and Social Workers

The distribution of physicians, nurses, and other health workers can be viewed from several perspectives: institutional, organizational structure, spatial, and gender. There is an element of interrelationship between these distributions. For example, the spatial distribution of medical personnel is closely related to the distribution of the various health institutions, which in turn reflects the socioeconomic status of a particular state or region.

Institutional Distribution

Table 11.6 shows the increases in the number of physicians in each of the three main public institutions between 1980 and 1994. The number working for the ISSSTE tripled; the number in the IMSS more than doubled, and the number in the SSA increased 1.6 times. The institutional distribution of physicians throughout the nation varied little over the years, with the IMSS being the largest employer. By far the larger of the two IMSS sections is the social security section, providing care to regularly employed wage workers in the formal sector and their families; the other section is the IMSS-Solidaridad, formerly IMSS-COPLAMAR, which attends the "open population," usually in rural areas. In 1994, 90 percent of IMSS physicians worked in the social security section.

In 1995, the social security systems of health care—IMSS, IMSS-Solidaridad, and ISSSTE—had 59.9 percent of all medical personnel and in theory attended 50.9 percent of the Mexican population. Institutionally, the social security systems of IMSS and ISSSTE command more personnel. The IMSS is by far the largest employer of medical staff, with 71 percent of all social security health staff. In 1995, IMSS and IMSS-Solidaridad attended to the needs of 49.95 percent of the population, with 46 percent of all national

**TABLE 11.6: GROWTH IN THE NUMBER OF PHYSICIANS
IN MEXICO SINCE 1980**

Year	No. Physicians[1]	SSA	IMSS[2]	ISSSTE
1980	61,084	19,927	28,552	7,738
1982	65,220	16,582	33,749	9,279
1984	66,958	19,206	31,973	10,488
1986	74,420	23,545	33,573	11,559
1988	89,130	23,933	45,329	12,555
1990	89,842	25,940	39,775	12,975
1992	103,354	29,529	48,369	14,002
1994[3]	110,255	32,786	50,042	14,376

Source: Secretaría de Salud (1994b).
[1] Includes dentists and *pasantes*.
[2] Includes physicians working in IMSS-COPLAMAR and IMSS-*Solidaridad*.
[3] Estimated figures.

medical staff. However, the distribution of staff between the two sections
was highly unequal. IMSS had 42.5 percent of all national medical staff, while
the IMSS-Solidaridad program had only 3.4 percent of all medical staff. And
IMSS-Solidaridad in theory was meeting the needs of 10 million Mexicans.

By way of contrast, the SSA, which covers 67.7 percent of the "open
population" (i.e., those without social security), had 29.3 percent of all national medical personnel in 1995. There are other institutions that serve the
"open population," but most are extremely small in size relative to the SSA.
The SSA employs 73.1 percent of all medical staff working in institutions
attending to the needs of the "open population."

Institutional distribution of physicians within the states reflects the level
of economic development in each state. For example, the poorer rural states
with fewer formal workers and a larger "open population," such as Oaxaca,
Guerrero, and Chiapas, have larger numbers of IMSS-Solidaridad and SSA
physicians.

A study carried out by the Secretaría de Salud (1993) as part of the Sistema Nacional de Salud estimated that there were over 46,000 physicians in
the private sector. At the same time, there were an estimated 94,227 physicians working in the three main public health institutions. In the equivalent
study of 1992 (Secretaría de Salud 1992), the private sector was considered

the second most important employer of physicians; only IMSS had more physicians. It should be recognized that many Mexican physicians operate in both the private and public sectors, thus making it extremely difficult to assess the overall size and influence of the private sector. The distribution of private medical professionals was highly concentrated; the D.F. and the states of Mexico and Jalisco accounted for 37 percent of all private physicians. Other minor concentrations occurred in the states of Guanajuato, Michoacán, Baja California, and Puebla.

A comparison of the institutional nursing distribution between 1980 and 1996 is given in Table 11.7. IMSS has by far the largest number of nurses. However, all institutions are highly dependent on auxiliary nurses. Indeed Martínez Benítez et al. (1993) found that auxiliary nurses dominate the institutions, while Valdez de Reyes and García Jiménez (1991) indicated that 58.4 percent of nurses are auxiliary nurses, with a great many working in urban areas. The data in Table 11.7 do not confirm this, however. Of these five types of nurses—general nurses, specialist, technical, auxiliary, and *pasantes*—auxiliary nurses could well be the largest group.

ORGANIZATIONAL STRUCTURE

The organizational distribution of physicians and nurses (no data are available on social workers) by level of care (primary, secondary, and tertiary) gives some indication of the balance between curative and preventive care. Primary care is widely distributed, whereas secondary care is located in urban areas, and tertiary (specialist) care is concentrated in the larger urban areas such as Mexico City, Guadalajara, Monterrey, and important state

TABLE 11.7: TOTAL NURSES AND AUXILIARY NURSES IN SSA, IMSS, AND ISSSTE IN 1980 AND 1996

Institution	Total Nurses		Auxiliary Nurses[1]	
	1980	1996	1980	1996
SSA	22,620	51,056	2,366	18,842
IMSS[2]	42,353	80,357	23,197	33,837
ISSSTE	8,012	18,203	4,855	7,210

Source: Secretaría de Salud (1994b:40–44; 1997:64).
[1] Those specifically identified as auxiliaries (19,407) are recorded as "Other."
[2] Includes IMSS-COPLAMAR and IMSS-Solidaridad.

capitals. With the development of PHC, and in particular the development of IMSS-COPLAMAR and later IMSS-Solidaridad, the organizational distribution of physicians and nurses changed. Statistics on human resources by level of activity are limited. However, in the Sistema Nacional de Salud annual yearbook, there are data available in very general terms. It should be noted that data concerning activity with patients are more readily available than data by level of operation.

Data for 1993 (see Table 11.8) demonstrate a concentration of physicians and nurses at the secondary level. In the case of nurses, more than half work at the secondary level, and more work in tertiary care than in primary care. In the case of physicians, the primary-level number includes *pasantes*, and a relatively small number of tertiary-level physicians indicates the small number of specialists. Most physicians are general practitioners or training to be general practitioners. Also, these figures are only for the public sector, and there is no IMSS-Solidaridad tertiary care. The study by Martínez Benítez et al. (1993:234) revealed that in 1982 over 89 percent of all professional nurses in the SSA were working in hospitals, with less than 4 percent working in communities. The rest were either teaching or in administrative positions. The situation in the SSA in 1996 was somewhat different, with less than 50 percent of nurses in hospitals.

The development of a selective PHC program in Mexico has caused some staff problems. In the program in marginal urban areas, physicians, nurses, and social workers are the basic operational team. Even in the smallest PHC unit—a T1 center—one physician, one nurse, and one social worker are the required team. It could be argued that placing a physician in the team was not essential in every location. However, an abundance of physicians in Mexico at the time meant that deployment in PHC centers was a justified use

TABLE 11.8: ORGANIZATIONAL DISTRIBUTION OF PHYSICIANS AND NURSES IN SSA, IMSS, IMMSS-SOLIDARIDAD, AND ISSSTE IN 1993

Level of Activity	Physicians	Nurses
Primary	36,512	30,555
Secondary	41,912	74,937
Tertiary	12,256	32,058
TOTAL	90,680	137,550

Source: Sistema Nacional de Salud (1993).

of trained personnel. What transpired was that some centers had a *pasante* physician while others had a fully qualified physician, and the *pasante* on completion of a year of social service often left the center to seek employment elsewhere or pursue further study. This possible annual staff turnover hinders PHC work. There is a lack of continuity and commitment to a community (Harrison 1991).

SPATIAL DISTRIBUTION

The spatial distribution of physicians, nurses, and paramedical staff (including social workers) is given in Table 11.9. There is an inequitable distribution between the states, with a relative "abundance" of medical personnel in those with large urban areas and the northern border states. Mexico, D.F. and Mexico state account for 22.2 percent of the Mexican population and have 34.3 percent of the physicians, 31.9 percent of the nurses, and 34.6 percent of the paramedical personnel. Of the two administrative units, Mexico, D.F. has twice as many physicians, nurses, and paramedics per unit of population as the state of Mexico. Note the apparent scarcity of nurses in the latter unit. The dominance of Mexico, D.F. is a reflection of the many tertiary-level hospitals and national institutions located in Mexico, D.F. More detailed data from the Sistema Nacional de Salud (1993) reveals that in 22 out of 32 states, the number of auxiliary and *pasante* nurses far exceeds the figure of nurses with a degree; indeed in 14 states auxiliary nurses exceed the number of nurses with a degree. The national SSA statistics for 1996 (unpublished data) reveal that there were 34,819 physicians, 47,637 nurses, and 2,643 social workers. More than one-third of social workers (940) worked in just two states: Mexico, D.F. (693) and Mexico state (247).

In the 1990 census INEGI (1992) obtained detailed information on the major professions in Mexico, including physicians. This was the first time INEGI systematically collected such specific data. Estimates of geographical distributions for previous years are based either on general data, with no detailed definition of what constituted a physician, or on small sample surveys like that of Nigenda and Najera (1996). The INEGI report highlights the relative abundance of physicians in the north—industrial—urban areas in contrast to the relative impoverishment of physicians in the south—agricultural—rural areas since the 1930s. Over time the absolute "gap" between these two areas has decreased. Between 1970 and 1990 the average annual rate of growth in the medical (physician) profession was 7.6 percent.

TABLE 11.9: GEOGRAPHICAL DISTRIBUTION OF POPULATION, PHYSICIANS, NURSES, AND PARAMEDICAL STAFF IN MEXICO IN 1990 AND 1993

State	% Pop. 1990	% Phys. 1990	% Nurses 1993	% Para. 1993
Aguascalientes	0.9	1.0	0.9	1.0
Baja California	2.0	2.2	2.2	2.2
Baja California Sur	0.4	0.4	0.6	0.4
Campeche	0.7	0.4	0.7	0.7
Coahuila	2.4	2.4	3.1	3.4
Colima	0.5	0.6	0.6	0.6
Chiapas	4.0	1.5	2.0	1.1
Chihuahua	3.0	2.6	3.0	3.4
Distrito Federal	10.1	24.3	24.6	25.1
Durango	1.7	1.3	1.6	1.0
Guanajuato	4.9	2.8	3.2	3.6
Guerrero	3.2	1.7	2.2	1.8
Hidalgo	2.3	1.5	1.7	1.2
Jalisco	6.5	7.9	6.7	7.0
Mexico	12.1	10.0	7.3	9.5
Michoacán	4.4	3.4	2.4	1.7
Morelos	1.5	1.4	1.4	1.3
Nayarit	1.0	0.8	1.0	0.7
Nuevo León	3.8	5.4	5.4	5.4
Oaxaca	3.7	1.7	2.0	1.2
Puebla	5.1	5.4	3.4	3.1
Querétaro	1.3	0.9	1.2	1.2
Quintana Roo	0.6	0.4	0.6	0.5
San Luis Potosí	2.5	1.4	1.9	1.5
Sinaloa	2.7	2.4	2.6	3.1
Sonora	2.2	2.0	2.8	2.5
Tabasco	1.8	1.4	2.0	2.0
Tamaulipas	2.8	3.0	3.3	3.7
Tlaxcala	0.9	0.7	0.6	0.6
Veracruz	7.7	7.0	5.2	5.8
Yucatan	1.7	1.7	1.7	1.5
Zacatecas	1.6	0.9	0.9	0.6

Source: INEGI (1992, 1995); Sistema Nacional de Salud (1993).

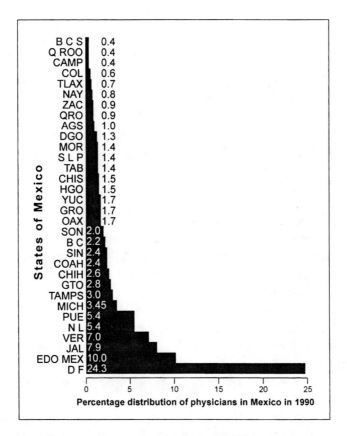

FIGURE 11.1: Percentage distribution of physicians in Mexico in 1990.

This is contrasted with a population growth rate of 2.7 percent (Frenk et al. 1995). By 1990 there were 489 inhabitants per physician nationally, whereas in Mexico, D.F. there were 213 inhabitants per physician and in Chiapas there were 1,213 inhabitants per physician. In 1970 the figures were 1,414 inhabitants per physician nationally, 474 in the D.F., and 4,601 in Chiapas.

The 1990 census statistics were used to develop an atlas of professionals (INEGI 1995). The distribution of physicians was far from equal; five states and the Federal District (D.F.) contained 60 percent of the nation's physicians. The six states were the D.F., Mexico, Jalisco, Veracruz, Nuevo León, and Puebla (see Figure 11.1). These states also contain just under 50 percent of the national population and are all highly urbanized. Over 80 percent of the population of the D.F., Mexico, Jalisco, and Nuevo León live in urban areas. Yet the presence of a physician does not mean people have increased access to physicians; INEGI results indicate that in five of the six states mentioned, 70 percent of the physicians are concentrated in urban areas. The exception is Veracruz state. From Table 11.9, it is clear there is a partial north/south, urban/rural divide in the overall distribution of physicians in Mexico. The southern states of Oaxaca, Guerrero, and Chiapas, the most rural and underdeveloped states, have fewer physicians per 10,000 inhabitants.

GENDER DISTRIBUTION

A key feature of health sector employment is the numerical dominance of female workers. Health sector work is seen as allowing women to combine their productive and reproductive roles. Women outnumber men in most health systems, but still most health systems "consist of an army of women managed by a relatively small number of males" (Mejia and Varju 1983 : 11). "Nursing is a woman's profession in almost every country of the world, with approximately 90 percent of all nurses being women" (Morrow 1986, cited by Douglas et al. 1996:496). The classic image of a nurse—Florence Nightingale—persists: most nurses work in curative medicine in hospitals (Norgueira and Brito 1986, Valdez de Reyes and García Jiménez 1991). Martínez Benítez et al. (1993) recognize nursing as a female profession, yet the work that is carried out does not make the profession specifically female. However, tradition and the linking of a woman's reproductive and productive roles in nursing have fostered the idea that nursing is a female activity. What is obvious is that most nurses do not have a high level of control and influence in the medical workplace; their work may be perceived as supportive rather than fundamental. Nurses carry out low-level manual work, are poorly paid, dependent, and have low social prestige. Nurses function in a subordinate position relative to physicians.

The numerical dominance of women is typified by social work and nursing student statistics. As already stated, details of employee statistics by gender are not readily available. Students studying for a social work degree are dominated by women. The male:female ratio is roughly 1:4; the figure is even more pronounced in nursing, with a ratio of 1:10 (ANUIES 1995). In nursing there are several specialities that can be taken. The areas of administration and teaching are dominated by men (ANUIES 1995).

The male:female ratio for students studying to be a physician are distinctly different—with more male students than female (see Table 11.4). There has, however, been a progressive shift; by 1994 there were nearly the same number of male and female students. In that same year, 50 percent of medical students completing their studies as a physician were female (ANUIES 1995). Over time, a small but increasing number of female physicians has become more important to the maintenance of the health sector. However, there is little evidence yet to suggest these female physicians are in positions of power and authority.

In 1993, an estimated 28 percent of physicians were female (Robledo Vera 1996). Robledo Vera went on to demonstrate that female physicians are more likely to be salaried workers for a public sector health institution than men, and women are less likely to work full time in the private sector. Public sector health employment statistics for 1995 reveal that proportionally more female physicians work in the "free" service of the SSA (31 percent) than in either of the other two major public social security systems— IMSS (28 percent) and ISSSTE (22 percent) (unpublished SSA, IMSS, and ISSSTE employment statistics 1995). The SSA and IMSS together employ 91 percent of all female physicians in the public sector. Also, the spatial distribution of female physicians is uneven. The metropolitan area of Mexico City (Federal District and state of Mexico) has relatively more female physicians than the provincial states. States with few SSA and IMSS female physicians (where less than 20 percent of physicians are female) are Colima, Sinaloa, and the Yucatan. However, well over 30 percent of IMSS and SSA physicians working in Oaxaca, Chiapas, and Guerrero are female, thus suggesting women are prepared to and do work in these poor, less developed states.

Case Study: Mexico, D.F., the Concentration of Medical Personnel

Mexico City has a concentration of health resources. Ward (1986) states that some concentration of resources in the capital city is both justifiable and desirable. It is sensible to locate centers of specialist surgery in the largest cities, which offer relatively easy access to a large hinterland population (p. 120). Thus, the citizens of Mexico City are in a privileged position, not only having an abundance of medical personnel but also a variety of health institutions. A subscriber to IMSS may also have access to SSA facilities in the capital as well as opt for private health care. Data in Tables 11.10 and 11.11 demonstrate the strength of Mexico, D.F. as a command center of health sector activities in Mexico in 1995. However, these figures also indicate that there are problems of oversupply or underusage of some Mexico, D.F. services. For example, daily medical consultations and hospital occupancy rates are relatively low, while the provision of physicians and nurses per 100,000 inhabitants is double the national average. Virtually 48 percent of the Mexico, D.F. population are classified as "open population" and should receive medical attention from the ssa. Yet imss and issste together employ 45 percent more staff than the ssa. Therefore, although the provision of medical

TABLE 11.10: HEALTH SECTOR INFRASTRUCTURE AND RESOURCES IN MEXICO AND MEXICO, D.F.

Infrastructure and Resources	National	D.F.	National Ranking
General hospitals	745	66	1
Specialist hospitals	146	47	1
External consultation units	14,634	667	9
Physicians in contact with patients	101,675	23,450	1
Paramedical staff	197,942	47,544	1
Hospital beds	76,642	18,207	1
Laboratories for clinical analysis	1,608	286	1

Source: INEGI (1997, Table 2.4.2, p. 33).

TABLE 11.11: MEDICAL SERVICE INDICATORS, 1995

Service	National	D.F.	National Ranking
Physicians per 100,000 inhabitants	111.5	276.2	1
Nurses per 100,000 inhabitants	184.5	477.9	1
Hospital beds per 100,000 inhabitants	84.1	214.5	1
General consultations per 100,000 inhabitants	1,376.0	1,709.4	11
Daily consultations per physician	8.4	5.5	23 out of 23
Nurses per bed	2.2	2.2	9 out of 13
Hospital occupancy (%)	65.4	61.4	27 out of 29

Source: INEGI (1997, Table 2.4.3, p. 34).

personnel in Mexico, D.F. may appear to be good, there is inequality between the major institutions. The SSA and the "open population" of Mexico, D.F. are in a "poor" position. Many inhabitants are theoretically covered by the SSA PHC marginal urban areas' program, and yet this PHC work has limited funds and is understaffed and underutilized (Harrison 1991).

A study (Secretaría de Salud 1992) of physicians, nurses, and social workers in PHC in the SSA in Mexico, D.F. in 1992 emphasized some of the characteristics of medical employment. The workforce was relatively young, female, and stable. More than half of those questioned were under forty years of age, and more than half of all nurses and social workers had worked more than ten years with the SSA and in the same health unit. Less than one-third of physicians had remained in the same health unit for more than ten years. Just over a half of all physicians, nurses, and social workers worked an eight-hour day. Pay levels for staff were poor and hence might explain why staff either sought a second job, and thus elected not to work an eight-hour shift, or, as in the case of physicians, sought to move out of PHC work (Harrison 1994).

> Throughout the brief history of the SSA PHC service in the Federal District, staff shortages and the loss of staff have been constant problems. Staff shortages can be explained by low pay levels, the availability of employment opportunities in other health institutions, and the overall lack of prestige of working at a PHC center. (Harrison 1994:403)

Having outlined the training, growth, and distribution of medical personnel in Mexico, I will now turn to some of the factors that influence employment and that thus account for the various distributions in the health sector workforce.

Factors Influencing Location of Employment in the Health Sector

In Mexico the tradition is to study for a professional degree in one's home state if the state has a university or technical institute. In the course of training, the aspirant physician, nurse, or social worker gains experience of medical institutions in the home state, and builds up contacts. Once someone has undertaken training, he or she needs to secure employment. Factors that influence where a person works in the health sector are as follows: contacts made during training, knowledge of local health institutions, health organizational structure, personal qualifications, an individual's ability or desire to work in a specific location, and the need to satisfy certain professional and personal aims and objectives (Harrison 1998). People seek employment to satisfy both practical and strategic needs. Practical needs are "usually a response to an immediate perceived necessity" (Moser 1989: 1803). On a day-to-day basis satisfaction of practical needs is paramount. However, long-term goals, such as career advancement (a strategic need), are also important. Satisfaction of a strategic need depends on personal circumstances, availability of work in a health institution, and organizational structure and opportunities (Harrison 1995).

Organizational structure clearly is an important influence on where health personnel work. As long as curative care remains the priority, health personnel will be attracted to work in curative health care units: general and specialist hospitals. These hospitals receive more funding, are perceived as prestigious, and are located in major urban areas. And any policy that aims to equalize the spatial, institutional, and organizational distribution of health sector workers must recognize that Mexican government policies and investment are directed at urban areas. Thus, medical employment will be concentrated in these areas (Yepes 1973).

In recent years there have been several analyses of the uneven spatial distribution of physicians in Mexico. Such studies (Nigenda and Najera 1996; Sandoval Navarrete 1986) have sought to explore the degree of mobility in the profession as well as the reasons for spatial fixity. For example, Sandoval Navarrete (1986) attempted to establish a theory of physician migration in Mexico. He identified several factors which may explain a physician's reluctance to migrate. These include (1) a lack of preparation at medical school (students are not sufficiently educated to consider the possibilities of working in unfamiliar environments, i.e., those beyond the immediate environment of the medical school), (2) the preference for hospital posts, (3) the inability of rural areas to satisfy personal needs, (4) the lack of economic incentives to attract physicians to less favored areas, and (5) the level of regional inequality in Mexico, which manifests itself in inferior social services in poorer regions. Sandoval Navarrete (1986) demonstrated that salary levels could influence physician mobility, and he concluded his study by outlining two strategies for the decentralization of physicians—incentives and coercion. Yet neither strategy would succeed; Yepes (1973) found government policy to be instrumental in determining where physicians are located. The two INSP studies of 1986 and 1993 attempted to identify how to attract physicians to rural and marginal areas as well as what factors keep or tie a person to a particular area and job (Frenk et al. 1994).

Analysis of the medical labor market has tended to focus on economic as well as institutional and organizational factors that influence employment patterns. However, social, cultural, and personal (including familial and household) factors are also important in accounting for employment location, distribution, and mobility. Harrison (1995) has demonstrated that a female physician's work location and career development are heavily influenced by an awareness of place, structures, opportunities, time, and familial support. The same issues probably apply to female nurses and social workers. Some of these influences will also be generic to male and female workers, whereas certain aspects, like childcare assistance, may be specific to female workers. Further, health sector workers may be reluctant to migrate for purely economic reasons: relocation may cause the employee to break equally important social, cultural, and institutional links—links which may be vital to the attainment of practical and strategic needs. It has been discovered that only a few female physicians have moved from their "known" home state environment to pursue work in another part of Mexico (Harrison 1998).

Other factors influencing work in the health sector, though not necessarily location of work, are flexible work patterns and a degree of job satisfaction. Work satisfaction for nurses was gained from self-fulfillment, service to others, and team membership (Douglas et al. 1996), while Harrison (1995) suggests that security of tenure and flexibility are highly prized by physicians in Mexico, D.F. Douglas et al. (1996) and Harrison (1994, 1995) reveal that those working in medicine are practicing what they want to do and in most cases have an aptitude for the work. In particular, those working in PHC valued their work with a community—the opportunity to go out into the community, to see lives and households change and improve, and to fight for the rights of a community. The varied nature of the work (Douglas et al. 1996; Harrison 1995) can both satisfy and frustrate workers. Certainly a lack of material resources—and not just in PHC work—can lead to stresses and strains in health care work. In PHC centers, workers may feel cut off from key decision makers and thus feel isolated and neglected. Low morale and absenteeism may prevail (Harrison 1991).

Tensions in Health Sector Employment in the Late 1990s

Since the start of the debt crisis in 1982 and continuing into the 1990s, the health sector and workforce have felt the effects of policies aimed at solving the debt burden. Qualified medical personnel are finding it increasingly difficult to secure employment. Restricted financial resources have led each institution to limit employment recruitment and engage workers on temporary contracts. These workers may wait years to secure a permanent post. The financial rewards of medicine are not great (Harrison 1994), yet work in one of the three major health institutions gives a person a degree of security, especially when a permanent post is gained. A permanent work contract ensures that workers will obtain a pension and provides employees with certain rights which are highly valued, such as annual leave. Nonpermanent contract workers have fewer benefits and are potentially less committed to the health institution where they work. However, if employees believe there is any chance of securing a permanent post, they may be willing to work extra hours.

Budget constraints also mean there is less money for in-house training and updating, as well as very limited funding for temporary cover for physicians taking a course. Due to institutional constraints and personal financial shortages, physicians find it increasingly difficult to update professional knowledge via further study, membership in learned bodies, and subscription to medical journals. Over time one is witnessing an academic "stagnation" within the profession. My research on physicians in provincial Mexico indicates that some physicians have not taken professional renewal courses for several years (Harrison, unpublished research results). The increased feminization of the profession has possibly exacerbated this problem. Women have to balance a career and family, and thus find it exceedingly difficult to attend a weekend course or one that takes them away from their home.

Employment in certain branches of health care is particularly precarious given the uncertainty of government funding in the future. IMSS-Solidaridad care schemes are notoriously vulnerable to fluctuations in available government funds. Nigenda (1995) has shown that if the funding for IMSS-Solidaridad work ceases, physicians will have no other option but to leave their health positions and seek work elsewhere. Thus, the more rural or larger the "open population" of a state, the more likely it is to suffer a periodic hemorrhage of physicians as well as an annual loss of *pasantes*. Other issues in PHC work, irrespective of where the PHC center is located, are limited resources and inadequate facilities, resulting in poor and difficult working conditions which are unlikely to attract workers to a particular area.

Economic difficulties, both individual and institutional, cause health workers to obtain two or more jobs, while others may migrate, and still others seek work in a more lucrative profession. In the 1993 INSP survey (unpublished results) an estimated 37.8 percent of all employed male physicians had two or more jobs and 20.6 percent of female physicians had two jobs. Only male physicians had three jobs. Many physicians come from the middle classes (Frenk 1990) and have a certain standard of living to maintain. Thus, as the value of the medical wage continues to decline, physicians must work longer hours to maintain that standard of living. Nigenda (1995) questions whether the traditional pattern of a physician working for a public institution and operating a private consultancy may be changing. Certainly some physicians seek out different forms of employment to increase their earnings. Robledo Vera (1996) highlights the importance of holding down more than one job for male physicians, yet Harrison (1994) discovered that a second job was not as important for female health workers in Mexico, D.F. In her more recent study of female physicians in provincial Mexico, she discovered that a second job is increasingly important, which could be due to the financial difficulties of the 1990s (Harrison 1998). Female health workers may provide either the main income or second income in the household. An increased household income is required to maintain the same standard of living during times of inflation.

The status of a career in medicine has declined in Mexico. In most countries medicine is perceived as a stable, secure profession which virtually guarantees work and an above-average wage. In Mexico, a medical career is no longer considered a prestigious profession. In 1990 a study of student preferences in higher education demonstrated that between 1977 and 1989 the relative popularity of medicine declined (Anonymous 1990). Elsewhere it was reported that men were leaving work in the sciences (including medicine) because of low wages (Shields 1990). Salary levels for engineering (chemical, mechanical, and industrial), administration, law, and architecture were higher than those for physicians (INEGI 1995); in fact the monthly wage level for physicians was the lowest of the ten most popular professions in Mexico. Wages for nurses and social workers have always been low (Martínez Benítez et al. 1993; Harrison 1994). The loss of men from the medical profession has allowed more women to secure work as physicians, but, as Butter et al. (1987) state, the increased entry of female physicians may negatively influence the status of the career. The decline in popularity of medicine is partly explained by increased competition from other "more attractive" disciplines but also the growing level of unemployment in the medical profession. For instance, Soberón-Acevedo (1987) stated that in 1984 only one in four physicians leaving medical school would be successful in obtaining work with a public health institute. The estimated level of unemployment and underemployment among physicians in 1993 was about 25 percent (INSP, unpublished statistics).

High levels of medical unemployment among physicians and other health workers (Frenk et al. 1991), increased workloads, no relative increase in resources (Harrison, unpublished research), more administrative work, and health sector restructuring have led to staff unease and increased stress. Douglas et al. (1996) identified the following as the principal work stresses in a sample survey of nursing auxiliaries in Mexico: interpersonal relations, "*angustia*," work overload, environment, and no resources. Harrison (unpublished survey results) found that SSA nurses and social workers in Mexico, D.F. also registered interpersonal relations and limited resources as problems in their work. Insufficient in-service staff training also leads to increased staff frustration and low morale.

Despite the national abundance of physicians, there are areas in Mexico that still need physicians and other medical personnel—the states of the southwest and many rural areas. For many years Mexico has aimed to achieve an equal spatial distribution of health services and equal access to physicians. Spatial equalization meant looking for gaps in distribution, *municipios* without physicians, and development of a strategy to remove the gaps (Collado Ardón and García Torres 1975; Nigenda 1995). As with Sandoval Navarrete's (1986) proposed strategy to increase physician mobility, the strategy is flawed because it does not take account of personal employee circumstances and the changing economic, social, and cultural context of Mexican development. Too little attention has been paid to how and where Mexico trains its physicians, its health institution structures, and the level of development in various parts of Mexico. In addition, insufficient notice is taken of individual professional preferences of where people wish to train, work, and live.

Frenk et al. (1991) suggested that by offering physicians financial and professional incentives, Mexico could possibly achieve a more even spatial distribution of physicians. However, Nigenda et al. (1990b) and Harrison (1998) suggest that physicians are not mobile. Training practices, strong family support systems, and association and familiarity with an area work against physician mobility regardless of the financial incentive to move. Also, physicians claim that the experience of the *pasante* year does not encourage them to remain in the rural area. With increased levels of unemployment in the medical profession, there is an urgent need to carry out studies of medical career developments across time, geographic region, and gender. Mobility both within and between the institutions and sectors, as well as geographic mobility, need to be analyzed in the attempt to work toward a more equitable and efficient health care system.

Future Developments

The state is "retreating" from areas traditionally under its control; this includes the provision of health services (Nigenda and Solorzano 1997). Starting in the 1980s and continuing in the 1990s, the Mexican government has been pursuing a policy of health sector reform emphasizing privatization and the development of new forms of private health care. Development of the Mexican private health service has consequences for the future of the health sector and medical profession. In recent years, various new hospitals and clinics have been established, and private companies, including those that were formerly state owned, prefer to purchase medical care for their workers rather than use IMSS services. Such schemes are attractive to employers because they control the quality, quantity, and availability of medical services. It is believed this form of health care, as well as more private group practices, will continue to grow in the future (Nigenda 1995). However, as private health care flourishes, which organization will ensure that the Mexican medical service does not become even more polarized and unequal?

An enlarged private health service would in theory lead to increased work opportunities for all medical professionals. The private sector might appear to be an attractive alternative area of employment for many workers, especially if wage levels are seen to be higher than in public institutions. However, the size of the private market is small and it is hard to see how this sector could absorb many medical personnel. Physicians who operate their own individual private consultancy are extremely vulnerable to changing economic circumstances, and thus the nurses and other paramedics they employ are equally vulnerable. Competition in the private sector is fierce, and as a result many physicians may find themselves underemployed.

The medical school curriculum and training practices should be reviewed with the aim of matching health care needs (at all three levels of operation) and student demand, and reducing if not eliminating physician unemployment. Professional "updating" is another key issue. The mechanisms by which Mexican physicians maintain and enhance their professional standards and knowledge should be studied. Also, the role of the health institutions, the state, professional bodies, and the individual in professional development must be reviewed.

As the provision of health care in Mexico changes, these changes and their impact on health care professionals need to be analyzed critically. The links between the private and public health sectors should be examined. Every aspect of private modern biomedical health care needs to be studied, in particular its resources (physical and human), structure, organization, quality, location, and access. In the public health sector, ways of overcoming its many problems (inefficiency, inadequacy, inequality, and insufficiency) need to be explored (Frenk et al. 1994). Running parallel to such investigations, work must continue in the analysis of Mexican epidemiology, for this should inform and influence the development of the Mexican health care system.

Conclusion

At the beginning of the twenty-first century the distribution of Mexican physical and human health resources, and access to those resources, is highly unequal. Inequality exists among institutions, levels of care, and states. Over 10 million Mexicans still do not have access to government-supported services, and yet an elite wealthy minority can buy some of the best health services in the Americas. The distribution of medical personnel is obviously related to the location of medical and technical schools and medical services.

In their quest for spatial equality, Mexican planners may have ignored the basic fact that the health service is hierarchical in structure. Physicians, nurses, and social workers seeking speciality training, promotion, and career advancement are concentrated in the main urban areas. If Mexico truly wishes to attend to all its population in the twenty-first century, realistic goals must be set and policies must be fully contextualized. The changing roles of the public and private health institutions and the state in determining the supply and distribution of health care services must be continually reviewed. Differences between areas and institutions should not be observed as problems but rather as opportunities. Geographic diversity can lead to new ways of seeing and alternative ways of providing a health service. If purely economic solutions persist, however, changing the uneven distribution of medical personnel will not be easy.

Despite the phenomenal growth of medical personnel—a threefold increase in physicians between 1970 and 1990 and an even more rapid rate of growth in the number of nurses—the national distribution of medical personnel in Mexico continues to be highly uneven. Yet, as Frenk et al. (1995) highlight, the numerical expansion of physicians has produced some paradoxical effects: a shortage of physicians in rural and marginal areas, and unemployment and underemployment in urban areas. The unequal geographic distribution of physicians has been a major concern for some time in Mexico (Nigenda et al. 1990a; Sandoval Navarrete 1986; Yepes 1973), yet not much attention has been paid to the distribution of nurses and social workers—possibly reflecting the prevailing attitude that paramedical staff are not as important as physicians.

The prospects for any medical profession, and for physicians in particular, do not appear to be good. Unemployment and underemployment appear to be here to stay. Health institutions are undermining the status of the medical profession through lack of investment, and the long-term prospects of a career in medicine are poor. The existing health service is proving hard to change; previous structural changes have achieved only partial success. If existing institutional and organizational structures do not change, Mexico will continue to witness the declining status of the profession. Similarly, the prospects of female physicians are not good. There may be more female physicians working in Mexico, but female health workers, including physicians, are always distributed at the bottom of the institution employment hierarchy (Butter et al. 1987). If female health workers are prepared to work for low wages, this does little to strengthen the cause for better wage levels for all medical personnel. Economic difficulties in Mexico make it highly unlikely that wage levels in the health sector will increase. Workers will be forced to work long hours in one job or secure two or more jobs.

Note

1. The author wishes to acknowledge that her research was funded by the Economic and Social Research Council (ESRC) Grant H52427502095.

CHAPTER 12

Mesoamerican Healers and Medical Anthropology
Summary and Concluding Remarks

Alan R. Sandstrom

Taken as a whole, medical healers and healing practices in Mesoamerica are products of a complex array of influences ranging from Native American traditions to beliefs and practices originating in Africa, ancient Greece and Persia, Arab and Spanish civilization, and Europe and the United States, as well as the modern biomedical system. Just as in Europe and the United States, many people in the Mesoamerican culture area seek relief from physical or mental "dis-ease" by embracing what has come to be known as alternative medicine, that is, medicine outside of the modern Western bio-medical system. In fact, it might be more accurate to say that in many cases sufferers see the biomedical model itself as the alternative to their complex, pervasive, and often ancient traditions of healing. Yet, as with all sociocul-tural phenomena—particularly phenomena having such diverse roots and occupying a place of such importance in the lives of so many people—how healing is accomplished in Mesoamerica can be difficult for outsiders to grasp. The sheer range of types of curers and medical strategies in the re-gion can be confusing even for the insider convinced of the efficacy of his or her own healing traditions.

My own introduction to Mesoamerican healing can serve as a brief ex-ample of what I mean. In 1970, as a graduate student in anthropology at Indiana University, I was asked to participate in an experimental field school in Mexico with three other students. The destination was the remote and isolated northern Veracruz region, where I was to be placed alone for two months in a Nahua (Nahuatl-speaking) village. Of course, I was anxious to experience Nahua culture firsthand and to try ethnographic field research among a group of people far removed from the influences of Europe and the United States. The community of six hundred people in which I found myself was almost one hundred miles from the nearest paved road and had no electricity, running water, stores, church, or apparent connection to the outside world. The people were largely monolingual in Nahuatl and, although there was a government school in the village with classes offered up to the third grade, the village—with its thatch-roofed houses grouped into patrilocal-extended family compounds, slash-and-burn horticultural practices, and people in striking traditional dress—seemed as far from the United States and from Mexican urban life as it could possibly be.

After an awkward arrival in the village, I was put under the charge of the *agente municipal*, whose job it was to look after my welfare while I was in residence. Within a few days I developed a feverish gastrointestinal disorder, almost certainly due to my own ignorance. I was drinking from the nearby *arroyo* (stream) rather than from springs, as the Nahuas did. I was also not accustomed to the sometimes searingly hot chile pepper dishes that, although I found quite good to eat, often caused severe distress afterward. One early morning when the *agente* came to take me to his house to eat, I complained that I was ill and could not go with him that day. He was concerned and thought for a while about the best course of action. The normal procedure, I later learned, would be to refer me to a *curandero* or perhaps to one of the old women in the village adept at curing with herbs. But he could see that I was clearly a foreigner and would probably balk at his suggesting either of these alternatives. Finally, he brightened up and said that I should take a cure that would surely help. He called it something like "*halcaset.*" At least that is how I wrote it down in my field notebook, convinced that it referred to some exotic leaf or root used in traditional curing. I was pleased that I had retrieved an interesting piece of ethnographic data that may even have practical application once I returned to the university and could have a sample analyzed. I said I would try it and he mysteriously asked for a peso and walked off toward one of the village *cantinas*. *Cantinas* are small stores, usually a corner of someone's house dedicated to selling a small variety of items for the convenience of other villagers. Shortly, he returned with a small item in his hand and told me to mix it with water and then drink the concoction and that I would soon feel better. I was taken aback when he handed me two Alka Seltzer tablets in an aluminum-foil packet. Clearly the appearance of *halcaset* meant that field research among the Nahuas was going to be more complicated than I had thought.

I have been returning regularly to the community for nearly thirty years now, and I have seen scores of occasions when villagers sought out the help of curing specialists. Village healers include midwives, bonesetters, herbalists, and *curanderos*, who are males or females struggling against diseases involving spirit entities. I have also had numerous occasions to speak with regional representatives of the biomedical establishment, including local physicians and staff members of clinics in the larger towns, as well as members of medical teams that visit remote Indian villages to vaccinate children. A clear divide exists between village curers and biomedical curers. Even the most conservative *curandero* occasionally recommends that people seek help for intractable diseases wherever they can get it. In my experience, village curers have an excellent grasp of what biomedical healers can do best and they do not hesitate to refer patients to a clinic or physician. *Curanderos* actively help insure that children are vaccinated by the visiting medical teams and see no contradiction in providing traditional cures alongside biomedical ones. Individual villagers see no contradiction in visiting a physician during the day and attending a curing ritual held by a *curandero* in the evening. For their part, the biomedical representatives with whom I have spoken have a very different attitude. They tend to dismiss village curers as quacks or superstitious charlatans. Their attitudes fit with those of many urban dwellers in Mexico who dismiss Indian society and culture as backward and in dire need of modernization.

As an anthropologist committed to science, I found the views expressed by the biomedical people to be incredibly arrogant and distressingly pervasive. There is no question that the application of science to problems of disease has revolutionized health care throughout the world. Few would argue with this statement. Certainly the Nahua villagers I know would not. But to then conclude that the biomedical approach to health care, with its exclusive focus on biological function, has reached its optimum with no further expansion necessary into additional poorly explored realms of the human condition strikes me as not only short-sighted but also antiscientific. Scientific formulations are frequently parochial and always provisional, particularly when it comes to the analysis of human beings. The door must always be left open to the possibility that an alternative idea or approach to a problem will prove to be of yet greater scientific value than unquestioned established truths. Scientific formulations are uncomfortably impermanent and do not serve well those seeking secure knowledge. At the point where arrogance sets in is often where true science stops.

Probably the most aggravating aspect of the facile dismissal of traditional medicine is an unspoken assumption that the people who seek such cures are fools who are easily duped by charlatans in the guise of *curanderos*. Ethnographers familiar with the people they study know better. I have found some Nahuas who are indeed true believers and easily fooled. But I also know people who are extremely insightful and as systematic and skeptical in their evaluation of curing procedures as any scientist. Like members of ethnic groups anywhere in the world, the Nahuas run the gamut of human types and they suffer the stereotyping of dominant groups. Most of the villagers that I know are interested in whether or not a certain type of cure works. They are quite empirical about it and evaluate the sometimes ambiguous evidence that accompanies medical treatment in any system. The *curandero*, midwife, or bonesetter who does not return the patient to health will find that fewer and fewer people will come to him or her for help. Every village has a number of trained curers who no longer practice because they could not maintain a clientele. How could this be so if the villagers were simpletons who were the easy marks of hucksters or charlatans? One man I have known for many years summed it up quite well. After discussing different curers and their various acknowledged talents or areas of weakness, I asked him about going to a physician or clinic. He said to me that in many cases—although not all—the medicines of the physician can cure a person. But then he added, "But you always feel much better after a ritual cleansing." Most Nahuas do not expect either physicians or *curanderos* to perform miracles. But they do not see the two approaches as mutually exclusive or contradictory. They constitute overlapping fields with the common goal of restoring well-being to the sufferer.

It is this expanded vision of health care—the restoration of a more authentic and open-minded scientific perspective on the biomedical enterprise as a whole—that is, and should be, the hallmark of medical anthropology. It is ironic how cutting-edge scientific medicine that aims to address the total human being in biological, psychological, and sociocultural terms—in short the new medicine—speaks very much against the scientific pretensions of so many contemporary biomedical practitioners. In expanding the field of theory and application, medical anthropology affirms medicine as scientific in the broadest and truest sense of the word.

The subfield specialty of medical anthropology has been well summarized in numerous publications. It has also been the subject of a number of texts and anthologies, many of which, unlike the present volume, attempt broad coverage of the field (for more recent works see Brown 1998; Loustaunau and Sobo 1997; Romanucci-Ross, Moerman, and Tancredi 1997; Sargent and Johnson 1996). It is a relatively new subfield, coming into its own only since World War II. In that short time, medical anthropology has become one of the most rapidly growing subfields in the discipline of anthropology (Trostle and Sommerfield 1996: 253). A number of researchers now hold the Ph.D. degree in anthropology as well as the M.D., and medical anthropologists in general have probably been the most successful of their colleagues in other anthropology subfields in securing employment outside of the university. They are in demand in several health-related fields both as permanent employees and as consultants. Rather than repeat what has been published elsewhere I would like to discuss four aspects or strengths of medical anthropology that help explain its current popularity and reveal something of its potential to both illuminate the human condition and alleviate some of the problems associated with that condition. In so doing, I hope to place the contributions in this volume in the broader context of medical anthropology as a whole.

First, medical anthropology shares with the discipline at large a commitment to holism in pursuit of its aims. It "encompasses the study of medical phenomena as they are influenced by social and cultural features, and social and cultural phenomena as they are illuminated by their medical aspects" (Lieban 1977: 15). By encouraging "consilience," the felicitous word revived by E. O. Wilson (1999) to signify unity among biological, cultural, linguistic, and archaeological phenomena, medical anthropology fulfills the promise of a unified study of health care in particular and human conduct in general. The adaptation that a group achieves to its geographic and social environment generates a disease load on the population that is then met by cultural means of coping. Anthropologists have known since the last century that human beings do not live in separate biological, cultural, or psychological realms but rather experience life as a totality. Separating levels of analysis is necessary for scientific investigation, but at some point the different levels have to be united into a single, coherent explanatory system.

Medical anthropology has made strides in the direction of unifying the study of disease as well as the general human condition, and it holds the promise of significant progress in this area in the future.

The second strength of medical anthropology derives from the first. By its very nature, the field is interdisciplinary and provides the opportunity for meaningful links among previously separate fields. It seems clear that in the near future we will witness an increase in mutual citing and conceptual overlap in published works produced by medical anthropologists, medical sociologists, epidemiologists, ecologists, evolutionary biologists, biomedical specialists, traditional social scientists, and even perhaps those affiliated with more humanities-oriented disciplines. Medical conditions often bring into play all of the complexities of human life, and solutions to problems in this area will require input from a number of hitherto separate fields of study (see, e.g., Trostle and Sommerfield's 1996 article on the new relationship between medical anthropology and epidemiology). This is not to advocate that disciplinary boundaries be eliminated. On the contrary. Despite much contemporary rhetoric extolling the virtues of the interdisciplinary approach, it is important to recognize that disciplines are deliberately distinct because they view their subject matter from a particular perspective. For example, in a real sense there is only one social science. But economists, cultural anthropologists, political scientists, historians, and sociologists each bring a unique perspective to their study of human beings. What is called for is cooperation and communication among disciplines, but not the homogenization of research efforts through the elimination of disciplinary boundaries.

A third strength of medical anthropology is that, probably more than any other component of anthropology, its findings and approaches have direct practical applicability to the solution of real-world problems. The stimulating insights and findings of other subdisciplines of anthropology certainly have potential for application, and they are increasingly used in applied programs, but medical anthropology has found an immediate home in hospitals, government medical programs, medical task forces, community health programs, and, increasingly, in medical schools. The early work of Foster (1952, 1955) and Paul (1955) represents pioneering efforts in the application of anthropology to the improvement of medical systems. Applied medical anthropology attracts funding for university programs as well as students who wish to use their knowledge to alleviate suffering. More important, it can increase the effectiveness of health programs by advocating that patients' perspectives and cultural orientations be taken into account, particularly if they are different from those of the caregivers. In addition, it can reveal to health care providers that the dominant biomedical model is a product of culture itself and that working with alternative systems of healing—those that fall outside of the biomedical purview—can significantly improve rapport between medical personnel and patients.

The fourth, and perhaps most controversial, strength of medical anthropology from my perspective derives from its applied nature. Because medical anthropologists often use their knowledge in situations where results of their work can be measured, they have been led to avoid the antiscientific and antiempirical aspects of postmodernism that have distorted other areas of anthropology, notably ethnology (see Kuznar 1997). If medical anthropologists are consulting on a governmental project to vaccinate children against whooping cough in rural Mexico, they are interested in empirical results and not in engaging in philosophical arguments that reject both anthropology and science as colonial enterprises and an imposition of Euro-American culture on the world's dispossessed peoples. From my experiences in the field, I can state that the people whose children are to be vaccinated have a critical interest in the empirical results of the vaccination program. The unity of theory and practice in medical anthropology is a powerful antidote to radical relativism and nihilism. For this reason, it may be medical anthropology, one of the youngest subfields in anthropology, that returns us to an empirical and scientifically based research program under whose influence the discipline was created in the first place.

We hope that the chapters included in this volume will provide the maturing field of medical anthropology with further impetus to continue its new direction. We anticipate a move away from generalized works introducing the new subfield to readers, or edited volumes that attempt to sample the entire subfield (except of course for use in the classroom). Medical anthropology is rapidly growing in the complexity and sophistication of its analyses, and the published literature in the subfield is exploding. We believe that in place of generalized texts, more specialized works will increasingly be published that explicate specific areas of interest or concern. In this volume, we have gathered together contributions from experts to help clarify the origin and role of the healer in the Mesoamerica culture area. We attempt to provide information in a coherent format on major traditions of healing in relation to their practitioners. Each chapter brings together information that is scattered in many different publication outlets, that appears in different languages, or that results from fresh field research on the part of the author. The bibliography is extensive and should be helpful to experts and novices alike.

As editors, we wanted to bring together chapters that cover major healing traditions often known to students of Mesoamerican history and culture but understood in a fragmentary or incomplete way. Coverage is not universal. For example, we have no chapter on herbalists. But we attempt to provide a systematic overview of those healers and healing traditions where adequate ethnographic and historical evidence exists to allow a synthetic and analytic summary of what is known. Although the amount of research published on medical systems in Mesoamerica has increased dramatically over the past decade or so, much work remains to be done. As the chapters gathered in this volume demonstrate, an exciting field awaits any researcher who wishes to investigate the medical systems of Mesoamerica. Nowhere is the ethnohistorical, historical, or archaeological record so complete, and nowhere is the contemporary ethnographic landscape so rich with such a long tradition of field investigation. And nowhere has the clash between European imperialist powers and the world's cultures been more catastrophically and devastatingly played out than in this region. If we are to clarify the coordinated effects of history, biology, and culture in human social life, there is no better place than Mesoamerica to initiate such an inquiry.

Our understanding of pre-Hispanic medical systems is based largely on the Aztecs because the ethnohistorical record is most complete for this group. Works by López Austin (1988) and Ortiz de Montellano (1990), for example, have contributed greatly to our knowledge of Aztec medicine. The medical systems of the many other groups in Mesoamerica are less well documented, and often we can only guess at their nature from ethnographic investigation of the practices of living descendants. For a majority of the population of Mesoamerica, the most important influence on healers was the European invasion in the early sixteenth century. Cortés and his soldiers and subsequent immigrants from Europe brought with them a complex system of beliefs and practices that has shaped much of the contemporary folk medical system. Luz María Hernández Sáenz and George M. Foster in their chapter have provided a superb overview of colonial medicine. They have shown that any understanding of European medicine must begin with the

Greek humoral beliefs, which arrived in Spain and then the New World via Persian and Moslem scholars. For a more extensive coverage of this important topic see Foster (1994). An important insight from Hernández Sáenz and Foster is that Spanish medical practices did not diffuse uniformly throughout the local population. There was elite medicine and popular medicine, the former under control of a royal tribunal, the Protomedicato, that tried to regulate recognized healers, while the latter was brought from Spain by soldiers and people occupying the lower rungs of the social ladder.

As Hernández Sáenz and Foster point out, the colonial elite medical system was simply not all that effective, and it was also quite expensive. The result is that most people turned first to the popular or informal system for their medical needs. The construction of hospitals and the activities of Catholic missionaries served to spread the Spanish system of medicine to the Indians, who ecumenically combined elements of their own medical systems with that of the strangers. In addition to the Spanish and Native American traditions must be added those of the Africans brought to Mesoamerica for slave labor. The authors point out that over time, both elite and popular systems combined to create a relatively uniform medical system among both Indians and mestizos. It is an evolved form of this system that we find among the urban poor and rural populations of contemporary Mesoamerica. Throughout the colonial period, elite healers added to their store of practical and empirical knowledge in their dealings with patients. This knowledge enriched but did not displace the dominant medical paradigm. For their part, popular healers added to the practical knowledge bequeathed to them from the pre-Hispanic era. Much of this knowledge, along with curative herbs and new sources of food, served to improve the health of European populations. On the other hand, diseases imported from Spain, along with a largely ineffective medical system to treat them, caused one of the most disastrous population declines in human history among Native Americans.

Carlos Viesca Treviño points out in his essay that pre-Hispanically trained curers were called "doctors" by the Spaniards in the years following the invasion and that they were doctors in the true sense of the word. Native practitioners were consulted by eminent Spaniards including Córtes and Viceroy Mendoza. The author makes the interesting observation that Spanish authorities tolerated Indian medical specialists, even issuing licenses to them, because they thought the natives were different by nature from Europeans and that indigenous doctors were better equipped to cure their own. This view was reinforced by obvious cultural differences such as language, dress, and food preferences. Of course, this tolerance excluded any curing procedures associated with religious belief. Viesca Treviño confirms that herbal remedies traveled from Mesoamerica to Europe. However, it was not long into the colonial period that indigenous doctors lost their status relative to their Spanish peers and became known as *curanderos,* a less prestigious designation. The author provides a pointed reminder that the status of *curandero* is a colonial creation.

Viesca Treviño searches the ethnohistorical record for information about *curanderos* and finds much that anticipates current practices and beliefs. In the area of northern Veracruz where I have worked, individuals are called to be healers through dreams or recovery from a serious illness, just as the author reports from the documents. He also notes the ambiguous status of curers because of their ability to consort with powerful spirits and the darker forces of the cosmos. It was not only Spanish authorities who persecuted *curanderos* suspected of causing harm, but also fellow Indians and mestizos. In the community where I work, I know personally of cases where local curers have been murdered in revenge for using their powers to cause disease and death. One key feature of the contemporary *curandero* that ethnohistorians have a difficult time seeing in the documentary record is the element of coercion present in the selection of new curers. Men or women who have certain disturbing dreams or who recover miraculously from illness often have little choice but to follow a curing career. *Curanderos* whom I know always comment on the danger inherent in resisting the call to heal. Several years ago when I returned to the field I was told about a young village boy (the son of a female curer) who renounced his gift of curing and was subsequently struck by a car and crippled while visiting relatives in Mexico City. Several people commented that his fate was clear punishment for resisting the directives of the spirits.

In their contributions to the volume, James Dow undertakes to generalize about the shamanic tradition of curing found in contemporary northern Mexico, while Frank Lipp does the same for southern Mexico and Guatemala. Dow tackles the difficult problem of defining the concept of shaman, and he concludes that shamans do exist in Mexico. He finds that their distinguishing features are that they heal by invoking the spirit world, they work within a Native American tradition, and they are called to their profession through dreams, visions, or spirit possession (see also Dow 1986a). He breaks with the orthodox position that limits use of the term "shaman" to those cultural traditions where spirits always take possession of the ritual specialist in the course of a cure. The published literature reports several different kinds of shamans operating in Mesoamerica, but Dow proposes that there are two basic types. The first he calls a "traditional shaman," which he defines as a person with religious authority who works in a coherent belief system based on myths with pre-Columbian connections. The second type is the "*curandero* shaman," defined as a more acculturated person who cures without the prestige of religious authority, basing his or her work on a diffuse mix of folk beliefs and myths deriving from Spanish colonial and to a lesser extent Native American sources. I would add here that successful shamans are often charismatic with powerful personalities. They are authoritative and have an air of danger about them combined with a strong sense of self-confidence. For example, shamans in northern Veracruz are sometimes reputed to have murdered people. Both traditional and *curandero* shamans would likely be called *curanderos* in Spanish by the people in the communities they serve, but the distinction that Dow draws serves to clarify their place in the context of Mesoamerican history.

From Dow's discussion of indigenous theories of disease etiology, diagnosis and identification of pathogenic forces, and therapeutic techniques it is clear that shamans in northern Mexico are heirs to a complex set of traditions that explain and control disease. It is also clear that many elements of shamanic practice derive from Native American traditions that preserve links to the pre-Hispanic era. However, as Dow recognizes, no shaman in Mesoamerica has avoided the influence of the Spanish presence. Many beliefs and practices, including the pervasive hot–cold syndrome used in diagnosing and curing, are probable imports from Europe. Trying to sort out which traits are native and which are imported can be a fruitless task, particularly when it is obvious that the shamans themselves do not apparently pay attention to whether a particular practice or belief is authentically aboriginal. Shamans in general are creative individuals—truly entrepreneurs— and to a certain extent each one produces idiosyncratic healing systems according to his or her own particularistic understandings. But, simultaneously, they partake of meanings, symbols, and practices that are common to all of Mesoamerica. Thus, the diagnostic and curing techniques of a shaman in one region will be different but basically comprehensible to a shaman in another region. Shamanic innovation is constrained by the set of under-standings about the nature of the causes and cures of disease shared widely throughout Mesoamerica (see Hunt 1976 for a detailed explication of the common pool of symbols that ties Mesoamerica into a single cultural sys-tem). Shamans must innovate enough to set themselves apart from their competitors but not so much that they fall outside of their clients' world-views and values. They can be seen as potentially dangerous and sometimes frightening, but they are often respected members of their communities whom people view as selfless warriors who do battle with the forces of dis-ease and disorder.

In his study of curers from southern Mexico and Guatemala, Lipp pro-vides statistical summaries of a number of factors relating to shaman-curers (see also Lipp 1991). He notes that curing is a part-time occupation for almost all practitioners and that most are female. And despite statements to the contrary, there is no evidence that they enjoy undue financial rewards from their practices. He shows that shamanic curers may be organized into hierarchies and undergo formal ritual initiation into the profession, or they may simply apprentice themselves to a master and work to create a clientele based on a successful cure rate. The social organization of healers reflects the social organization of the society at large. Lipp also discusses in some detail the widespread use of psychotropic plants among Mesoamerican folk healers. Hallucinatory experiences are used by healers to contact spirits and to diagnose and obtain information on curing a specific affliction. In all cases, whether in the southern or northern reaches of Mesoamerica, illness is interpreted by healers as a sign of sorcery or a disequilibrium in internal body processes or the social or cosmological order. Any deviation from the path of moderation such as drunkenness, envy, anger, or aggression can lead to illness that must be cured by a shaman.

Lipp calls for more research into trance, soul travel, and the nature of tutelary spirits before we can determine with precision whether Meso-american curers who restore harmony through control of spirits are sha-mans in the narrowest definition. In the end, he seems comfortable calling these healers shamans because of the way they are recruited, trained, and initiated. He points out that individual Mesoamerican shamans often take on multiple roles such as curer, diviner, priest, judge, sorcerer, myth teller, myth maker, consultant, and so on. In my experiences with shamans in northern Veracruz, it is the role of restorer of harmony and balance that is the defining characteristic of shamanic practice. The most commonly used term of reference for shamans in Nahuatl is *tlamatiquetl*, meaning "person of knowledge." It is knowledge of the spirit realm and the means to put it back in order after a disruption that defines this type of healer.

An interesting but neglected area of research related to shamanic symbolic curing in Mesoamerica that is hinted at by both Dow and Lipp are concepts of pollution and their relation to illness. Anthropologists normally associate elaborate pollution concepts with Asian societies, although it is recognized that pollution beliefs are found in all cultures. In northern Veracruz, shamans cut images of disease-causing wind spirits from paper and direct offerings to them as a means of removing the offending pathogens from the patient's body and surroundings. The names of these images often contain the word *tlasoli*, meaning "refuse" or "filth." The cuttings represent filthy, malevolent entities associated with death that originate in dirty water or tangled underbrush that pollute the body and cause disease (Sandstrom 1978, 1989; Sandstrom and Sandstrom 1986). Curing rituals throughout Mesoamerica are frequently called "cleansings" or "sweepings" to indicate that their purpose is to remove polluting and infectious agents from the body. Mary Douglas (1966) has shown that concepts of dirt and pollution are universally associated with areas in which there is a breakdown of cultural order. Clearly, curing in Mesoamerica fits this general idea quite well. Disruptions in the social, psychological, or spirit realms are associated in people's beliefs with pollution agents in the form of filthy winds. These elements of disorder are removed in cleansings and the threat to cultural systems of order are thereby eliminated and health is returned. It is interesting that the classical shamanic practice among the Inuit is often concerned with removing the effects of pollution caused by breaches of social norms and breaking of taboos.

The chapter by Kaja Finkler reveals that many of the alternatives to the biomedical healing system that exist in Mexico are relatively recent in origin. Her extensive and long-term study of the religious and healing movement known as Spiritualism is an excellent example of nonindigenous and noncolonial systems of healing that coexist with the dominant biomedical system (see Finkler 1994b). Of course, even Spiritualism has been influenced by Mexico's history, for example, in the beliefs that airs (winds) or anger can cause disease. She cautions the reader that the people attracted to Spiritualism are not all the same, although most are from urban, lower economic classes and most healers are women. Spiritualists usually attribute illness to invasion of the patient's body by an evil spirit, and healing is accomplished by removing the pathogen through a variety of techniques. Healers in the Spiritualist tradition specialize in afflictions that are not cured easily through biomedicine, and they have developed an interesting fail-safe mechanism. Those not cured by Spiritualism are said to have a special gift from God to become healers themselves. Thus, a failed cure is a major avenue of recruitment for Spiritualist healers.

A particularly instructive part of Finkler's chapter is the comparison from the perspective of the patient of alternative therapies—in this case, Spiritualism—with biomedicine. Lower economic class patients in Mexico find their interactions with physicians to be conflict-ridden, and they find diagnoses to be confusing and often contradictory and feel alienated by the inability of the physician to identify with their affliction. Spiritualist healers, by contrast, are viewed as knowing everything. They engage patients in their own recovery and they invite them to join a new social network and religious community that can alleviate dysfunctional marital or family relationships and ultimately heal by transforming their lives. What holds the greatest promise for increasing our understanding of the persistence of multiple systems of healing is focusing on the social factors that underlie people's choices of medical systems, as well as paying close attention to the actual experiences that people have with various systems of healing. In general, I would say that people do not continue to follow healing systems that do not work. Given the millions of Mesoamericans, and for that matter Europeans and North Americans, who search out alternatives to biomedicine, it is imperative that anthropologists and other researchers better understand what it is that afflicts people and how they are helped by systems that are too easily dismissed as mere quackery by members of the dominant group. Such studies would help explain the phenomenal growth throughout the region of religions such as Pentecostalism that purport to cure.

The contributions by Brad R. Huber and Alan R. Sandstrom, Sheila Cosminsky, and Elena Hurtado and Eugenia Sáenz de Tejada return us to more secular forms of healing in their discussions of midwifery. But in fact, no clear distinction exists between secular and sacred in any society and midwives in Mesoamerica often hold rituals or invoke spirits in the course of their duties. Huber and Sandstrom discuss midwives in northern Mexico, Cosminsky covers southern Mexico and Guatemala, and Hurtado and Sáenz de Tejada discuss relations between midwives and the dominant biomedical system in Guatemala. Midwifery is a key point of contention in the argument between the biomedical and alternative systems of healing. Even in North America, there is considerable debate as midwives seek official recognition of their work and the dominant medical establishment attempts to marginalize them and even criminalize their activities.

Many students of Mesoamerica have a general knowledge of the existence of midwives and their activities, but they often lack specific information from a cross-cultural perspective. Huber and Sandstrom provide summaries of the published literature covering forty-one groups in northern Mexico on this topic. The data are presented in tabular form and are accompanied by an in-depth look at midwives from a Nahuat-speaking community in the Sierra Norte de Puebla studied by Huber. It appears that population density, more than any other variable, determines whether or not a specific cultural group employs midwives to help in the birth process. Groups such as the Tarahumara, Huichol, and Tepehuani, with scattered populations and perhaps low birth rates, are apparently not able to support professional midwives. The authors document the distribution of various techniques employed by midwives and the multiple roles that they often play in their respective communities. One surprising finding is that male midwives exist in several of the societies surveyed. The finding is surprising because it is common in indigenous communities for male and female roles to remain quite distinct, with little overlap. Huber and Sandstrom also find the relationships between midwives and representatives of the biomedical establishment to be complex. Efforts are being made by rural health care teams to enlist midwives as allies by having them refer difficult cases to physicians or clinics. As agencies representing biomedicine penetrate the rural districts, the demand for midwife services has declined.

Cosminsky provides a summary of a wide range of published studies on midwifery for southern Mesoamerica combined with her own research on the topic. Much of what she reports regarding recruitment and training, prenatal care, the birth event itself, and postpartum care parallels findings from the northern region. Cosminsky affirms Dow's observation that ethnographers often report their data in such a way that makes comparison difficult. The author confirms the existence of male midwives in the southern region and notes an element of coercion among those called to their profession by spirits. She also underscores the ambiguous status of some midwives in the community because of their connection to the sacred and the potential for doing harm. As mentioned above, these last two features of midwives link them to shaman-curers, many of whom experience similar ambiguity of status and coercion in their calling. Just as with the Nahua shamans, discussed earlier, most midwives in this region appear to be tolerant of the biomedical system as long as they are shown respect for their knowledge. The clients of midwives are equally tolerant of multiple medical systems and happily use more than one. In many cases, however, biomedical personnel look down on midwives and clients both and criticize them for their practices and beliefs. Of course, as we move from culture to culture and from community to community, the situation grows complicated and individual cases may always be found to contradict such general statements.

Cosminsky goes on to review a number of studies on midwives conducted by government agencies and other representatives of the biomedical establishment. She contends that most such studies are flawed because they rely on self-reported behavior and contain no observations of actual behavior. Reliance on emic data alone reduces the validity of such studies. Cross-cultural misunderstanding is also rife, but little insight into the problem is evident in the published reports. Biomedical personnel often assume, for example, that the midwife has some kind of control or authority over his or her clients. They often accuse midwives of refusing to order their clients to hospitals or clinics if there are signs of trouble with the birth. However, in many rural communities the midwife is viewed more as an experienced colleague than an authority, with no power to issue orders. It is antiscientific arrogance on the biomedical side that seems to be at the root of the problem of communication across cultural divides. Providing instruction to midwives in their native language and showing respect for their experience and positive knowledge seem to be minimal first steps in bettering relations between proponents of the two different medical systems.

The Hurtado and Sáenz de Tejada chapter treats in detail the relations between midwives and the biomedical system in contemporary Guatemala. The country's Ministry of Health personnel face the reality that they have the human and financial resources to attend only 20 percent of all births in the country, and so working collaboratively with traditional midwives is an unavoidable necessity. The authors provide a brief but informative recent history of the development of biomedicine in Guatemala, including the government's plan to train midwives to report obstetrical problems to health authorities. They report on an extensive study of midwives and bio-medical health care providers conducted by Hurtado between 1995 and 1997. The study systematically reveals a long list of cross-cultural misunderstandings that prevent midwives from working in concert with the biomedical establishment. It is largely the Western-oriented representatives of biomedicine that bring to the problem their own difficult-to-break traditions of discrimination against women, Indians, and the poor, practically the defining characteristics of most midwives. This chapter amounts to a call for medical anthropologists to intervene and facilitate cross-cultural communication among the contending parties. Anthropologists with ethnographic experience in Guatemala possess the methods, empirical data, and the theoretical sophistication to identify problem areas and suggest solutions. The authors note that under anthropological guidance, tensions have been reduced between midwives and biomedical personnel in recent years. But there is much work to be done.

Other Mesoamerican healers who are much talked about but too little studied are bonesetters. Benjamin D. Paul and Clancy McMahon have contributed a chapter on Guatemalan bonesetting that relates an episode in which the second author had the opportunity to experience the therapy firsthand. In northern Veracruz and in most of northern Mesoamerica, bonesetting seems for the most part to be a secular therapy, but in some Maya groups in Guatemala it has a definite link to the sacred. One would think that broken or dislocated bones would require naturalistic therapies, but many bonesetters in Guatemala receive their gift to heal from spiritual forces. Healers in Mesoamerica, including bonesetters, avoid the disharmonic effects of egotism. Self-importance disrupts the pre-Hispanically derived mandate to maintain harmony with the psychological, social, and natural worlds. Shaman-curers, midwives, and Spiritualists credit their tutelary guardian spirits with successful cures, and the bonesetters described by Paul and McMahon attribute their healing powers to sacred objects. In this way, individuals are not credited with the ability to cure but are seen as vehicles for the sacred—"radio transmitters" for the spirits, in the words of the Spiritualists. Healers acquire social status because of their relations to the spirit world rather than any ability they have to alleviate suffering.

The authors describe a community known throughout Guatemala for its bonesetters which attracts people from afar to have their fractures healed. It is clear that bonesetting has become almost a way of life and that bonesetters in this community and elsewhere have built a significant body of knowledge about the musculoskeletal system that allows them to be effective and maintain a clientele. To repeat a point made earlier, people do not continue to follow a therapy that has no effect, particularly when alternatives are available, as they are throughout Mesoamerica. McMahon, who was treated by a bonesetter for a fractured ankle during the course of fieldwork, concluded that the treatment was effective. It is important to recognize the bonesetter's success at promoting healing, like the midwife's success at facilitating birth, because broken or displaced bones, like pregnancy, are concrete conditions with clear physical bases and prognoses, and the outcome of therapy is measurable. In both circumstances, traditional healers have proven their worth. The effectiveness of shaman-curers and Spiritualists is much harder for outsiders to measure.

Margaret E. Harrison discusses Western biomedical healers in her chapter in the context of the growth of scientific biomedicine in Mexico. She demonstrates that physicians, nurses, and social workers are an increasingly available source of therapy for the people of Mexico. Statistical measures of a number of variables reveal that biomedicine, with all of its flaws and faults, works remarkably well to effect cures and relieve suffering. As the result of the growth of a biomedical infrastructure, Mexicans live longer and are basically healthier than before. The author is able to trace the complex relations between biomedicine and the momentous changes taking place in Mexican society at large. She relates the evolution of health care in the context of such cataclysmic events as the Mexican Revolution, the massive population migrations from the rural areas to the cities, the transformation from an agricultural to industrial economy, subtle changes in male and female roles, and cyclical fluctuations in the economy. Her research helps to clarify the complex linkages between health care and social and historical factors. Harrison's analysis shows that problems in the health care system parallel those of other areas in modernizing Mexico, namely uneven development and distribution of benefits. For example, 10 million Mexicans do not have access to adequate biomedical services, while an elite minority has access to some of the best medical care in the world.

The author also clarifies the complex system that has grown up in Mexico to train medical personnel. She shows that overproduction of physicians and their concentrations in urban centers have reduced salaries and increasingly led students away from careers in medicine. There is also a feminization of the profession, with women constituting over one-quarter of practicing physicians. As a result of these and other factors, a medical career in Mexico is no longer considered to be a prestigious profession. At the end, Harrison is somewhat pessimistic about the future of the biomedical health care system in Mexico. While it has certainly been a success in some areas, it currently suffers from structural problems that must be corrected by government planners. The current economic crisis, coupled with the usual problems of a developing nation and region, do not bode well for significant reform. Again, here we witness a classic opportunity for social scientific methods and findings to inform planning efforts and produce results that benefit not only health care workers but also their potential patients.

The first step in any systematic inquiry (or in applying social scientific knowledge) is to assemble information on the problem in a coherent form. The basic objective of this volume has been to produce such a compilation on some of the important healers in Mesoamerica. Despite gaps in the ethnographic and historical record and sometimes incomparable findings in the published data, we are beginning to get a clearer picture of Mesoamerican healers and the complex interplay of cultural and historical factors and medical traditions in the region. If the purpose of anthropology as a whole—and medical anthropology in particular—is to produce broad-based, holistic, and scientific explanations of the human condition (and I believe that is the ultimate purpose of our efforts), then what we lack is an agreed-upon theoretical framework within which to pursue our goals. Although it is unpopular within some circles in anthropology to say so, I believe that we should pursue the goals of science set out during the Enlightenment to seek comprehensive explanations that incorporate as wide a field of phenomena as possible. Those of us in the human sciences should seek for the unity of knowledge that, albeit elusive, has been the promise of the natural sciences.

It seems to me that fruitful theoretical frameworks are already at hand in anthropology and its cognate fields that promise to bring us to new levels of understanding, but that these research strategies are in need of further elaboration, testing, and development. The most powerful approaches, and the ones with the greatest potential, in my view, are materialist and take into account the biological level of analysis. Proponents of these approaches agree that we should avoid idealist, meaning-centered, interpretivist, and radical relativist methodologies in the study of human social life because such research strategies are not holistic and they have not been, nor are they capable of being, productive of generalizing explanation. All seem to agree that we need to take care to avoid a biological determinism that would turn humans into "articulate chimpanzees" (Levins and Lewontin 1998:xi) controlled like robots by our genes. In this latter view, culture becomes a thin veil of illusion disguising preprogrammed biological machines. I would briefly like to discuss three important theoretical approaches that avoid these extreme, untenable positions and that show promise to take us to new biocultural frontiers of the human sciences.

First is the often unfairly dismissed perspective developed by Marvin Harris, called cultural materialism. Over several decades, Harris has worked to formulate a paradigm in anthropology that is rigorously scientific and maximally productive of explanations of cultural similarities and differences. The approach derives its inspiration from Karl Marx and from the cultural ecology of Julian Steward. Harris locates the dynamic of cultural evolution in the changing pragmatic material conditions of people's daily lives. Often falsely accused of ignoring values, ideas, and worldviews—or worse, of relegating these key elements of culture to the status of epiphenomena—cultural materialism has been dismissed as simplistic. However, though Harris assigns causal priority to material conditions, he has created a subtle, sophisticated approach to the complexities of human life that offers the possibility of taking into account and explaining socially shared beliefs and practices. Those who accuse Harris of oversimplifying have failed to understand the theory. Some of Harris' explanations of cultural phenomena have come under attack, and these controversies have given his critics another reason to dismiss his theoretical work. However, cultural materialist theories are generally testable, thus rendering them vulnerable to revision or even rejection, while rival theories are often impervious to empirical testing. From a scientific perspective, testability is a key feature of productive theory.

Harris continues in the tradition of Franz Boas and his students in his rejection of biological explanations of the specific content of culture. Thus, he would appear to close the door to the reconciliation of human biology and culture promised by medical anthropology. Yet, Harris remains a strong advocate of the four-field approach in anthropology, which includes bioanthropology. He fully recognizes the existence of a biologically based human nature (or biogram), but he chooses to minimize it in his explanations of human social life. Harris states that "the theoretical principles of cultural materialism hinge on the existence of certain genetically defined pan-human psychobiological drives that mediate between infrastructure and nature and that tend to make the selection of certain patterns of behavior more probable than others. Nothing I have said about the gene-free status of most cultural variation is opposed to the view that there is a human nature shared by all human beings. Hence the disagreement about the human biogram is entirely a matter of substance rather than of principle—that is, the precise identification of the content of the biogram" (1979:127). Harris is not anti-Darwinian but instead he struggles against the simplistic application of neo-Darwinian principles to explanations of cultural similarities and differences (Harris 1999:99–109). I would say that his critique has been basically correct.

A second development in theoretical frameworks is the new biocultural synthesis. This approach represents a conscious effort to remove barriers between culture and biology and to view them as continuous phenomena rather than dichotomous—as interpenetrating rather than occupying separate realms. The emphasis on biocultural links appears to distinguish this approach from cultural materialism. Specifically, this approach attempts to link political economy with biology in the context of an explicit political program that critiques capitalism (see Baer 1996; Singer and Baer 1995). Following Marx's formulation, the political economy approach views society as the product of class exploitation, unequal distribution of power and wealth, and self-interested manipulation of socially shared ideas and values by ruling elites. For proponents of this approach, biology enters into human social life not only in the sense of an underlying biogram but also in the interplay of unequal access to resources, differential disease loads on various groups in the population, nutritional differences, rates of infant mortality, demographic factors, levels of stress on a population, and so on.

The biocultural synthesis appears to be a response to the threatened breakup of anthropology as a unified, holistic discipline under the assault by staunch antiscientific postmodernists, radical relativists, and interpretivists. Proponents of the new synthesis see the split between culture and biology widening and fear that the gap will become unbridgeable. They rightly point out the power of a holistic approach in anthropology and to past successes that have made anthropology far more influential in the popular and scholarly world than its small size as a field would have predicted. A recent edited volume by Alan H. Goodman and Thomas L. Leatherman, entitled *Building a New Biocultural Synthesis: Political-Economic Perspectives on Human Biology* (1998), presents chapters that explore the possibilities of the new approach. Remarkably, aside from its added emphasis on biological variables such as rates of infant mortality or nutritional levels in a population, the approach does not significantly depart from cultural materialism. I see nothing in the reports of research that would cause a cultural materialist to take exception. Even more remarkably, Harris' work and that of adherents to his approach are barely mentioned in any of the chapters. Only Harris' well-known admonition to keep biology in the background when explaining cultural phenomena could account for such an omission. But as we saw above, Harris has no objection to recognizing the place of biology in human social life. He opposes using genetic variations among humans or biological mechanisms such as differential reproductivity as explanations for observed cultural differences and similarities. The authors in the Goodman and Leatherman volume would seem to have more in common with the intellectual lineage of cultural materialism than they acknowledge.

The third theoretical approach is by far the most radical in its use of biology to explicate culture. Much work in this area is inspired by E. O. Wilson and the new synthesis he called "sociobiology," which he defines simply as "the extension of population biology and evolutionary theory to social organization" (1978:x). Wilson and his followers propose that the human biogram creates tendencies for cultural development and that standard Darwinian mechanisms of differential reproduction account for many cultural similarities and differences. In attempting to apply Darwinian principles to explain human social behavior, the sociobiologists immediately ran into a firestorm of protest from a generation of social scientists raised on Boasian orthodoxy. One fear was that sociobiology heralded a return to turn-of-the-century scientific racism and possible rejuvenation of social Darwinism and the eugenics movement. Harris and the cultural materialists led the attack and the sociobiologists have scaled back their claims. Many sympathetic to the research program now reject the designation "sociobiology," preferring alternative labels for the approach such as "human behavioral ecology" or "evolutionary psychology."

Marvin Harris and E. O. Wilson share a commitment to science but differ radically in how the divide between biology and culture should be bridged. The cultural materialists may be surprised that Wilson is not the adamant hereditarian that he may at first have appeared to be. Perhaps as a result of cultural materialist critiques he states, "Nurturists and hereditarians generally agree that almost all the differences between cultures are likely to be the product of history and environment. . . . The culture of the Kalahari hunter-gatherers is very distinct from that of Parisians, but the differences between them are primarily a result of divergence of history and environment, and are not genetic in origin" (1999:155). In fact, the three perspectives outlined here that bridge the divide between biology and culture may be approaching a kind of consilience of their own. The dilemma of which level of analysis achieves causal priority can only be resolved empirically by branches of knowledge that are able to operate simultaneously in both realms. Medical anthropology, with its feet held to the ground by the need to resolve real-world problems with measurable results, is in the optimal position to contribute solutions to this greatest of all the problems in the unification of knowledge.

Mesoamerican healers are the cultural responses to the disease load that has been generated by the particular adaptations that groups have made to the social and natural environments in this intriguing world region. We are just now beginning to have adequate information on the shaman-curers, midwives, bonesetters, religious-based curing systems such as Spiritualism, biomedical specialists, and the historical processes that formed healers into what they are. We must know more in order to proceed to the next step of determining how curers are able to close the gap between the biological needs of their clients on the one hand and the cultures in which they operate on the other. By increasing our understanding of how healers succeed in reducing the suffering of their patients in the multiple cultural contexts in which they operate, medical anthropologists will have contributed not only to improving our ability to heal the afflicted, but also to solving one of the greatest mysteries of science, namely the emergence of human social life from the interaction of biology and culture.

Glossary

Agente municipal: In Mexico, this is the head of a committee that deals with the external relations of an *ejido* (a parcel of land granted to a community).

Audiencia: High administrative and judicial court in Spain's colonies.

Authoritative knowledge: Knowledge that is socially sanctioned, consequential, or "official" and that is regarded as the only basis for legitimate inferences and action (see Jordan 1993: 150).

Calmécac: Aztec temple-school attended chiefly by noble boys and used to educate high functionaries.

Cargo system: Ranked system of religious and political positions found in many Mesoamerican Indian communities.

Coordinación General del Plan Nacional de Zonas Deprimidas y Grupos Marginados: General Coordination of the Plan for Depressed Zones and Marginal Groups, or COPLAMAR, was created in 1977 to extend rural health programs to a wider group of rural people. It includes food subsidies, new schools, water systems, roads, and home improvement, as well as health care.

Creole: A Spaniard born in the New World.

Datura: A genus of poisonous and psychotropic plants that includes the species jimsonweed, a plant used by native peoples in North and South America.

Desarrollo Integral de la Familia: Mexico's program for the Integral Development of the Family, or DIF, is concerned with the health and social welfare of children and their parents.

Encomendero: Holder of an *encomienda*, an assignment of Indian tribute during the colonial period.

External (cephalic) version: Refers to the manipulative transabdominal conversion of a breech to a cephalic presentation, usually by a traditional birth attendant.

Hagiolatry: The invocation of saints to help the sick person, and the associated use of votive offerings.

IMSS-Solidaridad: This program was founded in 1988 and is administered by COPLAMAR (Coordinación General del Plan Nacional de Zonas Deprimidas y Grupos Marginados). The program provides health care to poor rural residents and also encourages improvements in sanitation, nutrition, housing, and health education.

Instituto de Seguridad y Servicios Sociales de los Trabajadores del Estado: Mexico's Institute for Social Security and Services for State Workers, or ISSSTE, provides health care and other services for public sector workers.

Instituto Mexicano de Seguro Social: The Mexican Social Security Institute, or IMSS, provides health care and social security primarily for urban industrial workers and their families. However, the IMSS greatly expanded its rural services in the 1970s and 1980s.

Instituto Nacional Indigenista: Mexico's National Indian Institute, or INI.

Mal aire or *Aire:* Refers to an illness produced by a tormented spirit roaming around and possessing the body of an individual; the spirit of a deceased person or restless spirit.

Mayordomo or *mayordoma:* A sponsor of a saint's feast day; a religious steward.

Medicalization: The process of defining and treating non-medical problems or normal life conditions as medical problems, e.g., the application of the biomedical model to obstetrics, which views pregnancy and birth as diseases or abnormal states.

Merthiolate: The registered brand name of a medication with antiseptic properties.

Mestizo, mestiza: A person regarded as of mixed white (Spanish) and Indian ancestry.

Ministerio de Salud Pública y Asistencia Social: Guatemala's Ministry of Public Health and Social Assistance, or MSPAS.

Mulato, mulata: A person regarded as of mixed white (Spanish) and African ancestry.

Ololiuhqui: Name of various psychotropic plants including *Rivea corymbosa*. Since the active principles are the alkaloids D-lysergic and D-isolysergic acids, their properties are very similar to those of LSD, producing visions and mystical experiences.

Orisha: In Africa, a spirit or deity that is thought to possess a person in order to act through him or her; a spirit in which is found a force of nature or a set of human-like behavioral characteristics.

Pasante: The term used in Mexico to refer to the new trainee doctor or nurse undertaking the one year of social service required by the Ley Federal de Profesiones.

Peyote: A small, gray-green hallucinogenic cactus found in Mexico and the southwestern United States which contains, among other alkaloids, mescalin.

Pomade: The term used to refer to a medicinal ointment.

Popol vuh: A Maya document originally written in Quiché with Spanish letters by a Mayan author or authors between 1554 and 1558 that chronicles the creation of man, the actions of the gods, and the origin and history of the Quiché.

Principal: A noble; an important leader.

Protomedicato: The colonial Spanish royal tribunal that regulated officially recognized healers such as physicians, surgeons, phlebotomists, and pharmacists. Members of the Protomedicato were known as *protomédicos.*

Pulque: An alcoholic beverage that is extracted from the agave plant.

Religious sodality: a lay religious association or brotherhood formed to carry on devotional or charitable activity. In Spanish the terms are *cofradía* or *hermandad.*

Santería: A term that is used to refer to a religion comprised of Roman Catholic elements mixed with African traditions.

Secretaría de Salubridad y Asistencia: Mexico's Ministry of Health, referred to as SSA, or as the Secretaría de Salud.

Syncretism: The process in which ideas, beliefs, and practices derived from two or more traditions are combined, reinterpreted, and transformed.

Temazcal: An underground or above-ground sweat house used for bathing, warming the body, and treating illness.

Tonales: Companion spirit animals that guard a person's animating force.

Tonalli: An animistic entity that can accidentally leave a person; an individual's destiny due to his or her date of birth.

References Cited

Archival Sources

Cárdenas Espinosa, Juan Timoteo

n.d.   Archivo General de la Nación (AGN), Protomedicato.

n.d.   Archivo General de la Nación (AGN), Ramo Inquisición.

1805   Petición de examen, Archivo Histórico de la Facultad de Medicina (AHFM), leg. 7, exp. 1, fols. 1–22.

Cervantes, Vicente

1808   Propuesta al fiscal, Archivo General de la Nación (AGN), Hospitales, vol. 29, exp. 2, fols. 68–82.

Consulta

1798   Consulta sobre el mejor arreglo del oficio de barberos y examen de los flebotomianos, AHFM, leg. 3, exp. 8, fols. 156–158.

Eguía y Muro Morales, Joaquín Pío Antonio de

1795   Solicitud de Joaquín Pío Muro para que se le nombre protomédico de merced, 1795, AGN, México, Ramo Hospitales, vol. 62, exp. 15, fols. 361–370.

Garfías, Antonio

1801   Permiso para abrir botica (1801), AHFM, leg. 2, exp. 14, fols. 1–10.

Gastos del Hospital de San Pedro

1811   Gastos del Hospital de San Pedro, AGN, Hospitales, vol. 58, exp. 15, fols. 332–338.

Lista de sueldos

1800   Lista de sueldos, AGN, Hospitales, vol. 19, exp. 24, fols. 452–456.

Moziño, Mariano

1795   Letter to Viceroy Branciforte (1795), AGN, Hospitales, vol. 72, exp. 11, fol. 292.

Published Sources

Acevedo, Dolores, and Elena Hurtado
1997   Midwives and Formal Providers in Prenatal, Delivery and Post-partum Care in Four Communities in Rural Guatemala: Complementarity or Conflict. *In* Demographic Diversity and Change in the Central American Isthmus, ed. Anne R. Pebley and Luis Rosero-Bixby, pp. 271–326. Santa Monica, Calif.: RAND.

Adams, Richard N.
1952   Un análisis de las creencias y prácticas médicas en un pueblo indígena de Guatemala. Instituto Indigenista Nacional, Publicaciones Especiales, no. 17. Guatemala: Editorial del Ministerio de Educación Pública.

Adams, Richard N., and Arthur J. Rubel
1967   Sickness and Social Relations. *In* Handbook of Middle American Indians. Vol. 6, ed. R. Wauchope, pp. 333–355. Austin: University of Texas Press.

Aguirre Beltrán, Gonzalo
1963   Medicina y magia: El proceso de aculturación en la estructura colonial. Colección de antropología social, no. 1. México, D.F.: Instituto Nacional Indigenista.

Alcorn, Janis B.
1984   Huastec Mayan Ethnobotany. Austin: University of Texas Press.

Alvarado, Neyra
1991   Medicina Mixe: Chupadores, adivinos y parteras. Ojarasca 3:23–26.

Álvarez Amézquita, J., M. Bustamante, A. López Picazos, and Francisco Fernández del Castillo
1960   Historia de la salubridad y de la asistencia en México. 4 Vols. México, D.F.: Secretaría de Salubridad y Asistencia.

Álvarez Heydenreich, Laurencia
1976   Breve estudio de las plantas medicinales en Hueyapan, Morelos. Estudios Sobre Etnobotánica y Antropología Médica 1:85–111.

1987   La enfermedad y la cosmovisión en Hueyapan, Morelos. Colección INI, no. 74. México, D.F.: Instituto Nacional Indigenista.

1992   Tipos de curanderos en Hueyapan, Morelos. *In* La antropología médica en México. Vol. 2, comp. Roberto Campos Navarro, pp. 127–138. México, D.F.: Universidad Autónoma Metropolitana.

Alzate, Antonio
1985   Memoria del uso que hacen los indios de los pipiltzintzintlis. México, D.F.: Universidad Nacional Autónoma de México. [1772]

Amaya Abad, Wellington
1994   R-6, residencia seis: Apuntamientos médico-históricos, 1689–1992. Guatemala: Editorial Óscar de León Palacios.

1995   Páginas de la historia de la oftalmología Guatemalteca. Guatemala: Editorial Óscar de León Palacios.

American Association for the Advancement of Science

1992 Health Professionals Persecuted in Violation of Their Human Rights: A Partial List of Cases. Journal of the American Medical Association 268 (5): 585–590.

Anderson, Arthur J. O., and Charles E. Dibble

1954 Book 8: Kings and Lords. Florentine Codex: General History of the Things of New Spain. Santa Fe, N.M.: Monographs of the School of American Research.

Anderson, Robert

1987 The Treatment of Musculoskeletal Disorders by a Mexican Bonesetter (Sobador). Social Science and Medicine 24 (1): 43–46.

1996 Magic, Science, and Health: The Aims and Achievements of Medical Anthropology. Fort Worth, Tex.: Harcourt Brace.

Anonymous

1990 La mujer en la educación superior en México. Uno Más Uno. December 9: 9, 11.

ANUIES [Asociación Nacional de Universidades e Instituciones de Educación]

1995 Sistema nacional de información para la educación superior. México, D.F.: ANUIES.

Anzures y Bolaños, María del Carmen

1989 La medicina tradicional en México: Proceso histórico, sincretismos y conflictos. México, D.F.: Universidad Nacional Autónoma de México. [1976]

————, ed.

1978 Juan de Esteyneffer, Florilegio medicinal de todas las enfermedades. 2 vols. La historia de la medicina en México, Colección nuestros clásicos, no. 2. México, D.F.: Academia Nacional de Medicina. [1712]

Argueta Villamar, Arturo, Leticia M. Cano Asseleih, and María Elena Rodarte

1994 Atlas de las plantas de la medicina tradicional mexicana. 3 vols. México, D.F.: Instituto Nacional Indigenista.

Argueta Villamar, Arturo, and Carlos Zolla, coords.

1994 Nueva bibliografía de la medicina tradicional mexicana. 2 vols. México, D.F.: Instituto Nacional Indigenista.

Arvigo, Rosita

1993 Jaguar Shamans and Mayan Spirits: My Apprenticeship with Don Eligio Ponti. Shaman's Drum 30: 21–28.

Asturias, Francisco

1958 Historia de la medicina en Guatemala. Serie Universidad de San Carlos de Guatemala. Vol. 28. Guatemala: Editorial Universitaria. [1902]

Asunción Lara, Ma. Acevedo, Maricarmen Lopez, and Elsa Karina

1993 La salud emocional y las tensiones asociadas con los papeles de género en las madres que trabajan y en las que no trabajan. Salud Mental 16 (2): 13–23.

Atkinson, Jane Monnig

1989 The Art and Politics of Wana Shamanship. Berkeley: University of California Press.

AvRuskin, Tara L.
1988   Neurophysiology and the Curative Possession of Trance: The Chinese Case. Medical Anthropology Quarterly 2 : 286–302.

Baer, Hans A.
1996   Bringing Political Ecology into Critical Medical Anthropology: A Challenge to Biocultural Approaches. Medical Anthropology 17 : 129–141.

Baer, Hans A., Merrill Singer, and Ida Susser
1997   Medical Anthropology and the World System: A Critical Perspective. Westport, Conn.: Bergin and Garvey.

Barabas, Alicia M.
1973   Messianismo chinanteco: El mediador de lo divino. Ninth International Congress of Anthropological and Ethnological Sciences, Chicago.

Barba de Piña Chan, Beatriz
1980   Curandería y magia en el Distrito Federal. Antropología e Historia 30 : 57–66.

Barrios E., Miguel
1949   Textos de Hueyapan, Morelos. Tlalocan 3 : 53–75.

Bartlett, Alfred V., Marco Antonio Bocaletti, and M. Elizabeth Paz de Bocaletti
1993   Use of Oxytocin and Other Injections during Labor in Rural Municipalities of Guatemala: Results of a Randomized Survey. Working paper no. 22. Washington, D.C.: MotherCare Project.

Bartlett, Alfred V., and M. Elizabeth Paz de Bocaletti
1991   Intrapartum and Neonatal Mortality in a Traditional Indigenous Community in Rural Guatemala. Acta Paediatrica Scandinavia 80 (3): 288–296.

Bartolache, José Ignacio
1979   Mercurio Volante. 3d ed. Biblioteca del Estudiante Universitario, no. 101. México, D.F.: Universidad Nacional Autónoma de México. [1772–1773]

Bartolomé, Miguel A., and Alicia M. Barabas
1996   Tierra de la palabra: Historia y etnografía de los chatinos de Oaxaca. México, D.F.: Instituto Nacional de Antropología e Historia. [1982]

Basauri, Carlos
1940   Tribu Chinantecos, H-me, Wan-mi. In La Población Indígena de Mexico. Vol. 2, pp. 545–568. México, D.F.: Secretaría de Educación Pública.

1990   La población indígena de México. Vol. 3. México, D.F.: Instituto Nacional Indigenista.

Baytelman, Bernardo
1986   De enfermos y curanderos: Medicina tradicional en Morelos. México, D.F.: Instituto Nacional de Antropología e Historia.

Beals, Ralph L.
1973a   Cherán: A Sierra Tarascan Village. New York: Cooper Square Publishers. [1946]
1973b   Ethnology of the Western Mixe. New York: Cooper Square Publishers. [1945]

Beltrán Morales, Filemon
1982   Medicina tradicional en la comunidad zapoteca de Zoogocho, Oaxaca. México,
       D.F.: Dirección General de Educación Indígena de la Secretaría de Educación
       Pública; Instituto Nacional Indigenista.

Benavides, Pedrarias de
1992   Secretos de Cirugía, ed. Francisco Fernández de Córdova. México, D.F.: Aca-
       demia Nacional de Medicina. [1567]

Benítez, Fernando
1964   Los hongos alucinantes. México, D.F.: Ediciones Era.

1968   En la tierra mágica del peyote. *In* Los indios de Mexico. México, D.F.: Edi-
       ciones Era.

Bennett, Wendell Clark, and Robert M. Zingg
1986   Los tarahumaras: Una tribu india del norte del Mexico. México, D.F.: Instituto
       Nacional Indigenista. [1935]

Benson, Herbert
1996   Timeless Healing: The Power and Biology of Belief. New York: Scribner's.

Betts, Robert C.
1993   Speaking with Dios: A Costumbre in Highland Guatemala. Shaman's Drum
       33:51–57.

Benzi, M.
1969   Voisins des Huichols sous l'effet du peyotl. Hygiéne Mentale 58 (3): 61–97.

Berlin, Elois Ann, and Brent Berlin
1996   Medical Ethnobiology of the Highland Maya of Chiapas, Mexico: The Gastro-
       intestinal Diseases. Princeton, N.J.: Princeton University Press.

Beyene, Yewoudbdar
1989   From Menarche to Menopause: Reproductive Lives of Peasant Women in Two
       Cultures. Albany: State University of New York Press.

Biersack, Aletta
1999   Introduction: From the "New Ecology" to the New Ecologies. American An-
       thropologist 101 (1): 5–18.

Boege, Eckart
1988   Los Mazatecos ante la nación. México, D.F.: Siglo Veintiuno Editores.

Bonfil Batalla, Guillermo
1968   Los que trabajan con el tiempo: Notas etnográficas sobre los graniceros de la
       Sierra Nevada, México. Anales de Antropología 5:99–128.

1969   Notas etnográficas de la región Huasteca, México. Anales de Antropología 6:
       131–151.

Boremanse, Didier
1998   Hach Winik: The Lacandón Maya of Chiapas, Southern Mexico. Institute
       for Mesoamerican Studies, monograph 11. Albany: Institute for Mesoamerican
       Studies, State University of New York Press. (Distributed by University of
       Texas Press)

Bortin, Sylvia
1993   Interviews with Mexican Midwives. Journal of Nurse-Midwifery 38 (3): 170–
          177.

Bossen, Laurel
1984   The Redivision of Labor: Women and Economic Choice in Four Guatemalan
          Communities. Albany: State University of New York Press.

Bossert, Thomas
1987   Sustainability of U.S. Government Supported Health Projects in Guatemala,
          1942–1987. Washington, D.C.: Center for Development Information and
          Evaluation, Bureau for Program and Policy Coordination, U.S. Agency for In-
          ternational Development.

Bourguignon, Erika
1989   Trance and Shamanism: What's in a Name? Journal of Psychoactive Drugs 21
          (1): 9–15.

Bower, Bethel
1946   Notes on Shamanism among the Tepehua Indians. American Anthropologist
          48:680–683.

Bronfman, Mario, Roberto Castro, Elena Zúñiga, Carlos Miranda, and Jorge Oviedo
1997   Del "cuánto" al "por qué": La utilización de los servicios de salud desde la
          perspectiva de los usarios. Salud Pública de México 39 (5): 442–450.

Brown, Michael Forbes
1988   Shamanism and Its Discontents. Medical Anthropology Quarterly 2 (2): 102–
          120.

Brown, Peter J.
1987   Microparasites and Macroparasites. Cultural Anthropology 2:155–171.

1998   Understanding and Applying Medical Anthropology. London: Mayfield.

Browner, C. H.
1985   Criteria for Selecting Herbal Remedies. Ethnology 24:13–32.

Bunzel, Ruth L.
1952   Chichicastenango: A Guatemalan Village. American Ethnology Society, publ.
          no. 22. Seattle: University of Washington Press.

Burke, Michael E.
1977   The Royal College of San Carlos: Surgery and Spanish Medical Reform in the
          Late Eighteenth Century. Durham, N.C.: Duke University Press.

Butler, James H., and Pedro Rocché Bixcul
1973   Ja Wecol Bak. Cuentos folklóricos y algunas experiencias personales en Tzu-
          tujil y en Español. Guatemala: Instituto Lingüístico de Verano.

Butter, Irene H., Eugenia S. Carpenter, Bonnie J. Kay, and Ruth S. Simmons
1987   Gender Hierarchies in the Health Labor Force. International Journal of
          Health Services 17 (1): 133–149.

Bye, Robert
1986   Medicinal Plants of the Sierra Madre: Comparative Study of Tarahumara and
          Mexican Garden Plants. Economic Botany 40:103–124.

Bye, Robert, and Edelmira Linares Mazari
1987 Usos pasados y presentes de algunas plantas medicinales encontradas en los mercados mexicanos. América Indígena 47:199–230.

Cabrera Perez-Arminan, Maria Luisa
1995 Otra historia por contar: Promotores de salud en Guatemala. Guatemala: Asociación de Servicios Comunitarios de Salud.

Cáceres, Armando
1996 Plantas de uso medicinal en Guatemala. Guatemala: Editorial Universitaria, Universidad de San Carlos de Guatemala.

Campos, Teresa
1983 El sistema médico de los Tojolabales. In Los Legítimos Hombres. Vol. 3, ed. Mario Humberto Ruz, pp. 195–224. México, D.F.: Universidad Nacional Autónoma de México.

Campos-Navarro, Roberto
1997 Nosotros los curanderos. México, D.F.: Nueva Imagen.

Cardeña, Etzel
1990 The Concept of Trance. Society for the Anthropology of Consciousness, annual conference, Pacific Palisades, Calif.

Cardona R., Rokael, and Gustavo Campos
1995 El caso de Guatemala. In Ajuste económico, políticas de salud y modelos de atención en centroamérica, ed. Luis Angel Garrido Sánchez and others. San José, Costa Rica: Instituto Centroamericano de Administración Pública.

Carlsen, Robert S., and Martin Prechtel
1994 Walking on Two Legs: Shamanism in Santiago Atitlán, Guatemala. In Ancient Traditions: Shamanism in Central Asia and the Americas, ed. Gary Seaman and Jane S. Day, pp. 77–111. Niwot: University Press of Colorado.

Carmack, Robert M., Janine Gasco, and Gary H. Gossen
1996 The Legacy of Mesoamerica: History and Culture of a Native American Civilization. Upper Saddle River, N.J.: Prentice-Hall.

Centro de Investigaciones Económicas Nacionales [CIEN]
1992 Lineamientos de política económica y social. Salud más que ausencia de enfermedad. Guatemala: CIEN. Unpublished manuscript.

Chant, Sylvia
1991 Women and Survival in Mexican Cities. Manchester: Manchester University Press.

Chaumeil, Jean-Pierre
1992 Varieties of Amazonian Shamanism. Diogenes 158:101–113.

Cheney, Charles Clark
1972 The Huaves of San Mateo del Mar: Cultural Change in a Mexican Indian Village. Ph.D. diss., University of California.

1979 Religion, Magic and Medicine in Huave Society. Kroeber Anthropological Society, Papers, no. 55–56:59–73.

Chimalpahin Cuauhtlehuanitzin, Domingo Francisco de San Antón Muñón
1965   Relaciones originales de Chalco Amaquemecan. México, D.F.: Fondo de Cultura Económica.

Cisneros, Diego
1618   Sitio, naturaleza y propiedades de la Ciudad de Mexico, aguas y vientos a que esta suieta, y tiempos del año: Necesidad de su conocimiento para el exercicio de la medicina, su incertidumbre y difficultad sin el de la astrologia assi para la curación como para los prognósticos. México, D.F.: Ioan de Blanco Alcaçar.

Coalition for Improving Maternity Services [CIMS]
1996   The Mother-Friendly Childbirth Initiative: Mission, Preamble and Principles. Washington, D.C.: CIMS.

Colburn, Forrest D.
1981   Guatemala's Rural Health Paraprofessionals. Ithaca, N.Y.: Rural Development Committee, Center for International Studies, Cornell University.

Colby, Benjamin N., and Lore M. Colby
1981   The Daykeeper: The Life and Discourse of an Ixil Diviner. Cambridge, Mass.: Harvard University Press.

Collado Ardón, Rolando, and José E. García Torres
1975   Los médicos en México en 1970. Salud Pública en México 17 (3): 309–324.

Comerford, Simon C.
1996   Medicinal Plants of Two Mayan Healers from San Andrés, Petén. Economic Botany 50: 327–336.

CONAPO [Consejo Nacional de Población]
1982   México demográfico. México, D.F.: CONAPO.

Congreso Nacional de Médicos Tradicionales Indígenas (Second)
1992   (August 11–15) Presente y futuro de la medicina tradicional. México, D.F.: Instituto Nacional Indigenista, Secretaría de Desarrollo Social.

Constituciones
1778   Constituciones y ordenanzas del Hospital Real de Indios. México, D.F.: D. Felipe Zúñiga y Ontiveros.

Cortés, Hernán
1991   Segunda carta de relación. In Los Cronistas: Conquista y Colonia. México, D.F.: Promexa.

Cortés, Jesús
1976   La medicina tradicional en la Sierra Mazateca. XLII International Congress of Americanists (Paris), Proceedings 6: 349–356.

Cosminsky, Sheila
1976a   Birth Rituals and Symbolism: A Quiche Maya-Black Carib Comparison. In Ritual and Symbol in Native Central America. Anthropological Papers, no. 9, ed. Philip Young and James Howe, pp. 107–123. Eugene: University of Oregon.

1976b   Introduction to reprint edition. *In* The Ethno-Botany of the Maya, ed. R. L.
         Roys. Reprint edition of Middle American Research Series no. 2. New Orleans:
         Institute for the Study of Human Issues, Tulane University.

1976c   The Role of the Midwife in Middle America. *In* Actas del XLI Congreso Inter-
         nacional de Americanistas, México, 2 al 7 de septiembre de 1974. México, D.F.:
         Instituto de Antropología e Historia.

1977a   Childbirth and Midwifery on a Guatemalan Finca. Medical Anthropology 1:
         69–104.

1977b   El papel de la comadrona en Mesoamerica. America Indígena 37:305–335.

1982a   Knowledge and Body Concepts of Guatemalan Midwives. *In* Anthropology of
         Human Birth, ed. Margarita Kay, pp. 233–252. Philadelphia: F. A. Davis.

1982b   Childbirth and Change: A Guatemalan Case Study. *In* Ethnography of Fertility
         and Birth, ed. Carole MacCormack, pp. 205–230. London: Academic Press.
         [Reissued by Waveland Press, 1994]

1987   Women and Health Care on a Guatemalan Plantation. Social Science and
         Medicine 25:1163–1173.

1997   Midwifery across the Generations. Paper presented at the annual meeting of
         the American Anthropological Association, Washington, D.C.

Cosminsky, Sheila, and Ira E. Harrison
1984   Traditional Medicine. Vol. 2, 1976–1981: Current Research with Implications
         for Ethnomedicine, Ethnopharmacology, Maternal and Child Health, Mental
         Health and Public Health. An Annotated Bibliography of Africa, Latin Amer-
         ica, and the Caribbean. New York: Garland.

Cosminsky, Sheila, and Mary Scrimshaw
1980   Medical Pluralism on a Guatemalan Plantation. Social Science and Medicine
         14B:267–278.

Crosby, Alfred W., Jr.
1972   The Columbian Exchange: Biological and Cultural Consequences of 1492.
         Westport, Conn.: Greenwood.

Csordas, Thomas
1994   The Sacred Self. Berkeley: University of California Press.

Dahlgren Jordan, Barbro
1994   Los Coras de la Sierra del Nayarit. México, D.F.: Universidad Nacional Autó-
         noma de México, Instituto de Investigaciones Antropológicas.

Dalton, Margarita and Guadalupe Musalem Merhy
1992   Mitos y realidades de las mujeres huaves. Oaxaca, México: IISUABJO-
         Comunicación Social.

Day, Michelle
1996   The Management of Reproduction and the Politics of Midwifery Practice in a
         Tzeltal (Maya) Speaking Community: Aguacatenango, Chiapas, Mexico. M.A.
         thesis, University of Chicago.

1997   Political Conflict, Economic Reform, and the Professionalization of Tzeltal Maya Midwives in Chiapas, Mexico. Paper presented at the annual meeting of the American Anthropological Association, Washington, D.C.

de Cárdenas, Juan
1591   Primera parte de los problemas y secretos maravillosos de las Indias. México, D.F.: Pedro Ocharte.

De la Cerda Silva, Roberto
1943   Los coras. Revista Mexicana de Sociología 5 (2): 89–117.

De la Fuente, Jesús
1949   Yalálag: Una villa zapoteca serrana. México, D.F.: Museo Nacional de Antropología.

De la Serna, Jacinto
1902   Manual de ministros de indios para el conocimiento de sus idolatrías y extirpación de ellas. *In* El alma encantada. Edited facsimile of Vol. 6 of the Anales del Museo Nacional, 1902. México, D.F.: Fondo de Cultura Económica.

De las Casas, Bartolomé
1967   Apologética historia sumaria. 2 vols. México, D.F.: Instituto de Investigaciones Históricas, Universidad Nacional Autónoma de México.

de Valverde, Christa
1989   La farmacia: Recurso de salud. Archivos Latino-Americanos de Nutrición 39 (3): 365–381.

De Vetancurt, Agustín
1982   Teatro mexicano. 2d ed. México, D.F.: Editorial Porrúa. [1698]

Del Pozo, Efrén C.
1965   La botánica medicinal indígena de México. Estudios de Cultura Náhuatl 5: 57–73.

Díaz del Castillo, Bernal
1955   Historia verdadera de la conquista de la Nueva España. 2 vols. México, D.F.: Editorial Porrúa.

Dibble, Charles E., and Arthur J. O. Anderson
1957   Book 4: The Soothsayers and Book 5: The Omens.

1961   Book 10: The People.

1963   Book 11: Earthly Things. *In* Florentine Codex: General History of the Things of New Spain. Santa Fe, N.M.: Monographs of the School of American Research.

Dienes, Istvan
1981   Shamanenaristokratie in den Nomadenstaaten. Congressus Quintus Internationalis Fenno-Ugristarum (Turku), pt. 8, ed. Osmo Ikola, pp. 326–338.

Douglas, Bill Gray
1969   Illness and Curing in Santiago Atitlán, a Tzutujil-Maya Town in the Southwestern Highlands of Guatemala. Ph.D. diss., Stanford University.

Douglas, Marilyn K., Afaf Ibrahim Meleis, Carmen Eribes, and Sulja Kim
1996 The Work of Auxiliary Nurses in Mexico: Stressors, Satisfiers and Coping Strategies. International Journal of Nursing Studies 33 (5): 495–505.

Douglas, Mary
1966 Purity and Danger: An Analysis of Concepts of Pollution and Taboo. London: Routledge and Kegan Paul.

Dow, James W.
1986a The Shaman's Touch: Otomí Indian Symbolic Healing. Salt Lake City: University of Utah Press.

1986b Universal Aspects of Symbolic Healing: A Theoretical Synthesis. American Anthropologist 88 : 56–69.

Durán-González, Lilia Irene, Martina Hernández-Rincón, and José Becerra-Aponte
1995 La formación del psicólogo y su papel en la atención primaria a la salud. Salud Pública de México 37 (5): 462–471.

Durrenberger, E. Paul
1975 Lisu Shamans and Some General Questions. Steward Anthropological Society Journal 7 (1): 1–20.

Earle, Duncan Maclean
1984 Night Time and Dream Space for a Quiche Maya Family. In Investigaciones Recientes en el Area Maya. Vol. 3, pp. 397–400. Sociedad Mexicana de Antropología, 17th Mesa Redonda. San Cristóbal de las Casas, Chiapas.

Eber, Christine
1995 Women and Alcohol in a Highland Maya Town. Austin: University of Texas Press.

Edmonson, Munro S., ed.
1974 Sixteenth-Century Mexico: The Work of Sahagún. Albuquerque: University of New Mexico Press.

Eger Valdez, Susana
1996 Wolf Power and Interspecies Communication in Huichol Shamanism. In People of the Peyote: Huichol Indian History, Religion, and Survival, ed. Stacy B. Schaefer and Peter T. Furst, pp. 267–305. Albuquerque: University of New Mexico Press.

Eisenberg, David, Roger B. Davis, Susan L. Ettner, Scott Appel, Sonja Wilkey, Maria Van Rompay, and Ronald C. Kessler
1998 Trends in Alternative Medicine Use in the United States, 1990–1997. Journal of the American Medical Association 280 (18): 1569–1575.

Eisenberg, David, Ronald C. Kessler, Cindy Foster, Frances Norlock, David Calkins, and Thomas Delbanco
1993 Unconventional Medicine in the United States. New England Journal of Medicine 328 (4): 246–283.

Eliade, Mircea
1974   Shamanism: Archaic Techniques of Ecstasy. Princeton, N.J.: Princeton University Press.

Elliott, Ray
1977   Nebaj Ixil Unitary Kin Terms. *In* Cognitive Studies of Southern Mesoamerica, ed. Helen L. Neuenswander and Dean A. Arnold, pp. 126–158. Dallas: Summer Institute of Linguistics, Museum of Anthropology.

Emboden, William A. Jr.
1972   Ritual Use of Cannabis Sativa L.: A Historical Ethnographic Survey. *In* Flesh of the Gods: The Ritual Use of Hallucinogens, ed. Peter T. Furst. New York: Praeger.

Emes Boronda, María, Cruz Ochurte Espinoza, Gloria Castañeda Silva, Benito Peralta González, Abigail Aguilar Contreras, Arturo Argueta Villamar, and Leticia M. Cano, coords.
1994   Flora medicinal indígena de México: Treinta y cinco monografías del atlas de las plantas de la medicina tradicional mexicana. 3 vols. México, D.F.: Instituto Nacional Indigenista.

Enge, Kjell I., and Polly Harrison
1988   Proveedores de salud materno infantil en Guatemala: Conocimientos, actitudes y prácticas. Hallazgos de la investigación y sugerencias para su aplicación. Report. Washington, D.C.: Primary Health Care Technology Project/U.S. Agency for International Development.

Engstrand, Iris W.
1981   Spanish Scientists in the New World: The Eighteenth-Century Expeditions. Seattle: University of Washington Press.

Fabila, Alfonso
1945   La tribu kikapoo de Coahuila. Biblioteca Enciclopedia Popular 50. México, D.F.: Secretaría de Educación Pública.

1959   Los huicholes de Jalisco. México, D.F.: Instituto Nacional Indigenista y Gobierno del Edo. de México.

Fabrega, Horacio, and Daniel B. Silver
1970   Some Social and Psychological Properties of Zinacanteco Shamans. Behavioral Sciences 15:471–486.

1973   Illness and Shamanistic Curing in Zinacantán: An Ethnomedical Analysis. Stanford, Calif.: Stanford University Press.

Farfán, Agustín
1579   Tractado breve de anathomía y chirugía y de algunas enfermedades que mas communmente suelen haber en esta Nueva España. México, D.F.: Antonio Ricardo.

Farfán Morales, Olimpia
1988   Los nahuas de la Sierra Norte de Puebla: El chamanismo entre los nahuas. *In* Estudios nahuas, ed. Efraín Cortés Ruiz et al., pp. 127–144. México, D.F.: Instituto Nacional de Antropología e Historia.

Faust, Betty
1988   When Is a Midwife a Witch? A Case Study for a Modernizing Maya Village. *In* Women and Health, ed. Patricia Whelehan, pp. 21–39. New York: Bergin and Garvey.

Favre, Henri
1973   Cambio y continuidad entre los mayas de México. México, D.F.: Siglo Veintiuno Editores.

Felger, Richard
1991   People of the Desert and Sea: Ethnobotany of the Seri Indians. Tucson: University of Arizona Press.

Fernández del Castillo, Francisco
1982   Antología de escritos histórico-médicos del Dr. Francisco Fernández del Castillo. 2 vols. México, D.F.: Departamento de Historia y Filosofía de la Medicina, Universidad Nacional Autónoma de México.

Findeisen, Hans
1957   Schamanentum. Stuttgart: Kohlhammer.
1960   Das Schamanentum als Spiritistische Religion. Ethnos 25 (3–4): 192–213.

Finkler, Kaja
1981   Dissident Religious Movement in the Service of Women's Power. Sex Roles 7:481–495.
1983   Dissident Sectarian Movements, the Catholic Church, and Social Class in Mexico. Comparative Studies in Society and History 25:277–305.
1984   The Nonsharing of Medical Knowledge among Spiritualist Healers and Their Patients: A Contribution to the Study of Intra-Cultural Diversity and Practitioner–Patient Relationship. Medical Anthropology 8:195–209.
1985   Spiritualist Healers in Mexico. Successes and Failures of Alternative Therapeutics. New York: Bergen and Garvey.
1991   Physicians at Work, Patients in Pain. Boulder, Colo.: Westview.
1994a   Sacred and Biomedical Healing Compared. Medical Anthropological Quarterly 8:178–197.
1994b   Spiritualist Healers in Mexico. Successes and Failures of Alternative Therapeutics. Salem: Sheffield Publishers. [1985]
1994c   Women in Pain. Philadelphia: University of Pennsylvania Press.
1996   Factors Influencing Patient Perceived Recovery in Mexico. Social Science and Medicine 42:199–207.
1997   Gender, Domestic Violence and Sickness in Mexico. Social Science and Medicine 45:1147-1160.

Follér, Maj-Lis
1996   The Construction of the Other: Knowledge, Culture and Medicine among the Maya Population in Yucatan. Unpublished manuscript, Department of Human Ecology, University of Göteborg.

Ford, Karen Cowen
1975   Las yerbas de la gente: A Study of Hispano-American Medicinal Plants. Anthropological Papers, no. 60. Museum of Anthropology, University of Michigan.

Foster, George M.
1952   Relations between Theoretical and Applied Anthropology: A Public Health Program Analysis. Human Organization 11 (3): 5–16.

1953   Relationships Between Spanish and Spanish-American Folk Medicine. Journal of American Folklore 66:201–217.

1955   Guide Lines to Community Development Programs. Public Health Reports 70:19–24.

1987   On the Origin of Humoral Medicine in Latin America. Medical Anthropology Quarterly 1:355–393.

1994   Hippocrates' Latin American Legacy: Humoral Medicine in the New World. Langhorne, Penn.: Gordon and Breach.

Fox, David J.
1972   Patterns of Morbidity and Mortality in Mexico City. Geographical Review 62: 151–185.

Francisco Velasco, Domingo, and Salvador Francisco
1985   Latamat (Vida). Cuadernos del Norte de Veracruz. México, D.F.: Dirección General de Culturas Populares.

Frank, Jerome D.
1979   Nonmedical Healing: Religious and Secular. In Ways of Health, ed. David S. Sobel, pp. 231–266. New York: Harcourt Brace Jovanovich.

Frankel, Stephen
1984   Peripheral Health Workers are Central to Primary Health Care: Lessons from Papua New Guinea's Aid Posts. Social Science and Medicine 19:279–290.

Frei, Barbara, Matthias Baltisberger, Otto Sticher, and Michael Heinrich
1998   Medical Ethnobotany of the Zapotecs of the Isthmus-Sierra (Oaxaca, Mexico): Documentation and Assessment of Indigenous Uses. Journal of Ethnopharmacology 62 (2): 149–165.

Frei, Barbara, Otto Sticher, Carlos Viesca Treviño, and Michael Heinrich
1998   Medicinal and Food Plants: Isthmus Sierra Zapotec Criteria for Selection. Angewandte Botanik 72:82–86.

Frenk, Julio
1985   Career Preferences under Conditions of Medical Unemployment: The Case of Interns in Mexico. Medical Care 23 (4): 320–332.

1990   La profesión médica en las áreas urbanas de México: Composición demográfica y origen social. Gaceta Médica de México 126 (2): 92–101.

Frenk, Julio, Javier Alagón, Gustavo Nigenda, Alejandro Muñoz del Rio, Cecilia Robledo, Luis A. Vasquez-Segovia, and Catalan Ramirez-Cuadra
1991   Patterns of Medical Employment: A Survey of Imbalances in Urban Mexico. American Journal of Public Health 81 (1): 23–29.

Frenk, Julio, Luis Durán-Arenas, Alonso Vázquez-Segovia, and Domingo Vázquez
1995   Los médicos en México 1970–1990. Salud Pública en México 37 (1): 19–30.

Frenk, Julio, Rafael Lozano, Miguel A. González Block, et al.
1994   Economía y salud: Propuestas para el avance del sistema de salud en México. Final report. México D.F.: Fundación Mexicana para Salud.

Freyermuth Enciso, Graciela
1988   Atención del parto, modificaciones en las prácticas tradicionales y su impacto en la salud. In Las mujeres en el campo, ed. J. Aranda, pp. 355–369. Oaxaca, Mexico: Universidad Autónoma Benito Juárez de Oaxaca.

1993   Médicos tradicionales y Médicos alópatas: Un encuentro difícil en los Altos de Chiapas. Tuxtla Gutierrez: Gobierno del Estado de Chiapas; Consejo Estatal de Fomento a la Investigaciones y Difusión de la Cultura; DIF-Chiapas, Instituto Chiapaneco de Cultura; Centro de Investigaciones y Estudios Superiores en Antropología-Sureste.

Fried, Jacob
1951   Ideal Norms and Social Control in Tarahumara Society. New Haven, Conn.: Yale University.

Frigerio, A.
1989   Levels of Possession Awareness in Afro-Brazilian Religions. Association of the Anthropological Study of Consciousness Quarterly 5 (2–3): 5–11.

Fuller, Nancy, and Brigitte Jordan
1981   Maya Women and the End of the Birthing Period: Postpartum Massage-and-Binding in Yucatan, Mexico. Medical Anthropology 5 : 35–50.

Furst, Peter T.
1972   To Find Our Life: Peyote among the Huichol Indians of Mexico. In Flesh of the Gods: The Ritual Use of Hallucinogens, ed. Peter Furst, pp. 136–184. New York: Praeger.

Furst, Peter T., and Barbara Myerhoff
1972   El mito como historia: El ciclo de peyote y la datura entre los huicholes. In El peyote y los Huicholes, ed. Salomón Nahmad Sittón, Otto Klineberg, Peter T. Furst, and Barbara G. Myerhoff, pp. 53–108. México, D.F.: Sep Setentas.

Galante, Cristina
1980   Plantas medicinales de la región istmena utilizadas en la reproducción. In Medicina tradicional, herbolaria y salud comunitaria en Oaxaca, ed. Paola Sesia, pp. 119–150. México, D.F.: Centro de Investigaciones y Estudios Superiores en Antropología Social.

Galinier, Jacques
1987   Pueblos de la Sierra Madre: Etnografía de la comunidad Otomí. México, D.F.: Instituto Nacional Indigenista.

1990   La mitad del mundo: Cuerpo y cosmos en los rituales otomíes, trans. Angela Ochoa and Haydée Silva. México, D.F.: Universidad Nacional Autónoma de México.

Gallegos Deveze, Marisela
1996   Chamanes y curanderos matlatzincas. *In* Historia de la salud en México, coord. María Elena Morales and Elsa Malvido, pp. 155–163. México, D.F.: Instituto Nacional de Antropología e Historia.

Garber, Missy
1996   That's Not Too Hard: Unassisted Birth among Mayans in Belize. Paper presented at the annual meeting of the American Anthropological Association, San Francisco.

García, Brigida, and Orlandina de Oliveira
1994   Trabajo femenino y vida familiar en México. México D.F.: El Colegio de México.

García Alcaraz, Agustín
1997   Tinujei: Los triquis de Copala. México, D.F.: Centro de Investigaciones y Estudios Superiores en Antropología Social.

García de Palacio, Diego
1576   Carta dirigida al Rey por el licenciado Diego García de Palacio en lo tocante a las provincias de Guazacapan, los Izalcos, Cuzcatlán y Chiquimula. *In* Relaciones geográficas del siglo XVI. Vol 1. Guatemala, ed. René Acuña, pp. 253–287. México, D.F.: Universidad Nacional Autónoma de México.

García Pastor de Domínguez, Eva, Aura Robles de Sandoval, and Olga Martínez Chopen
1988   Una modalidad de educación a distancia con auxiliares de enfermería del área comunitaria de Guatemala. Educación Médica y Salud 22 (1): 20–34.

García-Ruiz, Jesús F.
1984   El defensor y el defendido: Dialéctica de la agresión entre los Mochó (Motozintla, Chiapas). *In* Investigaciones Recientes en el Area Maya. Vol. 1, pp. 329–348. Sociedad Mexicana de Antropología, Seventeenth Mesa Redonda, San Cristóbal de las Casas, Chiapas.

Garduño-Espinosa, Juan, et al.
1995   Características del estudiante de medicina asociadas al éxito ulterior como médico. La Revista Investigación Clínica 47 (5): 355–364.

Garma Navarro, Carlos, Masferrer Kan, Elio, and Armando Alcántara Berumen
1995   Los totonacas. *In* Etnografía contemporánea de los pueblos indígenas de México: Región oriental, pp. 321–370. México, D.F.: Instituto Nacional Indigenista.

Garro, Linda C.
1986   Intracultural Variation in Folk Medical Knowledge: A Comparison Between Curers and Noncurers. American Anthropologist 88 (2): 351–370.

Gillin, John
1948   Magical Fright. Psychiatry 11:387–400.

1950   The Fear. Atlantic Monthly 186:68–72.

1951   The Culture of Security in San Carlos. Middle American Research Institute, publ. no. 16. New Orleans: Tulane University.

1956   The Making of a Witchdoctor. Psychiatry 19:131–136.

Girard, Rafael
1947   Farmacopea de los Indios Chortis. Boletín Indigenista 7 (4): 346–362.

Glaser, R., J. Rice, J. Sheridan, et al.
1987   Stress-Related Immune Suppression: Health Implications. Brain, Behavior, and Immunity 1:7–20.

Gómez Canedo, Lino
1982   La educación de los marginados durante la época colonial: Escuelas y colegios para indios y mestizos en la Nueva España. México, D.F.: Editorial Porrúa.

Gonzales, Nancie S.
1963   Some Aspects of Childbearing and Childrearing in a Guatemalan Ladino Community. Southwestern Journal of Anthropology 19:411–423.

González de la Rocha, Mercedes
1994   The Resources of Poverty. Oxford: Blackwell.

González Ramos, Gildardo
1992   Los coras. México, D.F.: Instituto Nacional Indigenista. [1972]

González-Ulloa, Mario
1959   La medicina en México. México, D.F.: Cyánimid de México.

González Villanueva, Pedro
1989   El sacrificio mixe: Rumbos para una antropología religiosa indígena. México, D.F.: Centro de Estudios Pastorales y Antropológicos de la Prelatura Mixepolitana.

Goodman, Alan H., and Thomas L. Leatherman
1998   Building a New Biocultural Synthesis: Political-Economic Perspectives on Human Biology. Ann Arbor: University of Michigan Press.

Goodman, Felicitas D.
1989   The Neurophysiology of Shamanic Ecstasy. In Shamanism: Past and Present, pt. 2, ed. Mihály Hoppál and Otto von Sadovsky, pp. 377–379. Los Angeles: ISTOR Books.

Goodrich, L. Carrington, ed.
1951   Japan in the Chinese Dynastic Histories: Later Han through Ming Dynasties, trans. Ryusaku Tsunoda. South Pasadena, Calif.: Perkins.

Gossen, Gary H.
1975   Animal Souls and Human Destiny in Chamula. Man 10:448–461.

Grajeda, Ruben, Rafael Perez-Escamilla, and Kathryn Dewey
1997   Delayed Clamping of the Umbilical Cord Improved Hematologic Status of Guatemalan Infants at Two Months of Age. American Journal of Clinical Nutrition 65:425–431.

Grambo, Ronald
1973   Sleep as a Means of Ecstasy and Divination. Acta Ethnographica (Budapest) 22:417–441.

Granados Ortiz, Roberto
1983   Semblanzas de médicos Guatemaltecos. Guatemala: Taller de Artes Gráficas, Ministerio de Salud Pública y Asistencia Social.

Greenberg, Linda
1982   Midwife Training Programs in Highland Guatemala. Social Science and Medicine 16:1599–1609.

Greene, Catherine
1988   Parteras, Partos, y Plantas: Isthmus Zapotec Childbirth, Ethnobotany, and Perinatal Traditions. M.A. thesis, Indiana University.

Griffen, William B.
1959   Notes on Seri Indian Culture, Sonora, Mexico. Gainesville: University of Florida Press.

Grimes, Joseph E., and Thomas B. Hinton
1972   Huicholes y coras. *In* Coras, huicholes y tepehuanes, ed. Thomas B. Hinton, pp. 73–97. México, D.F.: Instituto Nacional Indigenista.

Guarner Dalias, Vicente
1993   Contribución a la medicina de México de los médicos españoles de la inmigración de 1939. Gaceta Médica de México 129 (1): 87–92.

Güémez Pineda, Miguel
1989   Las parteras empíricas de Pustunich, Yucatan. Boletín de la Escuela de Ciencias Antropológicas de la Universidad de Yucatán 16 (91): 3–13.

1997   De comadronas a promotoras de salud y planificación familiar. *In* Cambio cultural y resocialización en Yucatán, ed. Esteban Katz, pp. 17–147. Merida: Ediciones de la Universidad Autónoma de Yucatán.

Guerra, Francisco
1969   The Role of Religion in Spanish American Medicine. *In* Medicine and Culture, ed. N. L. Poynter, pp. 179–188. London: Welcome Institute of the History of Medicine.

Guerra, Francisco, ed.
1982   El tesoro de medicinas de Gregorio López 1542–1596. Madrid: Ediciones Cultura Hispánica del Instituto de Cooperación Iberoamericana. [1672]

Guerrero Espinel, Eduardo, Rolando Eliseo Ortiz Rosales, Omer Robles, and Eva Sazo de Méndez
1992   Estudio básico del sector salud, Guatemala, 1991. Publicaciones científicas y técnicas de la Oficina Panamericana de la Salud, Guatemala, no. 4. Guatemala: Organización Panamericana de la Salud.

Guiteras Holmes, Calixta
1961   Perils of the Soul: The World View of a Tzotzil Indian. New York: Free Press of Glencoe.

1970   Sayula: Un pueblo de Veracruz. Havana: Editorial de Ciencias Sociales.

Hamburger, S.
1963   Profiles of Curanderos: A Study of Mexican Folk Practitioners. International Journal of Social Psychiatry 24:19–25.

Hanks, William F.
1984   Sanctification, Structure, and Experience in a Yucatec Ritual Event. Journal of American Folklore 97:131–166.
1990   Referential Practice: Language and Lived Space among the Maya. Chicago: University of Chicago Press.
1993   Copresencia y alteridad en la práctica ritual maya. In De palabra y obra en el nuevo mundo. Vol. 3, ed. Miguel León-Portilla and Edna Acosta Belén, pp. 75–117. Madrid: Siglo Veintiuno de España Editores.

Harner, Michael J., ed.
1973   Hallucinogens and Shamanism. New York: Oxford University Press.

Harris, Marvin
1979   Cultural Materialism: The Struggle for a Science of Culture. New York: Random House.
1999   Theories of Culture in Postmodern Times. Walnut Creek, Calif.: Altamira Press.

Harrison, Margaret E.
1991   Primary Health Care Operational Experience in Mexico City D.F. In Development Perspectives for the 1990s, ed. R. Prendergast and H. W. Singer, pp. 205–213. Houndmills: Macmillan.
1994   Hobby or Job? Mexican Female Health Workers. Health Care for Women International 15 (5): 397–412.
1995   A Doctor's Place: Female Physicians in Mexico D.F. Health and Place 1 (2): 101–111.
1998   Female Physicians in Mexico: Migration and Mobility in the Lifecourse. Social Science and Medicine 47 (4): 455–468.

Harrison, Polly
1977   Análisis del sector salud de Guatemala. Un estudio sobre las comadronas. Guatemala: U.S. Agency for International Development.

Heggenhougen, H. K.
1976   Health Care for the "Edge of the World": Indian Campesinos as Health Workers in Chimaltenango, Guatemala: A Discussion of the Behrhorst Program. Ph.D. diss., The New School for Social Research.

Heinrich, Michael
1994   Herbal and Symbolic Medicines of the Lowland Mixe (Oaxaca, Mexico). Anthropos 89:73–83.

Heinze, Ruth Inge
1988   Trance and Healing in Southeast Asia Today. Bangkok: White Lotus.

Hermitte, M. Esther
1970   Poder sobrenatural y control social en un pueblo maya contemporáneo. Ediciones Especiales, no. 57. México, D.F.: Instituto Indigenista Interamericano.

Hernández, Francisco

1942   Historia de las plantas de Nueva España. México, D.F.: Universidad Nacional Autónoma de México.

1959   Obras completas. México: Universidad Nacional Autónoma de México.

1984   Antigüedades de Nueva España. *In* Obras Completas de Francisco Hernández. Vol. 6. México, D.F.: Universidad Nacional Autónoma de México. [1574]

Hernández Sáenz, Luz María

1997   Learning to Heal: The Medical Profession in Colonial Mexico 1767–1831. New York: Lang.

Hines, Donald M.

1993   Magic in the Mountains, The Yakima Shaman: Power and Practice. Issaquah, Wash.: Great Eagle Publishing.

Hinojosa, Servando

1998   Spiritual Embodiment in a Highland Maya Community. Ph.D. diss., Tulane University.

Hobgood, John

1959   El curandera. *In* Esplendor del México antigua, coord. Carmen Cook de Leonard, pp. 861–876, 1271. México, D.F.: Centro de Investigaciones Antropológicas de México.

Holland, William R.

1963   Medicina maya en los altos de Chiapas. México, D.F.: Instituto Nacional Indigenista.

Holland, William R., and Roland G. Tharp

1964   Highland Maya Psychotherapy. American Anthropologist 64:41–52.

Holmberg, David

1993   The Shamanic Illusion. Journal of Ritual Studies 7 (1): 163–175.

Hondagneu-Sotelo, Pierrette

1994   Gender Transitions. Mexican Experiences of Immigration. Berkeley: University of California Press.

Hopkinson, Amanda

1988   Midwifery and Rural Health Care in Guatemala. *In* The Midwife Challenge, ed. Sheila Kitzinger, pp. 155–174. London: Unwin Hyman.

Howard, David

1980   The Royal Indian Hospital of Mexico City. Special Studies no. 20, Center for Latin American Studies. Tempe: Arizona State University.

Howells, William

1949   The Heathens: Primitive Man and His Religions. Garden City, N.Y.: Anchor/Doubleday.

Hrdlička, Aleš

1904   Notes on the Indians of Sonora, Mexico. American Anthropologist 6:51–88.

Hubbard, Joyce
1990   A Descriptive Study of the Developing Role of Village Health Workers in a Remote Tarahumara Pueblo. M.S. thesis, University of Arizona.

Huber, Brad R.
1990a   The Recruitment of Nahua Curers: Role Conflict and Gender. Ethnology 29 (2): 159–176.

1990b   Curers, Illness, and Healing in San Andrés Hueyapan, a Nahuat-Speaking Community of the Sierra Norte de Puebla, Mexico. Notas Mesoamericanas 12:51–65.

Huber, Brad R., and Robert Anderson
1996   Bonesetters and Curers in a Mexican Community: Conceptual Models, Status and Gender. Medical Anthropology 17:23–38.

Huber, Brad R., Alan R. Sandstrom, and Antonio Toribio Martínez
Forth.   Transformations in the Recruitment, Training, and Practice of Midwives in a Nahuat-Speaking Community of Mexico. *In* Mexican Midwives: Continuity, Controversy, and Change. Vol. 3. Austin: University of Texas Press.

Hughes, Dureen J.
1991   Blending with an Other: An Analysis of Trance Channeling in the United States. Ethos 19:161–184.

Hultkrantz, Åke
1973   A Definition of Shamanism. Temenos 9:25–37.

Hunt, Eva
1976   The Transformation of the Hummingbird: Cultural Roots of a Zinacanteco Mythical Poem. Ithaca: Cornell University Press.

Hurtado, Elena
1984   Estudio de las características y prácticas de las comadronas tradicionales en una comunidad indígena de Guatemala. *In* Etnomedicina en Guatemala. Colecciones monografías no. 1, ed. Elba M. Villatoro, pp. 251–264. Guatemala: Centro de Estudios Folklóricos.

1995   Percepción de las complicaciones maternas y perinatales y búsqueda de atención. Guatemala: Ministerio de Salud Pública y Asistencia Social and U.S. Agency for International Development/MotherCare.

1997a   La comadrona y los factores que influyen en la utilización de los servicios de salud pública para el embarazo, parto y post-parto en Guatemala. Guatemala: MotherCare Project.

1997b   Los conocimientos de comadronas tradicionales de Guatemala sobre complicaciones en el embarazo, parto y post-parto. Guatemala: MotherCare Project.

1998   Evaluación de la capacitación de comadronas tradicionales, Proyecto MotherCare/Guatemala. Unpublished final report.

Hurtado, Juan J.
1973   Algunas ideas para un modelo estructural de las creencias en relación con la enfermedad en el altiplano de Guatemala. Guatemala Indígena 8 (1): 7–22.

Ibach, Thomas J.
1981   The Temascal and Humoral Medicine in Santa Cruz Mixtepec, Juxtlahuaca, Oaxaca, Mexico. M.A. thesis, University of Tennessee.

Ichon, Alain
1973   La religión de los Totonacas de la Sierra. Serie de Antropología Social, no. 16. México, D.F.: Secretaría de Educación Pública y Instituto Nacional Indigenista.

Incháustegui, Carlos
1994   La mesa de plata: Cosmogonía y curanderismo entre los mazatecos de Oaxaca. México: Instituto Oaxaqueño de las Culturas.

Instituto Nacional de Estadística, Geográfica e Información [INEGI]
1986   Estadísticas históricas de México. Vols. 1 and 2. México, D.F.: INEGI.

1992   XI censo general de población (1990). Aguascalientes: INEGI.

1995   Atlas de los profesionistas en México. Aguascalientes: INEGI.

1997   Perspectiva estadística del Distrito Federal. Aguascalientes: INEGI.

Instituto Nacional de Estadística [INE], MSPAS, USAID, UNICEF, DHS, and Macro International, Inc.
1996   Encuesta nacional de salud materno infantil. Guatemala: INE.

Isaac, Claudia B.
1996   Witchcraft, Cooperatives, and Gendered Competition in a Purépecha Community. Frontiers 16 (2/3) :161–189.

Izquierdo, J. J.
1955   El Hipocratismo en México. México, D.F.: Imprenta Universitaria.

Jäcklein, Klaus
1974   Un pueblo Popoloca. Serie de Antropología Social, no. 25. México, D.F.: Secretaría de Educación Pública y Instituto Nacional Indigenista.

Jarcho, Saul
1957   Medicine in Sixteenth-Century New Spain as Illustrated by the Writings of Bravo, Farfán and Vargas Machuca. Bulletin of the History of Medicine 31: 425–441.

Johnson, Allen
1991   Regional Comparative Field Research. Behavior Science Research 25 (1): 3–22.

Johnson, Jean Bassett
1939a   The Elements of Mazatec Witchcraft. Ethnological Studies (Göteborg) 9: 128–150.

1939b   Some Notes on the Mazatec. Revista Mexicana de Estudios Antropológicos 3 (2): 142–156.

Jordan, Brigitte
1993   Birth in Four Cultures: A Crosscultural Investigation of Childbirth in Yucatan, Holland, Sweden, and the United States. 4th ed. Prospect Heights, Ill.: Waveland Press. [1978]

Katz, Esther
1992   Del frío al exceso de calor: Dieta alimenticia y salud en la mixteca. *In* Medicina
        tradicional, herbolaria y salud comunitaria en Oaxaca, ed. Paola Sesia, pp. 99–
        115. México, D.F.: Centro de Investigaciones y Estudios Superiores en Antro-
        pología Social.

Kay, Margarita Artschwager
1996   Healing with Plants in the American and Mexican West. Tucson: University of
        Arizona Press.

Kearney, Michael
1977   Oral Performance by Mexican Spiritualists in Possession Trance. Journal of
        Latin American Lore 3 (2): 309–328.

Kelly, Isabel Truesdell
1953   The Modern Totonac. Revista Mexicana de Estudios Antropológicos 13 (2–3):
        175–186.

1956   An Anthropological Approach to Midwifery Training in Mexico. Journal of
        Tropical Pediatrics 1:200–205.

Kestler, Edgar
1995   Guatemala: Maternal Mortality in Guatemala: Assessing the Gap, Beginning to
        Bridge It. World Health Statistics Quarterly 48 (1): 28–33.

Klein, Janice
1978   Susto: The Anthropological Study of Diseases of Adaptation. Social Science
        and Medicine 12:23–28.

Kloos, Peter
1968   Becoming a Piyei: Variability and Similarity in Carib Shamanism. Antropoló-
        gica 24:3–25.

Köhler, Ulrich
1977   Conbilal C'ulelal. Grundformen Mesoamerikanischer Kosmologie und Reli-
        gion in einem Gebetstext auf Maya-Tzotzil. Acta Humboldtiana, Series Geo-
        graphica et Ethnographica 5. Wiesbaden.

1990   Schamanismus in Mesoamerika? *In* Circumpacifica: Festschrift für Thomas S.
        Barthel, ed. Bruno Illius and Matthias Laubscher, pp. 257–275. Frankfurt:
        Peter Lang.

Kottak, Conrad P.
1999   The New Ecological Anthropology. American Anthropologist 101 (1): 23–35.

Krauze, Enrique
1997   Mexico: Biography of Power. New York: Harper Collins.

Krippner, Stanley
1989   The Use of Dreams in Shamanic Traditions. *In* Shamanism: Past and Present.
        Pt. 2, ed. Mihály Hoppál and Otto von Sadovsky, pp. 381–391. Los Angeles:
        ISTOR Books.

Kroeber, A. L.
1964   The Seri. Southwest Museum Papers, no. 6. Los Angeles: Southwest Museum.

Krumbach, Helmut
1977   Heilbäder bei den Maya und Azteken. Saeculum 28:145–156.

Kunow, Marianna Appel
1996   Curing and Curers in Pisté, Yucatán, México. Ph.D. diss., Tulane University.

Kuroda, Etsuko
1993   Bajo el Zempoaltépetl: La sociedad mixe de las tierras altas y sus rituales. México, D.F.: Centro de Investigaciones y Estudios Superiores en Antropología Social, Instituto Oaxaqueño de las Culturas. [1984]

Kuznar, Lawrence
1997   Reclaiming a Scientific Anthropology. Walnut Creek, Calif.: Altamira Press.

Kwast, Barbara
1996   Reduction of Maternal and Perinatal Mortality in Rural and Peri-Urban Settings: What Works? European Journal of Obstetrics, Gynecology, and Reproductive Biology 69:47–53.

Laderman, Carol
1991   Taming the Wind of Desire. Berkeley: University of California Press.

La Farge, Oliver
1947   Santa Eulalia: The Religion of a Cuchumatan Town. Chicago: University of Chicago Press.

La Farge, Oliver, and Douglas Byers
1931   The Year Bearer's People. Middle American Research Institute, publ. no. 3. New Orleans: Tulane University.

La Forgia, Gerard M., and Bernard Couttolenc
1993   Guatemala Health Sector Reform Lending Program: A Review of the Epidemiologic Context, Government Resource Allocation and Efficiency, and the Private Sector. Final report presented to the Inter-American Development Bank. Washington, D.C.: The Urban Institute.

Lagarriga Attias, Isabel
1975   Medicina tradicional y espiritismo: Los espiritualistas trinitarios marianos de Jalapa, Veracruz. México, D.F.: Secretaría de Educación Pública.

1978a   El papel del psicólogo en el campo de la medicina tradicional. Medicina Tradicional 1 (4): 55–60.

1978b   Técnicas catárticas en los templos espiritualistas trinitarios marianos. In Estudios sobre etnobotánica y antropología médica, no. 3, ed. Carlos Viesca Treviño, pp. 115–126. México, D.F.: Instituto Mexicano para el Estudio de las Plantas Medicinales.

Lagarriga, Isabel, and Carlos Viesca Treviño
1981   Diario de campo: El caso de Angela Guevara. Unpublished manuscript.

Lang, Jennifer, and Elizabeth Elkin
1997   A Study of the Beliefs and Birthing Practices of Traditional Midwives in Rural Guatemala. Journal of Nurse-Midwifery 42 (1): 25–31.

Lanning, John T.
1956   The University in the Kingdom of Guatemala. Ithaca, N.Y.: Cornell University Press.
1985   The Royal Protomedicato. *In* The Regulations of the Medical Professions in the Spanish Empire, ed. John Jay TePaske. Durham, N.C.: Duke University Press.

Larme, Anne C.
1985   The Changing Roles of Tarascan Healers and Midwives. M.A. thesis, University of North Carolina at Chapel Hill.

Laski, Marghanita
1961   Ecstasy in Secular and Religious Experience. Los Angeles: Tarcher.

Lassey, Marie L., William R. Lassey, and Martin J. Jinks
1997   Health Care Systems around the World. Upper Saddle River, N.J.: Prentice-Hall.

Latorre, Felipe A., and Dolores L. Latorre
1976   The Mexican Kickapoo Indians. Austin: University of Texas Press.

Laughlin, Robert M.
1969   The Tzotzil. *In* Handbook of Middle American Indians. Vol. 7, pt. 1, Ethnology, ed. Evon Z. Vogt, pp. 152–194. Austin: University of Texas Press.
1980   Of Shoes and Ships and Sealing Wax: Sundries from Zinacantán. Smithsonian Contributions to Anthropology, no. 25. Washington, D.C.: Smithsonian Institution Press.
1988   Mayan Tales from Zinacantán: Dreams and Stories from the People of the Bat, ed. Carol Karasik. Washington, D.C.: Smithsonian Institution Press.

Law, Howard W.
1960   Mecayapan, Veracruz: An Ethnographic Sketch. M.A. thesis, University of Texas.

Leacock, Seth, and Ruth Leacock
1975   Spirits of the Deep. Garden City, N.Y.: Anchor/Doubleday.

Leedam, E.
1985   Traditional Birth Attendants. International Journal of Gynaecology and Obstetrics 23:249–274.

León, Nicolás
1910   La obstetricia en México: Notas bibliográficas, étnicas, históricas, documentarias y críticas, de los orígenes históricos hasta el año 1910. México, D.F.: Tip. de la vda. de F. Díaz de Leon.
1911   La medicina entre los indios mazatecas del estado de Oaxaca, México. Crónica Médica Mexicana 14:215–216.

Levins, Richard, and Richard Lewontin
1998   Foreword. *In* Building a New Biocultural Synthesis: Political-Economic Perspectives on Human Biology, ed. Alan H. Goodman and Thomas L. Leatherman, pp. xi–xv. Ann Arbor: University of Michigan Press.

Lewis, I. M.
1971   Ecstatic Religion. Middlesex: Penguin.

1981   What is a Shaman? Folk 23:25–35.

Lewis, M. Paul
1993   Real Men Don't Speak Quiche: Quiche Ethnicity, Ki-che Ethnic Movement,
        K'iche' Nationalism. Language Problems and Language Planning 17 (1):
        37–54.

Lewis, Oscar
1963   Life in a Mexican Village: Tepoztlán Restudied. Urbana: University of Illinois
        Press.

Lewis, Walter H., and Memory P. F. Elvin-Lewis
1977   Medical Botany. Plants Affecting Man's Health. New York: Wiley.

Lieban, Richard W.
1977   The Field of Medical Anthropology. In Culture, Disease, and Healing: Studies
        in Medical Anthropology, ed. David Landy, pp. 13–31. New York: Macmillan.

Liebman, Amy King
1994   Health Care for All by the Year 2000? Guatemala: Health, Development, and
        State Repression. M.A. and M.P.A. thesis, University of Texas.

Lincoln, Jackson Steward
1935   The Dream in Primitive Culture. Baltimore: Williams and Wilkins.

1942   The Maya Calendar of the Ixil of Guatemala. Carnegie Institution of Wash-
        ington, publ. no. 528. Contributions to American Anthropology and History.
        Vol. 7, no. 38. Washington, D.C.: Carnegie Institution.

Lipp, Frank J.
1988   The Study of Disease in Relation to Culture: The Susto Complex among the
        Mixe of Oaxaca (Mexico). Dialectical Anthropology 12:435–442.

1991   The Mixe of Oaxaca: Religion, Ritual and Healing. Austin: University of Texas
        Press.

1992   Religion, Ritual and Medicine in Mixe Society. Journal of Latin American Lore
        18:15–27.

1996   Herbalism. New York: Little, Brown.

Litoff, J. B.
1978   American Midwives: 1860 to the Present. Westport, Conn.: Greenwood.

1986   The American Midwife Debate. Westport, Conn.: Greenwood.

Logan, Kathleen
1983   The Role of Pharmacists and Over the Counter Medications in the Health
        Care System of a Mexican City. Medical Anthropology 7 (1): 68–89.

Long, E. Croft, and Alberto Viau D.
1974   Health Care Extension Using Medical Auxiliaries in Guatemala. Lancet 1
        (843): 127–130.

López Acuña, Daniel
1980   La salud desigual en México. México, D.F.: Siglo Veintiuno Editores.

López Austin, Alfredo
1967   Cuarenta clases de magos del mundo náhuatl. Estudios de Cultura Náhuatl 7:87–117.
1973   El hombre-dios. México, D.F.: Universidad Nacional Autónoma de México.
1975   Textos de medicina náhuatl. 2d ed. México, D.F.: Instituto de Investigaciones Históricas, Universidad Nacional Autónoma de México.
1988   The Human Body and Ideology: Concepts of the Ancient Nahuas. 2 vols., trans. Thelma Ortiz de Montellano and Bernard Ortiz de Montellano. Salt Lake City: University of Utah Press.

López de Gómara, Francisco
1552   Historia de las indias y conquista de México. Zaragoza, México: Agustín Millán.

López Piñero, José María
1990   Las nuevas medicinas americanas en la obra (1565–1574) de Nicolás Monardes. Asclepio 42 : 3–67.

Lot-Falck, Eveline
1970   Psychopathes et Chamans Yakoutes. *In* Échanges et communications. Mélanges offerts à Claude Lévi-Strauss pour son 60*eme* anniversaire. Vol. 2, ed. Jean Pouillon and Pierre Maranda, pp. 115–129. The Hague: Mouton.

Loustaunau, Martha O., and Elisa J. Sobo
1997   The Cultural Context of Health, Illness, and Medicine. Westport, Conn.: Bergin and Garvey.

Lozoya Legorreta, Xavier, Georgina Velázquez Díaz, and Angel Flores Alvarado
1988   La medicina tradicional en México: Experiencia del programa IMSS-COPLAMAR, 1982–1987. México, D.F.: Instituto Mexicano del Seguro Social.

Lumholtz, Carl
1902   Unknown Mexico: A Record of Five Years Exploration of the Western Sierra Madre. *In* The Tierra Caliente of Tepic and Jalisco; and among the Tarascos of Michoacán. Vol. 1. New York: Charles Scribner's.
1904   El México desconocido. 2 vols. New York: Charles Scribner's.

McClain, Carol
1975   Ethno-Obstetrics in Ajijic. Anthropological Quarterly 48 (1): 38–56.

McCullough, John M.
1973   Human Ecology, Heat Adaptation, and Belief Systems: The Hot-Cold Syndrome of Yucatan. Journal of Anthropological Research 29 : 32–36.

MacDermot, Violet
1971   The Cult of the Seer in the Ancient Middle East: A Contribution to Current Research on Hallucinations Drawn from Coptic and Other Texts. Wellcome Institute of the History of Medicine, publ. n.s. 21. London.

McElroy, Ann, and Patricia K. Townsend
1996   Medical Anthropology in Ecological Perspective. Boulder, Colo.: Westview.

MacGregor, Ma. Teresa G. de
1984   Population Geography of Mexico. *In* Geography and Population, ed. J. I. Clarke, pp. 215–222. Oxford: Pergamon.

McKay, K.
1933   Mayan Midwifery. *In* The Peninsula of Yucatan: Medical, Biological, Meteorological and Sociological Studies. Carnegie Institution of Washington, publ. no. 431, ed. George Cheever Shattuck. Washington, D.C.: Carnegie Institution of Washington.

McMahon, Clarence Edward
1994   The Sacred Nature of Maya Bonesetting: Ritual Validation in an Empirical Practice. M.A. thesis, Texas A&M University.

Macro International, Inc. and INCAP
1997   Encuesta de proveedores de servicios de salud en cuatro departamentos de Guatemala. Guatemala: Ministerio de Salud Pública y Asistencia Social.

Madsen, Claudia
1968   A Study of Change in Mexican Folk Medicine. *In* Contemporary Latin American Culture, ed. Munro S. Edmonson, Claudia Madsen, and Jane F. Collier, pp. 92–137. Middle American Research Institute, publ. no. 25. New Orleans: Tulane University.

Madsen, William
1955   Shamanism in Mexico. Southwestern Journal of Anthropology 11:48–57.

1957   Christo-Paganism: A Study of Mexican Religious Syncretism. Middle American Research Institute, publ. no. 19. New Orleans: Tulane University.

1969   The Virgin's Children: Life in an Aztec Village Today. New York: Greenwood. [1960]

1983   Death of a Curandero. Notas Mesoamericanas 9:112–116.

Mak, Cornelia
1959   Mixtec Medical Beliefs and Practices. América Indígena 19 (2): 125–150.

Malinowski, Bronislaw
1948   Magic Science and Religion. *In* Magic Science and Religion and Other Essays. New York: Anchor/Doubleday.

Marshall, Mary Lynn
1986   Illness in a Guatemalan Maya Community. Ph.D. diss., Yale University.

Martínez, Maximino
1944   Las plantas medicinales de México. 3d ed. México, D.F.: Ediciones Botas.

1959   Plantas ultiles de la flora mexicana. México, D.F.: Ediciones Botas.

Martínez Benítez, Ma. Matilde, Pablo Latapi, Isabel Hernández Tezoquipa, and Juana Rodriguez Velázquez
1993   Sociología de una profesión. El caso de enfermería. México, D.F.: Centro de Estudios Educativos.

Martínez Cortés, Fernando
1993   De los miasmas y efluvios al descubrimiento de las bacterias patógenas. Los primeros cincuenta años del Consejo Superior de Salubridad. México, D.F.: Bristol-Myers Squib and Consejo de Salubridad.

Mata, Leonardo
1978   The Children of Santa Maria Cauqúe. Cambridge: MIT Press.

Mata Pinzón, Soledad, Diego Méndez Granados, Miguel Angel Marmolejo Monsivais, Jose Antonio Tascón Mendoza, Maritza Zurita Esquivel, Yolanda Galindo Manrique, and Gloria Irene Lozano Mascarúa. (Carlos Zolla, Director)
1994   Diccionario enciclopédico de la medicina tradicional mexicana. 2 vols. México, D.F.: Instituto Nacional Indigenista.

Mata Torres, Ramón
1982   Matrimonio huichol: Integración y cultura. Jalisco, México: Universidad de Guadalajara.

Maust, Marcia Good
1994   The Midwife or the Knife: The Discourse of Childbirth by Cesarean in Mérida, Yucatán. Latinamericanist 30 (1): 6–11.

1995   Childbirth and Conversations in Mérida, Yucatan. M.A. thesis, University of Florida.

1997   Parteras en Mérida: Una alternativa a la cesárea innecesaria. Nueva Época/ Salud Problema 2 (2): 21–33.

Mejia, Alfonso, and Livia Varju
1983   Women as Health Providers. World Health (September): 10–12.

Mellado Campos, Virginia, Armando Sánchez Reyes, Paolo Femia, Alfredo Navarro Magdaleno, Enrique Erosa Solana, Daisy Mary Bonilla Contreras, and Marina del Socorro Domínguez Hernández
1994   La medicina tradicional de los pueblos indígenas de México. 3 vols. México, D.F.: Instituto Nacional Indigenista.

Mellado Campos, Virginia, Carlos Zolla, and Xóchitl Castañeda. (with Antonio Tascón Mendoza)
1989   La atención al embarazo y el parto en el medio rural mexicano. México, D.F.: Centro Interaméricano de Estudios de Seguridad Social.

Mellen, George-Ann
1967   El uso de las plantas medicinales en Guatemala. Guatemala Indígena 9: 99–179.

Mendelson, Michael
1965   Ritual and Mythology. In Handbook of Middle American Indians. Vol. 6, ed. Manning Nash, pp. 392–415. Austin: University of Texas Press.

Méndez Domínguez, Alfredo
1983   Illness and Medical Theory among Guatemalan Indians. In Heritage of Conquest: Thirty Years Later, ed. Carl Kendall, John Hawkins, and Laurel Bossen, pp. 266–298. Albuquerque: University of New Mexico Press.

Méndez Morales, José Silvestre
1994   Problemas económicos de México. México, D.F.: McGraw-Hill.

Mendieta, Gerónimo de
1971   Historia eclesiástica indiana. México, D.F.: Editorial Porrúa.

Merrifield, William R.
1981   Proto Otomanguean Kinship. Dallas: International Museum of Cultures, Summer Institute of Linguistics.

Mesa-Lago, Carmelo
1992   Health Care for the Poor in Latin America and the Caribbean. Washington, D.C.: Pan American Health Organization; Arlington, Va.: Inter-American Foundation.

Metzger, Duane, and Gerald Williams
1972   Tenejapa Medicine I: The Curer. Southwestern Journal of Anthropology 19 (2): 216–234.

Miles, S. W.
1957   The Sixteenth-Century Pokom Maya. A Documentary Analysis of Structure and Archaeological Setting. Transactions of American Philosophical Society 47:731–781.

Ministerio de Salud Pública y Asistencia Social [MSPAS]
1993a   Lineamientos de política de salud 1994–1995. Guatemala: MSPAS. Unpublished manuscript.

1993b   Plan nacional de reducción de la mortalidad materna. Guatemala: MSPAS. Unpublished manuscript.

1999   Avances y Perspectivas. Extensión de cobertura con servicios básicos de salud. I: Nivel de atención. Guatemala: MSPAS, SIAS. Unpublished manuscript.

Mischel, Walter, and Frances Mischel
1958   Psychological Aspects of Spirit Possession. American Anthropologist 60:249–260.

Módena, María Eugenia
1990   Madres, médicos y curanderos: Diferencia cultural e identidad ideológica. Cuadernos de la Casa Chata, no. 37. México, D.F.: Centro de Investigaciones y Estudios Superiores en Antropología Social (CIESAS).

1992   Instituciones, médicos y paramédicos. In La antropología médica en México. Vol. 2, comp. Roberto Campos Navarro, pp. 43–68. México, D.F.: Universidad Autónoma Metropolitana.

Molina, Alonso de
1975   Confesionario mayor en lengua mexicana y castellana. Suplementos al Boletín del Instituto de Investigaciones Bibliográficas, México, D.F.: Universidad Nacional Autónoma de México. [1569]

Monaghan, John
1995   The Covenants with Earth and Rain: Exchange, Sacrifice, and Revelation in Mixtec Sociality. Norman: University of Oklahoma Press.

Monardes, Nicolás
1988   Historia medicinal de las cosas que se traen de nuestras Indias Occidentales que sirven en medicina. Sevilla: Padilla Libros. [1574]

Montero de Miranda, Francisco
1575?   Relación de la provincia de la Verapaz. *In* Relaciones geográficas del siglo XVI. Vol. 1, Guatemala, ed. René Acuña, pp. 223–248. México, D.F.: Universidad Nacional Autónoma de México.

Montoya Briones, José de Jesús
1964   Atla: Etnografía de un pueblo Nahuatl. México, D.F.: Instituto Nacional de Antropología e Historia.

Montoya Briones, José de Jesús, and Gabriel Moedano Navarro
1969   Esbozo analítico de la estructura socioeconómica y el folklore de Xochitlán, Sierra Norte de Puebla. Anales del Instituto Nacional de Antropología e Historia 2:257–299.

Morfit, Susan
1998   Portrait of a Birth. Unpublished manuscript.

Morrow, Helga
1986   Nurses, Nursing and Women. WHO Chronicle 40 (6): 216–221.

Morton, Julia Frances
1981   Atlas of medicinal plants of Middle America: Bahamas to Yucatan. Springfield, Ill.: Thomas.

Moser, Caroline O. N.
1989   Gender Planning in the Third World: Meeting Practical and Strategic Gender Needs. World Development 17 (11): 1799–1825.

Moser, Mary Beck
1982   Seri: From Conception through Infancy. *In* Anthropology of Human Birth, ed. Margarita Artschwager Kay, pp. 221–232. Philadelphia: F. A. Davis.

Münch Galindo, G.
1983   Etnología del istmo veracruzano. México, D.F.: Universidad Nacional Autónoma de México.

1984   Los presagios entre los grupos indígenas del Istmo de Tehuantepec. *In* Investigaciones recientes en el área Maya. Vol. 3, pp. 439–442. Sociedad Mexicana de Antropología, Seventeenth Mesa Redonda. San Cristóbal de las Casas, Chiapas.

Munn, Henry
1973   The Mushrooms of Language. *In* Hallucinogens and Shamanism, ed. Michael J. Harner, pp. 86–122. London: Oxford University Press.

Muñoz, Maurilio
1963   Mixteca, Nahua-Tlapaneca. Memorias del Instituto Nacional Indigenista. Vol. 9. México, D.F.: Instituto Nacional Indigenista.

Myerhoff, Barbara G.
1974   Peyote Hunt: The Sacred Journey of the Huichol Indians. Ithaca, N.Y.: Cornell University Press.

Nahmad, Salomon
1965   Los Mixes: Estudio social y cultural de la región del Zempoaltépetl y del Istmo de Tehuantepec. Memorias del Instituto Nacional Indigenista. Vol. 11. México, D.F.: Instituto Nacional Indigenista.

Nash, June
1967   The Logic of Behavior: Curing in a Maya Indian Town. Human Organization 26:132–140.

1970   In the Eyes of the Ancestors: Behavior in a Mayan Community. Prospect Heights, Ill.: Waveland Press.

Nava L., E. Fernando
1995   Los chichimecas. In Etnografía contemporánea de los pueblos indígenas de México, Región Centro, pp. 11–46. México, D.F.: Instituto Nacional Indigenista.

Nicolaidis, Christina
1993   Las comadronas. Journal of the American Medical Women's Association 48: 73, 92.

Nigenda, Gustavo
1995   The Medical Profession, the State, and Health Policy in Mexico, 1917–1988. Ph.D. diss., University of London.

Nigenda, Gustavo, Julio Frenk-Mora, Luis A. Vázquez, Catalina Ramírez-Cuadra, and Oscar Galván-Martínez
1990a   Distribución y utilización del personal médico. In Las profesiones en México. Vol. 3: Medicina, ed. D. Cardaci and D. Gonzalez de Leon, pp. 97–106. México, D.F.: Universidad Nacional Autónoma de México.

Nigenda, Gustavo, Julio Frenk-Mora, Cecilia Robledo Vera, Luiz A. Vázquez-Segovia, and Catalina Ramírez Cuadra
1990b   Los sistemas locales de salud y el mercado de trabajo médico: Resultados de un estudio de preferencias de ubicación geográfica. Educación Médica y Salud 24 (2): 115–135.

Nigenda, Gustavo, and Patricia Najera
1996   Outcomes of Physicians' Distributional Policy in Mexico (1930–1990): A Successful Story? Mimeograph.

Nigenda, Gustavo, and Armando Solorzano
1997   Doctors and Corporatist Politics: The Case of the Mexican Medical Profession. Journal of Health Politics 22 (1): 73–99.

Nishimura, Kho
1987   Shamanism and Medical Cures. Current Anthropology 28 (4): 59–64.

Nolasco, M.
1967   Los Seris, desierto y mar. Anales del Instituto National de Antropología e Historia 18:125–194.

Norgueira, Roberto P., and Pedro Brito
1986   Recursos humanos en salud de las Américas. Educación Médica y Salud 20 (3): 295–322.

Nutini, Hugo G.

1968   San Bernardino Contla: Marriage and Family Structure in a Tlaxcalan Municipio. Pittsburgh: University of Pittsburgh Press.

1993   Bloodsucking Witchcraft: An Epistemological Study of Anthropomorphic Supernaturalism in Rural Tlaxcala. Tucson: University of Arizona Press.

Nutini, Hugo G., and J. Forbes de Nutini

1987   Nahualismo, control de los elementos y hechicería en Tlaxcala rural. *In* La heterodoxia recuperada en torno a Angel Palerm, ed. Susan Glantz, pp. 321–346. México, D.F.: Fondo de Cultura Económica.

Nutini, Hugo G., and Barry L. Isaac

1974   Los pueblos de habla Nahuatl de la región de Tlaxcala y Puebla. México, D.F.: Instituto Nacional Indigenista.

Oakes, Maud

1969   The Two Crosses of Todos Santos. Princeton, N.J.: Princeton University Press. [1951]

Ocaranza, Fernando

1934a   Historia de la Medicina en México. México, D.F.: Laboratorios Midy.

1934b   El Imperial Colegio de Santa Cruz de Santiago Tlatelolco. México, D.F.

Ochoa Robles, Hector Antonio

1990   Medicina moderna en un mundo mágico: Un estudio médico-social en el Yaqui. Hermosillo, Sonora. México, D.F.: Gobierno del Estado de Sonora, Secretaría de Fomento Educativo y Cultura, Instituto Sonorense de Cultura.

Ochoa Zazueta, Jesús Angel

1992   Los Kiliwa y el mundo se hizo así. México, D.F.: Instituto Nacional Indigenista.

Orellana, Sandra L.

1987   Indian Medicine in Highland Guatemala: The Pre-Hispanic and Colonial Periods. Albuquerque: University of New Mexico Press.

O'Rourke, Kathleen

1995a   The Effect of Hospital Staff Training on Management of Obstetrical Patients Referred by Traditional Birth Attendants. International Journal of Gynaecology and Obstetrics 48:95–102.

1995b   Evaluación de un programa de capacitación de parteras tradicionales én Quetzaltenango. Boletín de la Oficina Sanitaria Panamericana 6:503–514.

Ortiz, Alfonso, ed.

1983   Southwest. Vol. 10. *In* Handbook of North American Indians, ed. William C. Sturtevant. Washington, D.C.: Smithsonian Institution.

Ortiz de Montellano, Bernard R.

1975   Empirical Aztec Medicine. Science 188 (4185): 215–220.

1990   Aztec Medicine, Health, and Nutrition. New Brunswick, N.J.: Rutgers University Press.

Ortiz Echániz, Sylvia
1977 Espiritualismo en México: ¿Quiénes y cuántos son los espiritualistas? Cuadernos de Trabajo, no. 20. México, D.F.: Departamento de Etnología y Antropología Social, Instituto Nacional de Antropología e Historia.

Pansini, Jude
1980 Plantation Health-Care in Guatemala: Aspects of the Problem. A study prepared for the U.S. Agency for International Development Mission in Guatemala by the Patronato Para el Mejoramiento de la Salud de Trabajadores Agrícolas (AGROSALUD) under contract no. USAID 520–470.

Parra, Pilar Alicia
1989 The Role of Midwives in Rural Mexico: An Analysis of Changing Health Policy. Ph.D. diss., University of Wisconsin, Madison.
1991 La mujer rural: Las comadronas y el sistema mexicano de salud. Estudios Demográficos y Urbanos 6 (1): 69–88.
1993 Midwives in the Mexican Health System. Social Science and Medicine 37 (11): 1321–1329.

Parsons, Elsie Clews
1931 Curanderos in Oaxaca, Mexico. Scientific Monthly 32:60–68.
1936 Mitla: Town of the Souls and Other Zapoteco-Speaking Pueblos of Oaxaca, Mexico. Chicago: University of Chicago Press.

Paul, Benjamin D.
1976 The Maya Bonesetter as Sacred Specialist. Ethnology 15 (1): 77–81.
———, ed.
1955 Health, Culture and Community: Case Studies of Public Reactions to Health Programs. New York: Russell Sage Foundation.

Paul, Lois
1974 The Mastery of Work and the Mystery of Sex in a Guatemalan Village. *In* Women, Culture, and Society, ed. Michelle Z. Rosaldo and Louise Lamphere, pp. 281–299. Stanford, Calif.: Stanford University Press.
1975 Recruitment to a Ritual Role: The Midwife in a Maya Community. Ethos 3 (3): 449–467.

Paul, Lois, and Benjamin D. Paul
1975 The Maya Midwife as Sacred Specialist: A Guatemalan Case. American Ethnologist 2 (4): 131–148.

Peck, H. Dudley, and Dorothy M. Peck
1966 Mam. *In* Languages of Guatemala, ed. Marvin K. Mayers, pp. 166–195. The Hague: Mouton.

Pelletier, Kenneth, and Denise L. Herzing
1988 Psychoneuroimmunology: Toward a Mind Body Model. Advances 5 (1): 27–56.

Pelliot, Paul
1913 Sur quelques mots d'Asie central attestés dans les textes chinois. Journal Asiatique Series 11 (1): 451–469.

Pennington, Campbell W.
1963   The Tarahumara of Mexico: Their Environment and Material Culture. Salt Lake City: University of Utah Press.

Perez, Roberto
1978   Folk Medicine and Medical Change in Acamixtla, Guerrero. Ph.D. diss., University of California, Riverside.

Pérez y López, Antonio Xavier.
1791–   Teatro de la legislación universal de España e Indias, por orden cronológico de
98   sus cuerpos y decisiones. Vol. 5. Madrid: M. González.

Peters, Larry G.
1982   Trance, Initiation, and Psychotherapy in Tamang Shamanism. American Ethnologist 9:21–46.

Peters, Larry G., and Douglas Price-Williams
1980   Towards an Experiential Analysis of Shamanism. American Ethnologist 7: 397–418.

Philips, George, ed.
1988   The Mexican Economy. London: Routledge.

Poder Ejecutivo Federal
1995   Programa de reforma del sector salud. México, D.F.: Estados Unidos Mexicanos.

Ponce de León, Pedro
1987   Breve relación de los dioses y ritos de la gentilidad. In El alma encantada. Facsimile of vol. 6 of the Anales del Museo Nacional, México, 1902. México, D.F.: Fondo de Cultura Económica. [1892]

Population Reference Bureau
1985   World Population Data Sheet. Washington, D.C.: Population Reference Bureau.

1995   World Population Data Sheet. Washington, D.C.: Population Reference Bureau.

Powell, John
1949   Bring Out Your Dead. Philadelphia: University of Pennsylvania Press.

Pozas, Ricardo
1959   Chamula: Un pueblo indio de los altos de Chiapas. Memorias del Instituto Nacional Indigenista. Vol. 8. México, D.F.: Instituto Nacional Indigenista.

Prado, Xóchitl
1984   Embarazo y parto en la medicina tradicional del área p'uhépecha. Relaciones (Colegio de Michoacán) 5 (20): 113–120.

Putney, Pamela, and Barry Smith
1989   Estudio acerca de las prácticas de las comadronas tradicionales en el altiplano de Guatemala. PRITECH Report prepared for U.S. Agency for International Development/Guatemala.

Quezada, Noemí
1976   La herbolaria en el México colonial. *In* Estado actual del conocimiento en plantas medicinales mexicanas, ed. Xavier Lozoya L., pp. 51–70. México, D.F.: IMEPLAM.

1989   Enfermedad y maleficio: El curandero en el México colonial. México, D.F.: Instituto de Investigaciones Antropológicas, Universidad Nacional Autónoma de México.

1991   The Inquisition's Repression of Curanderos. *In* Cultural Encounters: The Impact of the Inquisition in Spain and the New World, ed. Mary Elizabeth Perry and Anne J. Cruz, pp. 37–57. Berkeley: University of California Press.

Radin, Paul
1945   Cuentos de Mitla. Reprinted from Tlalocan 1 (1, 2, 3). Sacramento: House of Tláloc.

Ramírez, Axel
1978   Bibliografía comentada de la medicina tradicional mexicana (1900–1978). Monografías Científicas no. 3. México, D.F.: IMEPLAM.

Rätsch, Christian
1994   Indianische Heilkräuter: Tradition und Anwendung. Munich: E. Diederichs.

Ravicz, Robert
1960   La mixteca en el estudio comparativo del hongo alucinante. Instituto Nacional de Antropología e Historia, Anales 13:73–92.

Reales Ordenanzas
1804   Reales ordenanzas de los Colegios de Cirugía. Cádiz: Imprenta de D. Pedro Gómez de Requena.

Redfield, Margaret Park
1928   Nace un niño en Tepoztlán: A Child is Born in Tepoztlán. Mexican Folkways 4 (2): 102–108.

Redfield, Robert
1930   Tepoztlán, A Mexican Village: A Study of Folk Life. Chicago: University of Chicago Press.

1941   The Folk Culture of Yucatan. Chicago: University of Chicago Press.

Redfield, Robert, and Margaret Park Redfield
1940   Disease and Its Treatment in Dzitas, Yucatan. Carnegie Institution of Washington, publ. no. 523. Contributions to American Anthropology and History. Vol. 6, no. 32, pp. 49–81. Washington, D.C.

Redfield, Robert, and Alfonso Villa Rojas
1934   Chan Kom: A Maya Village. Chicago: University of Chicago Press.

Reinhard, Johan
1976   Shamanism and Spirit Possession: The Definition Problem. In Spirit Possession in the Nepal Himalayas, ed. John T. Hitchcock and Rex L. Jones, pp. 12–23. New Delhi: Vikas.

Relación de Antequera
1984   *In* Relaciones geográficas del siglo XVI. Vol 3, Oaxaca, ed. René Acuña, pp. 31–
        42. México, D.F.: Universidad Nacional Autónoma de México. [1579]

Relación de Michoacán
1977   Relación de las ceremonias y ritos y población y gobierno de los indios de la
        Provincia de Michoacán. Morelia, México: Balsal Editores. [1541]

Relación de Chilchotla
1987   *In* Relaciones geográficas del siglo XVI. Vol 9, Michoacán, ed. René Acuña,
        pp. 99–120. México, D.F.: Universidad Nacional Autónoma de México. [1579]

Relación de Santiago Atitlán
1982   *In* Relaciones geográficas del siglo XVI. Vol 1, Guatemala, ed. René Acuña,
        pp. 70–150. México, D.F.: Universidad Nacional Autónoma de México. [1585]

Relación de Tancítaro y su partido
1987   *In* Relaciones geográficas del siglo XVI. Vol 9, Michoacán, ed. René Acuña,
        pp. 288–296. México: Universidad Nacional Autónoma de México. [1580]

Relación de Tingüindín
1987   *In* Relaciones geográficas del siglo XVI. Vol. 9, Michoacán, ed. René Acuña,
        pp. 319–327. México, D.F.: Universidad Nacional Autónoma de México.
        [1581]

Relación de Tiripitío
1987   *In* Relaciones geográficas del siglo XVI. Vol 9, Michoacán, ed. René Acuña,
        pp. 339–376. México, D.F.: Universidad Nacional Autónoma de México.
        [1580]

Relación de Tlacolula y Miquitla
1984   *In* Relaciones geográficas del siglo XVI. Vol 3, Oaxaca, ed. René Acuña,
        pp. 255–264. México, D.F.: Universidad Nacional Autónoma de México.
        [1580]

Relación de Tuchpan y su partido
1987   *In* Relaciones geográficas del siglo XVI. Vol 9, Michoacán, ed. René Acuña,
        pp. 383–389. México, D.F.: Universidad Nacional Autónoma de México.
        [1580]

Relación de la Villa de Zacatula
1987   *In* Relaciones geográficas del siglo XVI. Vol 9, Michoacán, ed. René Acuña,
        pp. 449–462. México, D.F.: Universidad Nacional Autónoma de México.
        [1580]

Relación de Xiquilpan y su partido
1987   *In* Relaciones geográficas del siglo XVI. Vol 9, Michoacán, ed. René Acuña,
        pp. 409–418. México, D.F.: Universidad Nacional Autónoma de México.
        [1579]

Relación de Zapotitlán
1982   *In* Relaciones geográficas del siglo XVI. Vol 1, Guatemala, ed. René Acuña,
        pp. 23–52. México, D.F.: Universidad Nacional Autónoma de México. [1579]

Remesal, Antonio de
1966   Historia General de las Indias Occidentales. 2 vols. Madrid: Biblioteca de Autores Españoles, Ed. Atlas.

Reyes Gómez, Laureano
1992   Curanderismo popular entre los mixes de San Juan Guichicovi. *In* Medicina tradicional, herbolaria y salud comunitaria en Oaxaca, ed. Paola Sesia, pp. 55–75. México, D.F.: Centro de Investigaciones y Estudios Superiores en Antropología Social.

Riley, Carroll L.
1972   Los tepehuanes del sur y los tepecanos. *In* Coras, huicholes y tepehuanes, ed. Thomas B. Hinton, pp. 127–136. México: D.F.: Instituto Nacional Indigenista.

Risse, Guenter B.
1986   Hospital Life in Enlightenment Scotland: Care and Teaching at the Royal Infirmary of Edinburgh. Cambridge: Cambridge University Press.

Rita, Carla M.
1979   Concepción y nacimiento. *In* Los huaves de San Mateo del Mar, Oaxaca, ed. Italo Signorini, pp. 263–314. México, D.F.: Instituto Nacional Indigenista.

Rivera Álvarez, Ramiro
1996   Servicios de salud y asistencia social. *In* Historia General de Guatemala. Vol. 5. Época Contemporánea, 1898–1944, pp. 307–312. Guatemala: Asociación de Amigos del País, Fundación Para la Cultura y Desarrollo.

Robledo Vera, Celecia
1996   La feminización de la profesión médica en México a principios de los noventa. México, D.F.: El Colegio de México. Mimeograph.

Rodríguez Baciero, Gerardo, Francisco Javier Goiriena de Gandarias, and Pedro Manuel Ramos Calvo Bilbao
1987   El arte dental en el México prehispánico. Revista Española de Estomatología 35 (2): 113–119.

Rodríguez Rouanet, Francisco
1969   Prácticas tradicionales de los indígenas de Guatemala. Guatemala Indígena 4 (2): 51–86.

Rogoff, Barbara
1999   Personal communication.

Roldán Q., Luis Fernando
1990   Situación social, simbolismo y ritual en el matrimonio Totonaca: Estudio en dos comunidades de la Sierra de Puebla. *In* La Huasteca: Vida y milagros, ed. Ludka de Gortari Krauss and Jesús Ruvalcaba Mercado, pp. 79–99. Cuadernos de la Casa Chata, no. 173. México, D.F.: Centro de Investigaciones y Estudios Superiores en Antropología Social.

Romanucci-Ross, Lola, Daniel E. Moerman, and Laurence R. Tancredi
1997   The Anthropology of Medicine: From Culture to Method. Westport, Conn.: Bergin and Garvey.

Romney, A. Kimball
1967   Kinship and Family. *In* Social Anthropology, ed. Manning Nash, pp. 207–237. Vol. 6 of Handbook of Middle American Indians. Austin: University of Texas Press.

Romney, A. Kimball, and Romaine Romney
1966   The Mixtecans of Juxtlahuaca, Mexico. Huntington, N.Y.: Robert E. Krieger.

Rouse, Roger
1978   Talking about Shamans. Anthropological Society of Oxford Journal 9 (2): 113–128.

Roux, Jean-Paul
1959   Le Chaman Gengiskhanide. Anthropos 54:401–432.

Rubel, Arthur J., and Jean Gettelfinger-Krejci
1976   The Use of Hallucinogenic Mushrooms for Diagnostic Purposes among some Highland Chinantecs. Economic Botany 30:235–248.

Rubel, Arthur J., Carl W. O'Nell, and Rolando Collado
1985   The Folk Illness Called Susto. *In* The Culture-Bound Syndromes: Folk Illnesses of Psychiatric and Anthropological Interest, ed. Roland C. Simons and Charles C. Hughes, pp. 333–350. Boston: D. Reidel.

Rubio, Miguel Ángel
1995   La morada de los santos: Expresiones del culto religioso en el sur de Veracruz y en Tabasco. México, D.F.: Instituto Nacional Indigenista.

Ruebush, Trenton II, and Hector A. Godoy
1992   Community Participation in Malaria Surveillance and Treatment I: The Volunteer Collaborator Network of Guatemala. American Journal of Tropical Medicine and Hygiene 46 (3): 248–260.

Ruíz de Alarcón, Hernando
1987   Tratado de las supersticiones y costumbres gentilicias que oy viuen entre los indios naturales desta Nueva España. *In* El Alma Encantada. Edited facsimile of vol. 6 of Anales del Museo Nacional, 1902. México, D.F.: Fondo de Cultura Económica. [1629]

Ruiz-Matus, Cuauhtémoc, Eloísa Dickinson, Jaime Sepúlveda, and Harrison Stetler
1990   Experiencia de México en el adiestramiento de personal en epidemiología aplicada. Educación Médica y Salud 24 (3): 222–236.

Ruz, Mario Humberto
1983   Médicos y loktores: Enfermedad y cultura en dos comunidades Tojolabales. *In* Los legítimos hombres. Vol. 3, ed. Mario Humberto Ruz, pp. 143–186. México, D.F.: Universidad Nacional Autónoma de México.

1992   Los profesionales de la medicina. *In* La antropología médica en México. Vol. 2, comp. Roberto Campos Navarro, pp. 182–201. México, D.F.: Universidad Autónoma Metropolitana.

Sahagún, Bernardino de
1969   Historia General de las cosas de Nueva España. 4 vols. México, D.F.: Editorial Porrúa.

Saler, Benson
1962   Unsuccessful Practitioners in a Bicultural Guatemalan Community. Psycho-
         analytic Review 49 (2): 103–118.

Sanchez Flores, Guillermo
1982   Estudio de comunidad: Hueyapan, Puebla. Unpublished manuscript.

Sandoval Navarrete, Rafael J.
1986   Hacia una teoría de la migración médica en México. Ciencia y Desarrollo 69:
         43–58.

Sandstrom, Alan R.
1975   Ecology, Economy and the Realm of the Sacred: An Interpretation of Ritual in
         a Nahua Community of the Southern Huasteca, Mexico. Ph.D. diss., Indiana
         University.

1978   The Image of Disease: Medical Practices of Nahua Indians of the Huasteca.
         Monographs in Anthropology, no. 3. Columbia: University of Missouri.

1989   The Face of the Devil: Concepts of Disease and Pollution among Nahua Indi-
         ans of the Southern Huasteca. In Enquetes sur l'Amerique moyenne: Mélanges
         offerts à Guy Stresser-Péan, ed. Dominique Michelet, pp. 357–372. Etudes
         Mésoaméricaines. Vol. 16. México, D.F.: Instituto Nacional de Antropología e
         Historia, Consejo Nacional para la Cultura y las Artes and Centre d'Etudes
         Mexicaines et Centroaméricaines.

1991   Corn Is Our Blood: Culture and Ethnic Identity in a Contemporary Aztec
         Indian Village. Norman: University of Oklahoma Press.

Sandstrom, Alan R., and Pamela E. Sandstrom
1986   Traditional Papermaking and Paper Cult Figures of Mexico. Norman: Univer-
         sity of Oklahoma Press.

Sapper, Karl
1924   Über Brujería in Guatemala. International Congress of Americanists, Proceed-
         ings (Göteborg) 21 (2): 391–405.

Sapper, Karl, and Vincente A. Narciso
1904   Sitten und Gebräuche der Pokonchí Indianer. International Congress of Amer-
         icanists, Proceedings (Stuttgart) 14 (2): 403–414.

Sargent, Carolyn F., and Grace Bascope
1997   Ways of Knowing about Birth in Three Cultures. In Childbirth and Authori-
         tative Knowledge, ed. Robbie Davis-Floyd and Carolyn F. Sargent, pp. 183–
         208. Berkeley: University of California Press.

Sargent, Carolyn F., and Thomas M. Johnson
1996   Handbook of Medical Anthropology: Contemporary Theory and Method.
         Westport, Conn.: Greenwood.

Sarton, George
1954   Galen of Pergamon. Lawrence: University of Kansas Press.

Scheffler, Lilian
1977   Medicina folk y cambio social en un pueblo nahuatl del Valle de Tlaxcala. Boletín del Departamento de Investigación de las Tradiciones Populares 4:83–107.

Schendel, Gordon
1968   Medicine in Mexico: From Aztec Herbs to Betatrons. Austin: University of Texas Press.

Schieber, Barbara, Kathleen O'Rourke, C. Rodriguez, and A. Bartlett
1994   Risk Factor Analysis of Peri-neonatal Mortality in Rural Guatemala. Bulletin of the Pan American Health Organization 28 (3): 229–238.

Schmid-Dolan, Lora
1995   Social Work Community Practice in Mexico and the United States: A Comparative Analysis. M.S. thesis, University of Texas, Arlington.

Schröder, Dominik
1955   Zur Struktur des Shamanismus. Anthropos 50:848–881.

Schroeder, Susan
1990   Tijuana's Elite Healers: The Blending of Western Medicine with Ritualistic Cures. Journal of Latin American Lore 16 (2): 233–258.

Schulman, Diane Plamordon
1975   Childbearing Behavior and Modern Medicine in a Traditional Culture in Yucatan. Ph.D. diss., University of Texas Health Science Center, Houston School of Public Health.

Schultze-Jena, Leonhard
1933   Leben, Glaube und Sprache der Quiché von Guatemala. Indiana. Vol. 1. Jena: Fischer.

Schutz, Alfred
1962   On Multiple Realities. In Collected Papers I: The Problem of Social Reality, ed. Maurice Natanson, pp. 207–259. The Hague: Martinus Nijhoff.

Schwartz, Norman B.
1974   Dreaming and Managing the Future: Notes on a Guatemalan Ladino (non-Indian) Theory of Dreams. Sociologus 24:16–36.

Secretaría de Salud
1992   Unidades médicas privadas: Recursos físicos, materiales y humanos. México, D.F.: Secretaría de Salubridad y Asistencia.

1993   Medicina privada. Encuesta de unidades médicas con hospitalización. Resultados por Entidad Federativa. Subsecretaría de Planeación. Dirección General de Estadística e Información (DGEI). México D.F.: Secretaría de Salubridad y Asistencia.

1994a   Encuesta nacional de salud II. México D.F.: Secretaría de Salubridad y Asistencia.

1994b   Brevario estadístico, Sistema Nacional de Salud 1980–1994. México, D.F.: Secretaría de Salubridad y Asistencia.

1997   Boletín de información estadística. Recursos y servicios. Sistema Nacional de Salud, Año 1996. Vol. 16, no. 1. México D.F.: Secretaría de Salubridad y Asistencia.

Sepúlveda y H., María Teresa

1973   Petición de lluvias en Ostotempa. Boletín-Instituto Nacional de Antropología e Historia 4:9–20.

1988   La medicina entre los Purépecha prehispánicos. México, D.F.: Universidad Nacional Autónoma de México.

Serrano, Antonio

1946a   Carta al virrey José de Iturrigaray. *In* La cirugía mexicana en el siglo XVIII, ed. Rómulo Velasco Ceballos, pp. 307–314. México, D.F.: Archivo Histórico de la Secretaría de Salubridad y Asistencia. [1804]

1946b   Carta al virrey Félix María Calleja. *In* La cirugía mexicana en el siglo XVIII, ed. Rómulo Velasco Ceballos, pp. 345–387. México, D.F.: Archivo Histórico de la Secretaría de Salubridad y Asistencia. [1815]

Sesia, Paola

1992   La obstetricia tradicional en el Istmo de Tehuantepec: Marco conceptual y diferencias con el modelo biomédico. *In* Medicina tradicional, herbolaria y salud comunitaria en Oaxaca, ed. Paola Sesia, pp. 17–54. México, D.F.: Centro de Investigaciones y Estudios Superiores en Antropología Social.

Shaara, Lila, and Andrew Strathern

1992   A Preliminary Analysis of the Relationship between Altered States of Consciousness, Healing and Social Structure. American Anthropologist 94:145–160.

Sharon, Douglas

1976   The Distribution of the Mesa in Latin America. Journal of Latin American Lore 2 (1): 71–95.

Shaw, Mary, and Helen Neuenswander

1966   Achí. *In* Languages of Guatemala, ed. Marvin K. Mayers, pp. 15–48. The Hague: Moutons.

Sherwin, Susan

1996   Cancer and Women: Some Feminist Ethic Concerns. *In* Gender and Health: An International Perspective, ed. Carolyn F. Sargent and Caroline B. Brettell, pp. 187–204. Upper Saddle River, N.J.: Prentice-Hall.

Shi, Kun

1996   An Introduction to Manchu and Mongol Shamans. Shamanism 9 (1): 6–11.

Shields, David

1990   Crece la participación de la mujer en la ciencia. El Nacional. April 20, p. 5.

Shirokogoroff, Sergei M.
1935   Psychomental Complex of the Tungus. London: Routledge and Kegan Paul.

Sibley, Lynn
1993   Traditional Birth Attendants, Their Training, and Maternal Health in Belize. Ph.D. diss., University of Colorado.

Siegel, Morris
1941   Religion in Western Guatemala: A Product of Acculturation. American Anthropologist 43:62–76.

Signorini, I.
1979   Los huaves de San Mateo del Mar, Oaxaca. México, D.F.: Instituto Nacional Indigenista.

1982   Patterns of Fright: Multiple Concepts of Susto in a Nahua-Ladino Community of the Sierra de Puebla (Mexico). Ethnology 21 (4): 313–323.

Simeon, George
1973   The Evil Eye in a Guatemalan village. Ethnomedizin 2:437–441.

Singer, Merrill, and Hans Baer
1995   Critical Medical Anthropology. Amityville, N.Y.: Baywood.

Sistema Nacional de Salud
1993   Boletín de información estadística. Recursos y servicios. Vol. 13, no. 1. México, D.F.: Secretaría de Salubridad y Asistencia.

Soberón-Acevedo, Guillermo
1987   El cambio estructural en la salud, III. La investigación y los recursos humanos como instrumentos del cambio. Salud Pública en México 29 (2): 155–165.

Soberón-Acevedo, Guillermo, Ana Langer, and Julio Frenk
1988   Requerimientos del paradigma de la atención primaria a la salud en los albores del siglo XXI. Salud Pública de México 30 (6): 791–803.

Soberón-Acevedo, Guillermo, and R. M. Najera
1988   Recursos humanos de enfermería en el sector salud. IX Congreso Nacional de Enfermería y Obstetricia. México, D.F. Mimeograph.

Somolinos d'Ardois, Germán
1966   Capítulos de historia médica mexicana. Vol. 2. México, D.F.: Sociedad Mexicana de Historia y Filosofía de la Medicina.

1978   Capítulos de historia médica mexicana. Vols. 3 and 4. México, D.F.: Sociedad Mexicana de Historia y Filosofía de la Medicina.

Soustelle, Georgette
1958   Tequila: Un village nahuatl du Mexique oriental. Paris: Institut d'Ethnologie.

Starr, Frederick
1900   Notes upon the Ethnography of Southern Mexico. Davenport, Ia.: Putman Memorial Publication Fund.

Starr Sered, Susan
1994   Priestess, Mother, Sacred Sister. New York: Oxford University Press.

Stebbins, Kenyon Rainier
1984   Second-Class Mexicans: State Penetration and Its Impact on Health Status and
        Health Services in a Highland Chinantec Municipio in Oaxaca. Ph.D. diss.,
        Michigan State University.

Steggerda, Morris
1943   Remedies for Disease as Prescribed by Maya Indian Herb-Doctors. Bulletin of
        Historical Medicine 13:54–82.

Steinbeck, John
1941   The Forgotten Village. New York: Viking.

Tanck de Estrada, Dorothy
1982   La colonia. *In* Historia de las profesiones en México, ed. Lilia Cárdenas Tre-
        viño. México, D.F.: El Colegio de México.

Tapia García, Fermin
1985   Las plantas curativas y su conocimiento entre los amuzgos: Arboles grandes y
        arbustos. México, D.F.: Centro de Investigaciones y Estudios Superiores en
        Antropología Social.

Taub, Bonnie
1992   Calling the Soul Back to the Heart: Soul Loss, Depression and Healing Among
        Indigenous Mexicans. Ph.D. diss., University of California.

Tedlock, Barbara
1983   Knowledge That Comes in the Dark: Highland Maya Dream Epistemology.
        Revista Mexicana de Estudios Antropológicos 29:115–123.

1992a   Time and the Highland Maya. Albuquerque: University of New Mexico Press.

1992b   The Role of Dreams and Visionary Narratives in Maya Cultural Survival.
        Ethos 20:453–476.

Tenzel, James H.
1970   Shamanism and Concepts of Disease in a Mayan Indian Community. Psychia-
        try 33:372–380.

Termer, Franz
1930   Zur Ethnologie und Ethnographie des Nördlichen Mittel-Amerika. Ibero-
        Amerikanisches Archiv 4 (3). Berlin.

Thomas, Nicholas, and Caroline Humphrey
1994   Introduction. *In* Shamanism, History and the State, ed. Nicholas Thomas and
        Caroline Humphrey, pp. 1–12. Ann Arbor: University of Michigan Press.

Thompson, J. Eric. S.
1930   Ethnology of the Mayas of Southern and Central British Honduras. Field Mu-
        seum of Natural History, Anthropological Series. Vol. 17, no. 2. Chicago: Field
        Museum of Natural History.

1941   Apuntes sobre las supersticiones de los Mayas de Socotz, Honduras Británica.
        In Los Mayas Antiguos, ed. Carlos Lizardi Ramos, pp. 99–110. México, D.F.:
        El Colegio de México.

Tousignant, Michel
1979   Espanto: A Dialogue with the Gods. Culture, Medicine and Psychiatry 3:347–361.

Tranfo, Luigi
1974   Vida y magia en un pueblo otomí del Mezquital, trans. Alejandra Ma. A. Hernández. México, D.F.: Dirección General de Publicaciones del Consejo Nacional para la Cultura y las Artes: Instituto Nacional Indigenista.

Trostle, James A., and Johannes Sommerfield
1996   Medical Anthropology and Epidemiology. Annual Review of Anthropology 25:253–274.

Turner, Paul R.
1984   The Highland Chontal. New York: Irvington. [1972].

Tuynman-Kret, Martine
1982   The Development of Health Care in the Process of Modernization: Sociological Research in the Villages of Chiconcuautla and Cuacuila, Two Rural Societies in the Sierra Norte de Puebla in Mexico. Instuut voor Culturele Antropologie en Sociologie der Niet-westerse Volken, publ. no. 56. Leiden: Instituut voor Culturele Antropologie en Sociologie der Niet-westerse Volken.

Unidad Regional de Acayucan
1983   Ciclo de vida de los nahuas. Cuadernos de Trabajo, Acayucan, no. 22. México, D.F.: Dirección General de Culturas Populares.

Universidad Nacional Autónoma de México
1995   Guía de carreras. México, D.F.: Universidad Nacional Autónoma de México.

U.S. Agency for International Development/Guatemala–Central American Programs.
1995   Family and Community Health Strategy. Guatemala. Unpublished manuscript.

Valdez de Reyes, María Elena, and María Alberta García Jiménez
1991   Perspectivas de la profesión de enfermería en el contexto de la meta de salud para todos en el año 2000: Prospectiva de la enfermería en México. Educación Médica y Salud 25 (4): 410–431.

Valladares, Leon
1957   El hombre y el maíz. México, D.F.: Editorial Costa-Amic.

Varela, Francisco, ed.
1997   Sleeping, Dreaming and Dying. Boston: Wisdom.

Vargas, Luis Alberto, and Leticia E. Casillas
1989   Medical Anthropology in Mexico. Social Science and Medicine 28 (12): 1343–1349.

Vargas Melgarejo, Luz María
1994   Biblio-hemerografía sobre antropología médica (1900–1990). México, D.F.: Centro Regional de Investigaciones Multidisciplinarias, Universidad Nacional Autónoma de México.

Vargas Ramírez, Jesús

1995   Los nahuas de la huasteca veracruzana. *In* Etnografía contemporánea de los pueblos indígenas de México, Región Oriental, pp. 105–164. México, D.F.: Instituto Nacional Indigenista.

Vargas Ramírez, Jesús, and María del Refugio Vargas

1983   Ahuateno: "Al pie de los encinos." 2 vols. Cuadernos del Norte de Veracruz. México, D.F.: Dirección General de Culturas Populares.

Vázquez Rojas, Gonzalo

1995   Los Matlatzincas. *In* Etnografía contemporánea de los pueblos indígenas de México, Región Centro, pp. 49–84. México, D.F.: Instituto Nacional Indigenista.

Velasco, Luis de

1551   Mandato en relación con la autorización que se da a Martín de la Cruz para ejercer como curandero, 27 de mayo de 1551. Microfilm copy of document no. 140 of the Hans P. Krauss Collection of Hispanic American Manuscripts, Library of Congress, Washington, D.C.

1553   Licencia para curar y examinar otorgada a Antón Martín y Graviel Mariano, octubre de 1553. Manuscript no. 1121, Ayer Collection, Newberry Library, Chicago.

Venegas, Carmen

1973   Régimen hospitalario para indios en la Nueva España. México, D.F.: Secretaría de Educación Pública/Instituto Nacional de Antropología e Historia.

Vexler, Mona Jill

1981   Chachahuantla, A Blouse-Making Village in Mexico: A Study of the Socio-Economic Roles of Women. Ph.D. diss., University of California.

Viesca Treviño, Carlos

1984   El médico mexica. *In* México antiguo. Vol. 1, coord. Alfredo López Austin and Carlos Viesca Treviño, pp. 217–230, México, D.F.: Universidad Nacional Autónoma de México; Academia Nacional de Medicina.

1990   Los médicos indígenas frente a la medicina europea. *In* La medicina novohispana del siglo XVI. Vol. 2, coord. G. Aguirre Beltrán and R. Moreno de los Arcos, pp. 132–153. México, D.F.: Universidad Nacional Autónoma de México; Academia Nacional de Medicina.

1995   Y. Martín de la Cruz, autor del Códice de la Cruz Badiano, era un médico tlatelolca de carne y hueso. Estudios de Cultura Náhuatl 25:480–498.

1996   Sitio, naturaleza y propiedades de la ciudad de México . . . de Diego Cisneros. Boletín del Instituto de Investigaciones Bibliográficas 1 (1): 183–206.

Villa Rojas, Alfonso

1945   The Maya of East Central Quintana Roo. Carnegie Institution of Washington, publ. no. 559. Washington, D.C.: Carnegie Institution of Washington.

1955   Los mazatecos y el problema indígena de la cuenca del papaloapan. Memorias del Instituto Nacional Indigenista. Vol. 7. México, D.F.: Instituto Nacional Indigenista.

1969   The Maya of Yucatan. *In* Handbook of Middle American Indians. Vol. 7, pt. 1, ed. Evon Z. Vogt, pp. 244–275. Austin: University of Texas Press.

Villatoro, Elba M.
1994   La comadrona a través de la historia en las prácticas obstétricos pediátricas: Una experiencia en el área Ixil, Quiche. La Tradición Popular 97 : 1–21.

Vitebsky, Piers
1995   The Shaman. Boston: Little, Brown.

Vogt, Evon Z., ed.
1966   H?iloletik: The Organization and Function of Shamanism in Zinacantan. *In* Summa anthropológica en Homenaje a Roberto J. Weitlaner, pp. 359–369. México, D.F.: Instituto Nacional de Antropología e Historia.

1969a   Ethnology. Vols. 7 and 8. *In* Handbook of Middle American Indians, ed. Robert Wauchope. Austin: University of Texas Press.

1969b   Zinacantan: A Maya Community in the Highlands of Chiapas. Cambridge, Mass.: Harvard University Press.

1970   Human Souls and Animal Spirits in Zinacantan. *In* Échanges et Communications. Mélanges Offerts à Claude Lévi-Strauss pour son 60eme Anniversaire. Vol. 2, ed. Jean Pouillon and Pierre Maranda, pp. 1148–1167. The Hague: Mouton.

1976   Tortillas for the Gods: A Symbolic Analysis of Zinacanteco Ritual. Cambridge, Mass.: Harvard University Press.

Voigt, V.
1984   Shaman—Person or Word? *In* Shamanism in Eurasia. Pt. 1, ed. Mihály Hoppál, pp. 13–20. Göttingen: Edition Herodot.

Voigts, Linda E., and Michael R. McVaugh
1984   A Latin Technical Phlebotomy and Its Middle English Translation. Transactions of the American Philosophical Society 74, pt. 2.

Wagley, Charles
1949   The Social and Religious Life of a Guatemalan Village. American Anthropologist 51 (4), pt. 2, Memoir 71.

1957   Santiago Chimaltenango. Seminario de Integración Social Guatemalteca, publ. no. 4. Guatemala.

Walt, Gill
1994   Health Policy. An Introduction to Process and Power. London: Zed.

Ward, Peter M.
1986   Welfare Politics in Mexico: Papering over the Cracks. London: Allen and Unwin.

Wasson, R. Gordon, George Cowan, Florence Cowan, and Willard Rhodes
1974   María Sabina and Her Mazatec Velada. New York: Harcourt Brace Jovanovich.

Watanabe, John M.
1992   Maya Saints and Souls in a Changing World. Austin: University of Texas Press.

Weimann, Claudia, and Michael Heinrich
1998   Concepts of Medicinal Plants among the Nahua of the Sierra de Zongolica, Veracruz (Mexico). Angewandte Botanik 72:87–91.

World Health Organization-United Nations Children's Fund [WHO-UNICEF]
n.d.   The Baby-Friendly Initiative. Pamphlet.

Willats, Amy
1995   Midwives and Community Workers in Conflict: Exploring the Cultural Appropriateness of Family Planning Programs. M.A. thesis, Vanderbilt University.

Williams García, Roberto
1957   Ichcacuatitla. La Palabra y el Hombre 1:51–63.

1963   Los tepehuas. Xalapa, Veracruz, México: Instituto de Antropología, Universidad Veracruzana.

Wilson, E. O.
1978   On Human Nature. Cambridge, Mass.: Harvard University Press.

1999   Consilience: The Unity of Knowledge. New York: Vintage.

Wilson, Kevara
Forth.   Midwives and Childbirth in Nahualá. *In* Diverging Roads: Culture, Access, and Differential Development in Two Kiche Maya Communities, ed. John P. Hawkins and Walter R. Adams.

Winkelman, Michael
1986   Trance States: A Theoretical Model and Cross-Cultural Analysis. Ethos 14:174–204.

1990   Shamans and Other "Mágico-Religious" Healers: A Cross-Cultural Study of Their Origins, Nature, and Social Transformations. Ethos 18:308–352.

Wisdom, Charles
1940   The Chorti Indians of Guatemala. Chicago: University of Chicago Press.

1952   The Supernatural World and Curing. *In* Heritage of Conquest, ed. Sol Tax, pp. 119–141. Glencoe, Ill.: The Free Press.

Withnall, E.
1993   Birth Customs in Guatemala. Midwifery Today and Childbirth Education 25:25.

Woods, Clyde M., and Theodore D. Graves
1973   The Process of Medical Change in a Highland Guatemalan Town. Los Angeles: University of California Press.

Wright, Peggy A.
1989   The Nature of the Shamanic State of Consciousness: A Review. Journal of Psychoactive Drugs 21 (1): 25–33.

1994   A Psychobiological Approach to Shamanic Altered States of Consciousness. ReVision 16 (4): 164–172.

Yepes, F.
1973   Distribución geográfica de los médicos: Factores que los afectan. Educación, Médica y Salud 7:3–4.

Young, James Clay
1978   Health Care in Pichátaro: Medical Decision Making in a Tarascan Town of Michoacán, Mexico. Ph.D. diss., University of California.

Zayas, Maritere
1992   Tres mujeres curanderas yoremes. *In* Símbolos del desierto, ed. María Eugenia Olavarría, pp. 103–122. México, D.F.: Universidad Autónoma Metropolitana.

Zedillo Castillo, Antonio.
1984   Historia de un hospital: El Hospital Real de Naturales. México: Instituto Mexicano del Seguro Social.

Zeki, Semir
1993   A Vision of the Brain. Oxford: Blackwell Scientific Publications.

Zingg, Robert M.
1982   Los huicholes: Una tribu de artistas. 2 vols. México, D.F.: Instituto Nacional Indigenista. [1937]

Contributors to the Volume

SHEILA COSMINSKY is associate professor of anthropology at Rutgers, in Camden, New Jersey. She has conducted research in Guatemala, Belize, Kenya, Zimbabwe, and Japan, and has published numerous articles in medical and nutritional anthropology, especially maternal and child health. She is currently completing a study of cross-generational midwifery on a Guatemalan plantation.

JAMES W. DOW is professor of anthropology at Oakland University. He has worked with the Ñähñu- (Otomí) speaking people of eastern Mexico since 1967. He is a past president of the Central States Anthropological Society and a board member of the Anthropology of Religion Section of the American Anthropological Association. He is editor of *Volume 8, Middle America and the Caribbean*, of the *Encyclopedia of World Cultures*, and an author and editor of other books and articles.

KAJA FINKLER is professor of anthropology at the University of North Carolina at Chapel Hill. In addition to her work on Spiritualism, she has published on biomedical practice and patient response in Mexico (*Physicians at Work, Patients in Pain*, Westview) and on women's health (*Women in Pain*, University of North Carolina, Chapel Hill). She recently completed a book entitled *Experiencing the New Genetics: Consequences for Family and Kinship in American Society* (University of Pennsylvania Press, 2000).

GEORGE M. FOSTER is professor emeritus in the UC-Berkeley Department of Anthropology. His current interest is trying to mop up a lot of loose ends from his Tzintzuntzan research as well as in the field of anthropology, which has been his second love since 1934. (His first love is his wife, Mary, and that love dates from the same time. They met in Herskovits' introductory anthropology course in 1934 at Northwestern). On a more formal level, he continues his long-time interest in medical anthropology, especially international health and ethnomedicine. Among his principal books are: *A Primitive Mexican Economy*, 1942; *Empire's Children: The People of Tzintzuntzan*, 1948;

Culture and Conquest: America's Spanish Heritage, 1960; *Traditional Cultures and the Impact of Technological Change*, 1962; *Tzintzuntzan: Mexican Peasants in a Changing World*, 1967; *Applied Anthropology*, 1969; (with Barbara Anderson) *Medical Anthropology*, 1978; (Ed., with T. Scudder, E. Colson, and R. Kemper) *Long-Term Field Research in Social Anthropology*, 1979; and *Hippocrates' Latin American Legacy: Humoral Medicine in the New World*, 1994.

MARGARET E. HARRISON is a principal lecturer in geography at Cheltenham and Gloucester College of Higher Education. She has published widely on medical geography with a particular emphasis on the supply, distribution, and employment of physicians and nurses in the Mexican health care service. Her article on female physician migration and mobility in the lifecourse in Mexico was published in the journal *Social Science and Medicine* in 1998.

LUZ MARÍA HERNÁNDEZ SÁENZ is assistant professor, Department of History, University of Western Ontario. She is the author of *Learning to Heal: The Medical Profession in Colonial Mexico, 1767–1831* and is presently researching the development of health policies and institutions in Mexico during the nineteenth century.

BRAD R. HUBER is associate professor of anthropology at the College of Charleston. His main interests are in medical anthropology, research methods, cross-cultural studies, and Mesoamerican cultures, especially the Nahua. He has undertaken research in the United States, Costa Rica, and Mexico and has worked in the Sierra Norte de Puebla since 1983. His publications have appeared in the journals *Ethnology* and *Medical Anthropology*, and include works on Nahua shamans, midwives, and bonesetters.

ELENA HURTADO, B.S., M.P.H., is a Guatemalan social scientist. Her research has focused on health-seeking behavior throughout Central America, and includes studies of emic classifications of illness, nonbiomedical and biomedical treatments of disease, reasons for the under-utilization of rural health systems, and relations between traditional and modern health providers. She codeveloped "Rapid Assessment Procedures," a combination of qualitative techniques used by health and nutrition programs for assessment before, during, and after program implementation. She works as an independent consultant and is currently an investigator associated with the Instituto de Nutrición de Centro América y Panamá (INCAP).

FRANK J. LIPP is research director of the New York State Office of Children and Family Services. He taught at Pace University and the Universidad de las Américas in Puebla, Mexico. Since 1992 he has been a field associate of the Foundation for Shamanic Studies. His publications include works on ethnobotany, Mesoamerican agriculture, ethnomedicine, and religion. His current research interest is kinship and religion in the southern Philippines. His publications include *The Mixe of Oaxaca: Religion, Ritual and Healing* and *Herbalism: Living Wisdom*.

CLANCY MCMAHON was born in 1967 in Oklahoma City. He graduated with a B.A. in biology from Hendrix College in Conway, Arkansas, in 1989. He earned an M.A. in anthropology at Texas A&M University in 1994. As part of his graduate work, he studied traditional medicine and farming practices of the Maya in the Guatemalan highlands near Lake Atitlán. Today, Clancy is in the home building business in northwest Arkansas and lives with his wife and two children on a small farm. His M.A. thesis is entitled *The Sacred Nature of Maya Bonesetting: Ritual Validation in an Empirical Practice.*

BENJAMIN D. PAUL is professor emeritus, Department of Anthropology, Stanford University. He founded and directed the social science program at the Harvard School of Public Health (1951–62) and in 1955 published the influential volume *Health, Culture and Community: Case Studies of Public Reactions to Health Programs* (fourteen printings, 1955–1990). Together with Lois Paul, he made a community study of San Pedro la Laguna, Guatemala, in 1941 and has returned periodically for twenty-five seasons of follow-up fieldwork (1956–98) to observe sociocultural changes in the same Tz'utuhil-Maya community.

EUGENIA SÁENZ DE TEJADA has a *licenciatura* in anthropology from the Universidad del Valle de Guatemala. She is currently working as a consultant for PAHO (Pan American Health Organization), training teams in five Latin American countries to undertake research related to blood donation. During the past five years, she has worked on a variety of projects related to health, nutrition, and education. She has worked for BASICS (Basic Support for Institutionalizing Child Survival), Guatemala's Ministry of Health, CESSIAM (Centro de Estudios en Sensioropatías, Senectud e Impedimentos y Alteraciones Metabólicas), INCAP (Instituto de Nutrición de Centroamérica y Panamá), and the International Eye Foundation. She is the author or coauthor of a number of books, book chapters, and articles on Maya infant health and nutrition, economic development in Guatemala, and traditional Guatemalan Maya dress.

ALAN R. SANDSTROM is professor of anthropology at Indiana University-Purdue University Fort Wayne. He conducted ethnographic field research for one year among Tibetans in exile in the Himalaya region of northern India, and for twenty-nine years among Nahuatl speakers in northern Veracruz, Mexico. His interests include cultural ecology, medical anthropology, economic anthropology, religion and symbol, and history and theory of anthropology. Major publications include *Corn Is Our Blood: Culture and Ethnic Identity in a Contemporary Aztec Indian Village* (University of Oklahoma Press, 1991), and "Contemporary Cultures of the Gulf Coast," in *Supplement to the Handbook of Middle American Indians* (University of Texas Press, 2000). He is current editor of the *Nahua Newsletter*, a biannual publication begun by Brad Huber, and now in its fourteenth year.

CARLOS VIESCA TREVIÑO, M.D., is professor of history and philosophy of medicine and medical anthropology and chair of the Department of History and Philosophy of Medicine at the Universidad Nacional Autónoma de Mexico. He is the author or editor of 12 books and some 150 published papers about ancient Mexican medicine and medical anthropology.

Index

rifice in, 23, 77–92, 100, 101, 102,
107, 111, 121, 146; postpartum, 154,
176n.24–25, 200; prenatal, 189; public, 69, 91–92, 97, 99, 101, 106; shamanic, 66–67, 73, 78, 97. *See also*
calendar; cleansing; harmony; paper
figures
ritual specialists. *See curanderos* or curers;
healers; shamans; *and types of healers*
rivers or streams, 75, 93
Royal and Pontifical University, 50, 54
Royal Hospital of Madrid, 32
Royal Indian Hospital (Mexico), 30, 32,
34, 39–40
Royal Scientific Expedition of New
Spain and Guatemala, 29
Royal Surgical College of San Carlos in
Madrid, 33
Ruíz de Alarcón, Hernando, 62, 63
Rush, Benjamin, 46

Sáenz de Tejada, Eugenia, 17, 320, 322
Sahagún, Fray Bernardino de, 21, 22, 25,
45 n.2, 55
saints, 23, 45, 77, 81, 85; and angels, 103;
talking, 109
salves, 264
San Andrés Hueyapan (Puebla), 139,
146–147, 149–150, 151, 155, 157,
158–160, 161, 162, 163, 165, 166–
168, 169, 173 n.7, 174 n.16, 175 n.17,
177 n.30, 178 n.38, 247, 257
San Cristobal, 195
Sandstrom, Alan R., 15, 17, 320–322
Santa Fe (New Mexico), 62
Santa Rita de Casia, 193
santería, 60
Santorio, Santorio, 28
Schutz, Alfred, 113
séances, 107, 115
Second National Health Survey (Mexico), 278–279
Secretaría de Educación Pública (SEP),
271
Secretaría de Salubridad y Asistencia

(SSA), 168, 169, 274, 279, 281, 287–
288, 289–290, 291, 295, 296, 297,
302
seeds: blessing of, 91; divinatory, 102
semen, 199
Sered, Starr, 130
Sessé, Martín, 29
sexual abuse, rumors of, 224
shadow, 57
shamanism: and animism, 71; in central
and north Mexico, 66–94; defined,
112–115; description and analysis of,
67–68; in southern Mexico and Guatemala, 95–116; urban, 113–114. *See
also curanderismo*
shamans, 2, 15–16, 41, 66–116, 143,
201, 244, 316–319, 323; Asiatic, 112,
114, 115; Cakchiquel, 97, 102; calling
of, by supernatural means, 71, 93;
Chatino, 105; Chichimec, 61, 66;
Chinantec, 100, 102, 105; Chocho,
97; Chontal, 97; Chorti', 101, 102;
Chuj, 101; Chukchi, 113, 114; Cora,
70, 72, 74, 78, 82, 85, 86, 93; defined
and compared to other healers, 66–
70, 73, 88, 90–94, 96, 102–104, 112–
115, 316–318; distribution of, 68–
70; ethics of, 88; and hierarchy of
spiritual attainment, 69, 72, 91; Huave, 99, 115; Huichol, 70, 72, 76, 82,
86, 91, 92, 176 n.24; Ixcatec, 97; Ixil,
101, 102, 105, 106; Jakalteko, 101,
102; K'iche', 98, 101, 102, 106, 109,
114, 115; male, compared to female,
13, 87, 92–93, 98; Mam, 100, 101,
102, 104, 108, 109; Matlazinca, 75,
78, 86; Maya, 97, 98, 101, 102, 103,
105; Mazatec, 97, 98, 100, 105, 107,
111; Mixe, 2, 97, 98, 102, 105, 107,
108, 115; Mixtec, 97, 176 n.24; Mochó, 102, 107; Ñähñu (Otomí), 2, 70,
72–75, 77–86, 88–92, 154; Nahua,
70, 73, 76–77, 79–80, 82, 85, 91–
93, 154, 322; Papago, 78, 80, 88, 90;
Popoloca, 77, 78, 89, 105; Poqom-

Breinigsville, PA USA
08 July 2010
241399BV00003B/1/P